Handbook of Emergency
Neurology

Handbook of Emergency Neurology

Edited by
Thomas P. Campbell
Department of Emergency Medicine, Allegheny General Hospital, Pittsburgh
Kevin M. Kelly
Department of Neurology, Allegheny General Hospital, Pittsburgh

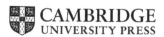
CAMBRIDGE
UNIVERSITY PRESS

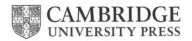

Shaftesbury Road, Cambridge CB2 8EA, United Kingdom

One Liberty Plaza, 20th Floor, New York, NY 10006, USA

477 Williamstown Road, Port Melbourne, VIC 3207, Australia

314–321, 3rd Floor, Plot 3, Splendor Forum, Jasola District Centre,
New Delhi – 110025, India

103 Penang Road, #05–06/07, Visioncrest Commercial, Singapore 238467

Cambridge University Press is part of Cambridge University Press & Assessment,
a department of the University of Cambridge.

We share the University's mission to contribute to society through the pursuit of
education, learning and research at the highest international levels of excellence.

www.cambridge.org
Information on this title: www.cambridge.org/9781009439893

DOI: 10.1017/9781316338513

First published 2023

A catalogue record for this publication is available from the British Library.

A Cataloging-in-Publication data record for this book is available from the Library of Congress.

ISBN 978-1-009-43989-3 Paperback

Cambridge University Press & Assessment has no responsibility for the persistence
or accuracy of URLs for external or third-party internet websites referred to in this
publication and does not guarantee that any content on such websites is, or will
remain, accurate or appropriate.

....

Every effort has been made in preparing this book to provide accurate and up-to-date information that
is in accord with accepted standards and practice at the time of publication. Although case histories are
drawn from actual cases, every effort has been made to disguise the identities of the individuals involved.
Nevertheless, the authors, editors, and publishers can make no warranties that the information
contained herein is totally free from error, not least because clinical standards are constantly changing
through research and regulation. The authors, editors, and publishers therefore disclaim all liability for
direct or consequential damages resulting from the use of material contained in this book. Readers are
strongly advised to pay careful attention to information provided by the manufacturer of any drugs or
equipment that they plan to use.

Contents

Additional videos can be found at:
http://www.cambridge.org/campbellkelly

Contributors

At the time of writing all authors were physicians at Allegheny Health Network.

Deeksha Agrawal

Mara Aloi

Khaled Aziz

Susan Baser

Randy Beatty

Margaret S. Blackwood

Jon S. Brillman

Matthew Brucks

James Burgess

Thomas P. Campbell

Russell Cerejo

Melani S. Cheers

Roseann Covatto

Sheilah M. Curran-Melendez

Moira Davenport

Kate DeAntonis

Troy Desai

Richard Feduska

Charles J. Feronti

Dan Geary

Michael F. Goldberg

Erik Happ

David Jho

Diana J. Jho

Richard M. Kaplan

Kevin M. Kelly

Lauren King

Evelina Krieger

Timothy Leichliter

Jody Leonardo

Charles Q. Li

Ye Vivian Liang

Arthur Alcantara Lima

Molly A. McGraw

Melody Milliron

Zaw Min

Raj Nangunoori

Chadd E. Nesbit

John O'Neill

Austin Oblack

Michael Oh

Paul S. Porter

Timothy A. Quezada

Timothy Quezada

Sandeep Rana

Tulika Ranjan

Brent Rau

Brian Rempe

Bertram Richter

Dolores Santamaria

Thomas F. Scott

George A. Small

Kristen Stabingas

Matthew Stripp

Andrea Synowiec

Ronald L. Thomas

Nestor Tomycz

Chris Troianos

James P. Valeriano

Arvind Venkat

Rade Vukmir

Donald Whiting

James E. Wilberger

Crystal Wong

Alexander K. Yu

Emergency Neurologic Examination

Melani S. Cheers, Thomas F. Scott, and Kevin M. Kelly

1.1 Introduction

The human nervous system contains more than 100 billion neurons. Each has a unique function enabling taste, smell, touch, sight, hearing, movement, respiration, cognition, and much more. In the setting of a neurologic emergency, patients may lose these unique capacities. It is the emergency physician's responsibility to complete a neurologic history and examination to determine the type of deficit and the neuroanatomical location of the abnormality.

A unique aspect of neurology is that anatomical localization of lesions is of paramount importance. Localizing lesions is a multiphase process: The initial history, general physical examination, and neurological examination integrate symptoms and signs that provide clues to the suspected anatomical location of the abnormality. This localization of neuro-anatomical abnormality informs an ordinally ranked differential diagnosis. If the localization process suggests multiple lesions in the nervous system, the implications of each lesion are considered separately and in combination. It is often said that neurologic diagnosis is based 90% on history and 10% on examination. Prior to examining the patient, the physician often has a clear understanding of likely disease processes to explain the patient's chief complaint from the history alone.

A comprehensive neurologic examination is often impractical in the emergency setting and therefore an examination targeted to the patient's presenting symptoms and neurologic deficits is required. If a patient presents with a fever, confusion, and generalized weakness, the primary considerations are very different than those of a patient who presents with sudden-onset aphasia and right hemiparesis. In the first example, the history and physical examination aim to uncover clues involving multiple organ systems that may point to infection or toxic-metabolic syndromes. The second example points to a primary neurologic disease process, but the emergency physician must explore all of the possibilities for systemic disease that may also contribute. The goal of the emergency department (ED) neurologic evaluation is to determine if a neurologic condition exists, to identify possible causes, to intervene in a timely fashion, and to establish the proper disposition of the patient.

The stepwise process of the ED neurologic evaluation is:

1. Identify and characterize the neurologic symptoms (e.g., loss of sensation, ataxia, weakness, aphasia) through a detailed history.
2. Complete an initial neurologic examination (mental status, cranial nerves, motor, sensation, and reflexes) focusing on relevant symptoms.
3. Localize the lesion(s) (central or peripheral: focal, multifocal, or diffuse).

4. Generate a differential diagnosis in the order of the most likely to the least likely consideration.
5. Determine a diagnostic plan with appropriate testing as directed by the differential diagnosis and order consultations as indicated.
6. Initiate treatment when there is clinical urgency.
7. Determine disposition from the ED.

1.2 History

A thorough history is key to determining the cause of neurologic disease or dysfunction and making an accurate diagnosis in the ED. It is also a useful tool to evaluate the patient's mental status by their presentation of the history of their present illness. While obtaining the neurologic history, the physician may also assess the patient's speech, mood, affect, and general appearance. A bystander or family member's description of the patient's behavior is often helpful in making a diagnosis. Obtaining a detailed neurologic history is essential to determine the anatomic localization, tailor the differential diagnosis, and streamline the neurologic examination.

1.3 Key Elements of a Focused Neurologic History

1. Symptoms (location, quality, radiation, severity)
2. Onset (exact time of onset, precipitating events, last time known normal)
3. Duration (minutes, hours, days, intermittent, chronic)
4. Progression (slowly progressing, acute onset, gradual resolution, intermittent)
5. Associated symptoms (recent illness, fever, headache, trauma, loss of consciousness)
6. Aggravating or alleviating factors (movement, hot or cold, light)
7. Distribution of process (unilateral, bilateral, dermatomal)
8. Medical history (previous episodes, medication use or ingestions, occupation, family history)

After obtaining a thorough neurologic history and performing a neurologic examination, physicians should not hesitate to revisit and refine the patient's neurologic history. Examination findings may change the understanding of the case and create new questions for the patient and family members.

1.4 Neurologic Examination

The neurologic examination is a bedside tool that helps to localize the origin of the patient's symptoms to either the central or peripheral nervous system. This includes assessment of the patient's mental status, language, cranial nerves, sensory and motor function, and reflexes. A complete neurologic examination in the emergency setting is often neither necessary nor appropriate given the time constraints and the rapidity with which a diagnosis must be made. Therefore, a neurologic examination tailored to the patient's history and symptoms is most useful.

1.5 Brief Neurologic Examination

1. Mental status (assessed through history-taking, concise mental status examination, and/or Glasgow Coma Score in altered patients)
2. Cranial nerve function
3. Motor function

4. Sensation
5. Coordination and balance
6. Reflexes (both deep tendon and pathologic)

Video 1.1: Emergency Neurologic Exam. Video 1.1 can be accessed at http://www.cambridge.org/campbellkelly

---

1.6 Mental Status

Mental status is a key part of the neurologic examination as it frequently impacts the patient's ability to cooperate with evaluation. Consider the patient's general appearance, behavior, attention, orientation, speech, dress, memory, mood, affect, and attitude. Is the patient disheveled? Do they have rapid pressured speech? Do they require constant stimulation or are they able to carry on a normal conversation? If there is evidence of severe encephalopathy, the patient is unlikely to be able to follow commands and participate in a thorough assessment of strength and sensory function. If they are able to provide information about their medical history and the history of present illness clearly and in a consistent manner, then they have normal mental status. If not, then a more thorough mental status examination is necessary and there are tools such as the OMIHAT Mnemonic (Table 1.1) or the Mini-Mental Status Exam. In altered patients, the Glasgow Coma Scale (GCS) (Table 1.2) may be the best assessment tool to assess responsiveness and mental status.

1.6.1 Cranial Nerves

Evaluation of cranial nerves II–XII can be completed in a few simple steps:

Check visual acuity, pupillary light reflex, and visual fields (CN II).

Look for ptosis and evaluate ocular motion, conjugate gaze, and nystagmus by asking the patient to follow a target moved in the shape of an "H" with only their eyes (CN III, IV, VI).

Softly touch the face in the three divisions of the trigeminal nerve bilaterally (CN V).

Ask the patient to smile, raise their eyebrows, shut their eyes, and puff out their cheeks (CNVII).

Evaluate hearing bilaterally with whispered word or finger rub (CN VIII).

Assess for gag reflex and ensure that the uvula is midline (CN IX, X).

Have the patient shrug their shoulders and turn their head against resistance (CN XI) and protrude and move the tongue (CN XII).

Table 1.1 Rapid Mental Status Exam OMIHAT

O	Orientation
M	Memory
I	Intellect
H	Hallucinations
A	Affect
T	Thought

Table 1.2 Glasgow Coma Scale

Eye opening	Spontaneously	4
	To verbal command	3
	To pain	2
	Do not open	1
Verbal response	Alert and oriented	5
	Disoriented	4
	Nonsensical speech	3
	Unintelligible	2
	Unresponsive	1
Motor response	Follows commands	6
	Localizes pain	5
	Withdraws from pain	4
	Decorticate flexion	3
	Decerebrate extension	2
	No response	1
Total score		3–15

1.6.2 Motor Examination

The motor examination can be difficult if movement is limited by pain or if the patient is uncooperative. If the patient is able to walk, evaluation of the patient's gait can be very helpful. If the patient is unable to ambulate, assess pronator drift to identify subtle weakness of the upper extremities. To do so, ask the patient to hold their arms out, palms up, for 10 seconds. If pronation and downward drift occurs, this indicates motor weakness. Test the strength of several muscle groups and record the strength assessment with a five-point scale (Table 1.3).

Proceed head to toe, examining strength at multiple levels (deltoid flexion, biceps flexion, wrist extension/flexion, bilateral grip strength). In the lower extremities, test hip flexion, knee extension/flexion, and ankle dorsi/plantar flexion to evaluate strength bilaterally.

1.6.3 Sensory Examination

Sensory findings are difficult to interpret particularly during a concise ED examination. Traditionally, a full sensory evaluation is done by examining light touch, pinprick, position sense, vibration, temperature, and pain. Evaluate sensation in a rapid fashion in the ED by asking a patient to close their eyes and identify simple letters or numbers written on the palm of their hand. A cooperative patient can be asked to outline the area of sensory deficit or change. There are many references to use on your phone, Internet, or text to identify the dermatome assigned to the symptoms as detailed in Table 1.4.

Table 1.3 Five-point scale for muscle strength testing

5 = normal strength

4 = movement against some resistance

3 = movement against gravity

2 = unable to move against gravity

1 = muscles contract, but no motion follows

0 = no muscle contraction

Table 1.4 Sensory examination and dermatomes

Cervical nerves and their dermatomes

C2: the base of the skull and behind the ear
C3: the back of the head and the upper neck
C4: the lower neck and upper shoulders
C5: the upper shoulders and the two collarbones
C6: the upper forearms, thumbs, and index fingers
C7: the upper back, back of the arms, and middle fingers
C8: the upper back, inner arms, and ring and pinky fingers

Thoracic nerves and their dermatomes

T1: the upper chest, back, and upper forearm
T2, T3, and T4: the upper chest and back
T5, T6, and T7: the mid-chest and back
T8 and T9: the upper abdomen and mid-back
T10: the midline on the abdomen and the mid-back
T11 and T12: the lower abdomen and mid-back

Lumbar nerves and their dermatomes

L1: the groin, upper hips, and lower back
L2: the lower back, hips, and tops of the inner thighs
L3: the lower back, inner thighs, and inner legs just below the knees
L4: the backs of the knees, inner sections of the lower legs, and the heels
L5: the tops of the feet and the fronts of the lower legs

Sacral nerves and their dermatomes

S1: the lower back, buttocks, backs of the legs, and the outer toes
S2: the buttocks, genitals, backs of the legs, and heels
S3: the buttocks and genitals
S4 and S5: the buttocks

1.7 Reflexes

Reflex testing is an objective method to test patency of simple neural connectivity from the periphery to the spinal cord to the effector muscle. To test deep tendon reflexes (DTRs) – actually, muscle stretch reflexes (MSRs) – the limb should be relaxed and in a symmetric

Table 1.5 Muscle stretch reflexes

Biceps	C5–C6
Supinator brachioradialis	C6
Triceps	C7
Knee	L4
Ankle	S1
Cutaneous reflexes	
Abdominal – upper umbilicus	T8–T10
Abdominal – lower umbilicus	T10–T12
Cremasteric	L1–L2
Anal	S2–S5

position. Check one side and then immediately compare the reflex response with that of the contralateral side. Reflexes are graded on a scale of 0–4: no reflex elicited (0), hypoactive reflexes (1), normal reflexes (2), hyperactive reflexes (3), and clonic reflexes (4). Reflexes graded 1–3 are not considered to be abnormal. However, clonus, gross asymmetry between arms and legs or a substantial difference between contralateral sides should warrant further investigation. Many conditions such as age, electrolyte abnormalities, thyroid dysfunction, toxic ingestions, diabetes, and even anxiety can influence reflexes. However, testing the biceps (C5–C6), brachioradialis (C6), triceps (C7), patellar (L4), and Achilles (S1) tendons can help to identify the spinal nerve roots involved in a particular injury (Table 1.5).

It is also important to check for pathologic reflexes. The Babinski reflex can be elicited by running a dull object (such as a pen) up the lateral aspect of the plantar surface of the foot to the toe. If an extensor plantar response is obtained (i.e., an "up-going toe") this indicates an upper motor neuron lesion.

The absence of normal cutaneous reflexes such as the anal wink or perineal reflex (S2–S4) and cremasteric reflex (L1–L2) can be helpful in identifying pathology, such as a conus medullaris or cauda equina lesion or an epidural hematoma.

1.7.1 Coordination and Balance

The ability of the body to balance and coordinate movement is referred to as equilibrium. If the patient exhibits ataxia, has difficulty with tandem gait, or has a positive Romberg sign, this indicates disequilibrium. Truncal ataxia is recognized by a wide-based gait and poor balance while sitting or standing. Limb ataxia can be identified by testing the finger–nose–finger and heel–knee–shin movements of bilateral upper and lower extremities, respectively. Ataxia, tremor, and impairment of rapid alternating hand movements are classic indicators of cerebellar lesions.

1.7.2 Language

Dysarthria and aphasia are the two most common speech abnormalities. Dysarthria is caused by a deficit in the motor production of speech. Slurring of words may be caused by oral or facial lesions as well as central lesions affecting the posterior circulation or neurologic disorders such as multiple sclerosis, Parkinson's disease, or amyotrophic lateral sclerosis.

Aphasia arises from injury to the language centers of the brain resulting in disordered communication. Aphasia is characterized by the inability to speak, read, write, or comprehend. Aphasia is most frequently caused by stroke, traumatic brain injuries, tumors, or progressive neurologic disorders. During the history and physical examination, it is critical to determine the onset, progression, and type of aphasia (either receptive or expressive) as these will provide strong clues to localize the disease process.

1.7.3 Using the Results of the Neurological Exam

The findings of the neurologic examination must be incorporated in the context of the patient's overall history and general physical examination to determine the appropriate course of investigation (e.g., CT, MRI, lumbar puncture) and to rapidly determine the most appropriate therapy (e.g., hydration, antibiotics, transfusion, TPA) to treat the disease. Physicians should expand upon specific elements of the history and physical examination as the stepwise process unfolds. Physicians often need to return to the bedside to perform more detailed examinations as part of the diagnostic process and rapidly evolving symptoms often require repeating the examination at regular intervals.

Pearls and Pitfalls

- History is critical and should be obtained in all manners possible, including the patient, family, friends, and electronic records, and often requires repeated attempts.
- Similar to the history, serial examinations are critical to determine any rapid changes or progression of abnormal neurologic signs.
- The chaotic environment of the ED may necessitate interrupted evaluations and it is important not to forget the progression of the evaluation.
- History-taking and the neurologic examination are as important as, and often more so than, imaging studies, which should not be considered a replacement for a thorough history and examination.

Bibliography

Aghababian R. *Emergency Medicine: The Core Curriculum Illustrated.* Lippincott-Raven, 1998.

Cydulka RK, Fitch MT, Joing SA, et al. *Tintinalli's Emergency Medicine Manual,* 8th ed. McGraw Hill, 2017.

Goldstein JN, Greer DM. Rapid focused neurological assessment in the emergency department and ICU. *Emerg Med Clin North Am* 2009;27(1):1–16.

Mahadevan S, Garmel G (eds.). *An Introduction to Clinical Emergency Medicine.* Cambridge University Press, 2012.

Pangman VC, Sloan J, Guse, L. An examination of psychometric properties of the Mini-Mental State Examination and the Standardized Mini-Mental State Examination: implications for clinical practice. *App Nurs Res* 2000;13(4): 209–213.

Rosen P, Hockberger RS, Walls RM, et al. *Rosen's Emergency Medicine: Concepts and Clinical Practice.* Vols. 1–2. Elsevier, 2018.

Chapter 2

Neuroradiology

Sheilah M. Curran-Melendez, Margaret S. Blackwood, and Michael F. Goldberg

2.1 Introduction

Nearly half of all emergency department (ED) visits in the United States result in some type of imaging study, a large number of which are performed for neurologic complaints. Common presenting neurologic complaints include headache, weakness, stroke, and trauma. Often the initial study performed for the evaluation of these complaints is an unenhanced computed tomography (CT) of the brain. However, as will be discussed below, certain presentations and clinical history can warrant magnetic resonance imaging (MRI) as a superior first-line imaging test. This chapter seeks to provide guidance in imaging modality selection and to discuss imaging findings in common clinical presentations to the ED. When pertinent, alternative and recommended follow-up studies are also discussed.

2.2 CT vs MRI

CT is the primary imaging modality employed in the evaluation of patients presenting to the ED with neurologic complaints. This is due to its ubiquity, relative low cost, rapid image acquisition time, and few contraindications. Unenhanced CT is very sensitive in the evaluation of acute intracranial hemorrhage and may detect even small amounts of blood. It is less sensitive in the evaluation of subacute and chronic blood products, which may appear isodense to brain parenchyma. In the case of suspected subacute hemorrhage, MRI, particularly fluid-attenuated inversion recovery (FLAIR) and T2*-weighted sequences, may be of benefit as a noninvasive adjunct to lumbar puncture.

CT is also the primary imaging modality used to evaluate patients with symptoms of acute ischemic stroke (AIS) primarily due to its sensitivity for acute hemorrhage, the latter a contraindication to thrombolytic therapy. In the subacute setting, the patient is often scheduled for nonemergent MRI evaluation to confirm the size and location of the infarct as well as response to therapy. The role of additional imaging modalities used in the assessment of stroke, such as multiphase CT angiography (CTA) and CT perfusion (CTP), is discussed later in this chapter.

In the setting of trauma, CT is the preferred imaging modality due to its speed of acquisition, sensitivity for hemorrhage, and ability to depict osseous traumatic abnormalities. In suspected vascular trauma, CTA and CT venography (CTV) may be employed to further evaluate arterial and venous structures.

In patients with suspected subarachnoid hemorrhage (SAH), initial imaging evaluation is performed with unenhanced CT which, if positive, is often followed by CTA to evaluate for a ruptured aneurysm as a source of bleeding. Of note, the American College of Radiology (ACR) in its Appropriateness Criteria does not recommend routine imaging in the evaluation of patients with chronic headache in the absence of new features or a neurologic deficit. In those patients who meet these criteria, MRI with contrast is the recommended imaging modality for the evaluation of underlying pathology. Likewise, evaluation of suspected CNS malignancy, whether due to patient symptoms or suspicious CT findings, is best performed with enhanced MRI. In patients for whom MRI is contraindicated or difficult to obtain, enhanced CT is the alternative.

MRI, although not as readily available as CT, demonstrates superior soft tissue detail and is preferable in the work-up of spinal complaints as the spinal cord is difficult to evaluate on CT. Specifically, for stat indications, including spinal cord compression and cauda equine syndrome, MRI is the preferred imaging modality. Contrast-enhanced imaging is only recommended in the setting of suspected malignancy or infection. For patients requiring evaluation of the spinal cord who have contraindications for MRI, CT myelography is an alternative imaging test.

2.3 Cerebrovascular Accident

The purpose of imaging the patient presenting with AIS is to rapidly identify those patients who may benefit from therapy, either intravenous thrombolytic therapy and/or intra-arterial therapy (IAT). This has become particularly important recently given the publication of several trials, specifically the DAWN and DEFUSE 3 trials, which have led to the expansion of the treatment window for AIS to 24 hours from symptom onset.

The imaging work-up of AIS is an ever-evolving process that has undergone multiple iterations in the recent past, and often differs between institutions. These variations aside, initial evaluation of a patient with symptoms of stroke is, with few exceptions, an unenhanced CT. This modality is primarily employed to identify contraindications to acute thrombolytic therapy, including intracranial hemorrhage (Figure 2.1) and large, established infarct. CT can also evaluate for other, nonischemic causes of an acute neurologic deficit (i.e., "stroke mimics").

Findings of acute ischemia include hypoattenuation of the brain parenchyma within the affected territory with loss of gray–white differentiation. Intravascular hyperdensity indicative of thrombus, most notably the "hyperdense middle cerebral artery (MCA) sign" (Figure 2.2a) is a specific but insensitive sign of acute ischemia. The unenhanced head CT is relatively insensitive in the setting of hyperacute AIS with a sensitivity of only 31% within 3 hours of symptom onset.

The Alberta Stroke Program Early CT Score (ASPECTS) is a 10-point quantitative score applied to brain CT performed at initial presentation (<3 hours) of patients with stroke symptoms. The patient score is determined by dividing the brain parenchyma supplied by the MCA on the affected side into 10 segments. A single point is subtracted from the initial score of 10 for every segment demonstrating early changes of ischemia. The final score can then be used to predict patient outcome, with a final score of 7 or less portending a poor outcome even in patients treated with thrombolysis.

Many institutions choose to pursue vascular examination by performing CTA of the head and neck vessels immediately after the initial unenhanced CT in patients who are within the window of treatment. This study can evaluate for the presence of intracranial proximal arterial occlusion, which may guide further intervention, including IAT. This can also be used to evaluate for other etiologies of AIS, including dissection.

Prospective clinical trials, including the MR CLEAN and ESCAPE studies, have shown improved outcomes in AIS patients from rapid IAT with the latest generation of

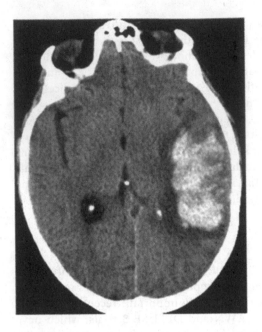

Figure 2.1 Unenhanced axial CT demonstrating a hemorrhagic infarction involving the left temporal and parietal lobes.

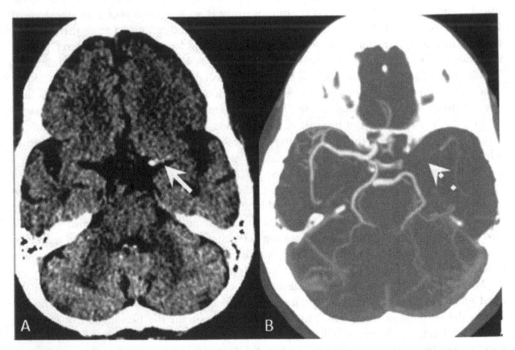

Figure 2.2 Axial CT images demonstrating a hyperdense left MCA (solid arrow) consistent with acute embolus within the left MCA (a). Complete occlusion (dashed arrow) of the artery is confirmed by subsequent CTA (b).

endovascular devices. Treatment decisions are based on clinical findings as well as the imaging findings, most commonly CT and CTA findings. Additionally, the 2018 Guidelines for Management of Acute Ischemic Stroke from the American Heart Association/American Stroke Association have expanded their recommendations to include evaluation with CT perfusion, diffusion-weighted imaging MRI, and/or MRI perfusion in patients presenting within 6–24 hours of symptom onset. Given that MRI is not often readily accessible for emergent evaluation, the brunt of expanded assessments will likely be performed with CTP rather than MRI.

The most common finding in early AIS is loss of gray–white differentiation due to cytotoxic edema and sulcal effacement due to gyral swelling. As the infarct evolves and becomes subacute, parenchymal hypoattenuation and sulcal effacement become more pronounced with worsening mass effect. As mentioned above, a specific but insensitive sign of AIS is intravascular hyperdensity, most often within the MCA, which represents intravascular embolus. Intracranial CTA may demonstrate complete occlusion of the involved vessel (Figure 2.2b); evaluation of the neck vessels may identify a potential source of embolus.

Additional imaging tools are available in the evaluation of acute infarction although there is little consensus among specialists in their utility, and their current role in the evaluation of patients varies between institutions. Two such tools are multiphase CTA and CTP. Multiphase CTA evaluates collateral circulation by acquiring CT images of the entire brain at three time points (peak arterial, peak venous, and late venous phases) after the administration of intravenous contrast. Pial vessel enhancement of the affected cerebral hemisphere is then compared to the contralateral (normal) hemisphere and the level of pial filling is then scored (Figure 2.3). Menon et al. (2015) have proposed that multiphase CTA may be used as an adjunct in clinical decision-making as a better means to select patients who may benefit from IAT and exclude those patients in whom IAT would be futile. They have also suggested that multiphase CTA is superior to unenhanced CT alone or CTP in the risk stratification of stroke patients for treatment decision-making purposes.

Although the role of CTP varies widely at different institutions, it has been used to help identify the penumbra, the at-risk but salvageable brain, and the core, the infarcted and irretrievable portion of the brain. This can better stratify patients who would benefit from acute intervention from those who would not benefit, and perhaps be adversely affected, by acute intervention.

In AIS, the amount of potentially salvageable tissue is determined by comparing the penumbra, which demonstrates a prolonged mean transit time (MTT) but only moderately reduced CBF and normal to increased cerebral blood volume (CBV), to the infarcted core of brain parenchyma, which demonstrates a prolonged MTT, but decreased CBV and CBF (Figure 2.4). The role of CTP may increase, as its use in two recent clinical trials demonstrated the benefit of IAT in AIS patients who were selected, in part, on the basis of CTP data.

On MRI, the earliest sign of acute ischemia is restricted diffusion identified on diffusion-weighted sequences (Figure 2.5a). Diffusion-weighted images and their corresponding apparent diffusion coefficient (ADC) maps are positive within 6 hours after the initial insult and may become positive as early as a few minutes after onset of an acute infarct. Later in the acute period, usually greater than 6 hours, there will be increased T2/FLAIR signal in the affected territory (Figure 2.5b). Parenchymal swelling will cause mass effect; if severe, this can lead to midline shift, herniation, and ventricular entrapment.

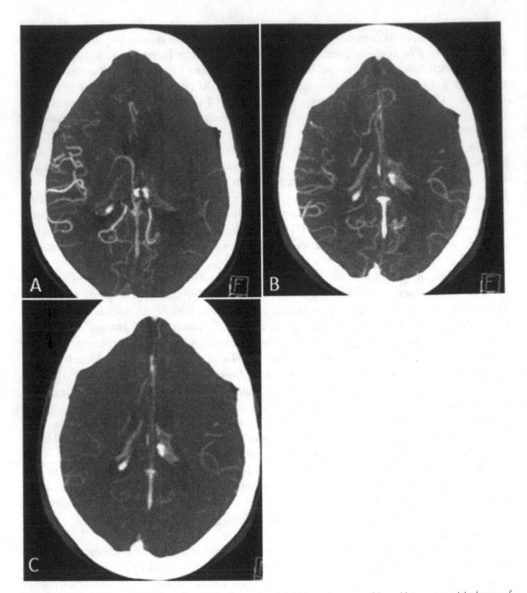

Figure 2.3 Multiphase axial CTA performed in the peak arterial (a), peak venous (b), and late venous (c) phases of contrast enhancement demonstrating poor pial collateral supply to the left frontal lobe, consistent with left MCA infarction.

In the subacute setting, AIS patients are often evaluated with nonemergent MRI. In some instances, if a patient is not considered to be a candidate for intervention, clinicians may forgo emergent arterial evaluation with CTA and instead choose to perform MR angiography (MRA) of the head and neck at the time of nonemergent MRI. MRA may also be performed as an alternative to CTA in patients who cannot receive contrast, due to allergy or renal insufficiency, as the study can be performed without contrast.

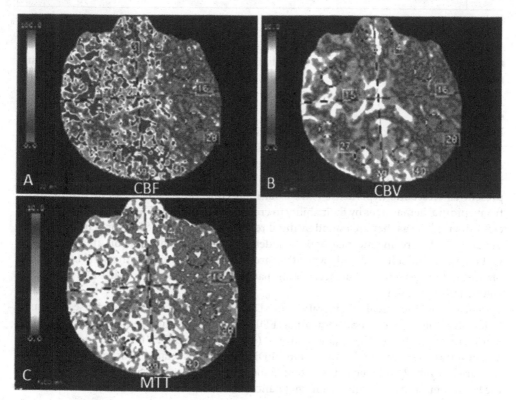

Figure 2.4 CT perfusion study demonstrating matched decreased cerebral blood flow (CBV) (a), decreased cerebral blood volume (CBV) (b), and prolonged mean transit time (MTT) (c) involving the majority of the left MCA territory. This matched defect demonstrates a large infarct with absent penumbra which portends a poor outcome. This patient would not be considered a good candidate for thrombolytic therapy.

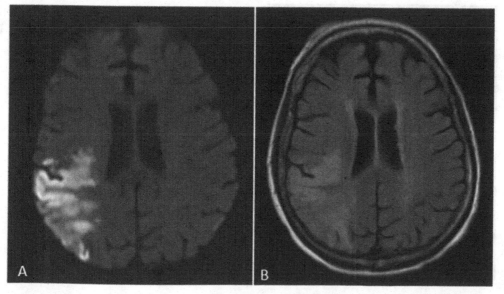

Figure 2.5 Diffusion-weighted image of the brain (a) demonstrating restricted diffusion. FLAIR image (b) of the brain demonstrating corresponding increased T2 signal in the right parietal lobe. Findings represent an AIS.

The imaging and treatment of this disease is rapidly evolving and it is best to coordinate regularly updated care plans and protocols in conjunction with your site radiology and neurology teams.

2.4 Trauma

Emergent unenhanced CT is the standard imaging tool for intracranial evaluation in the setting of trauma, primarily in search of acute intracranial hemorrhage (ICH) but also in the evaluation of fracture. The most common type of ICH is subdural hematoma (SDH), which is often secondary to venous hemorrhage from tearing of bridging cortical veins. SDHs present as crescentic hyperdense extra-axial fluid collections, which can be distinguished from epidural hematomas by their ability to cross cranial sutures (Figure 2.6) but inability to cross the midline as they are bound by dural reflections. Subacute SDH, or acute hematoma in patients who are anemic, may appear isodense to brain parenchyma on unenhanced CT, making them difficult to identify when they are small in size. If a subacute SDH is suspected, often due to mass effect on adjacent brain parenchyma, unenhanced MRI may be used as confirmatory imaging.

The major differential consideration for SDH in the presence of a hyperdense extra-axial fluid collection is the epidural hematoma (EDH), which classically demonstrates a biconvex lentiform shape bound by cranial sutures (Figure 2.7a). EDH is caused by tearing of a meningeal artery or dural venous sinus. EDH is often associated with underlying cranial fractures (Figure 2.7b). Due to the potential for rehemorrhage and subsequent expansion of the hematoma, repeat imaging with unenhanced CT is recommended within 36 hours after the initial injury.

Special attention should be paid to patients who are being treated with anticoagulants as they are at increased risk of ICH and evaluation with CT is recommended even with mild

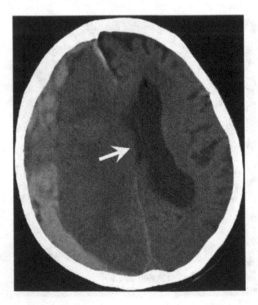

Figure 2.6 Axial CT demonstrating a hyperdense crescentic extra-axial collection consistent with an acute subdural hematoma. Mass effect causes leftward midline shift and effacement of the right lateral ventricle (arrow).

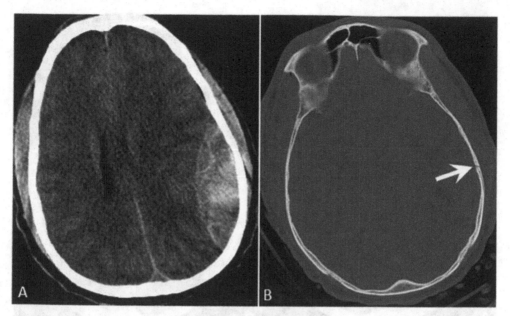

Figure 2.7 Unenhanced CT in soft tissue window demonstrating a lenticular-shaped hyperdense extra-axial collection bound by cranial sutures consistent with an EDH (a). The same CT in bone window demonstrating an underlying calvarial fracture (arrow) (b).

head trauma. Delayed hemorrhage, defined as new hemorrhage within 2 weeks of head trauma in a patient with a negative CT scan on initial evaluation, should be a consideration in these patients. As this post-traumatic complication is rare, estimated to be <1% on a recent study, close clinical follow-up is recommended with follow-up imaging only in the case of acute mental status changes or other concerning clinical findings.

SAH can be identified as hyperdense material within the subarachnoid space and is described later in this chapter.

Parenchymal hemorrhagic contusions are most commonly the result of contrecoup injury caused by contact of brain parenchyma with the inner table of the calvarium. Contusions most commonly involve the inferior frontal lobes and temporal lobes (Figure 2.8) due to the irregularity of adjacent calvarium. A contusion may initially present as an area of hypodensity that may or may not also contain internal foci of hemorrhage. Intraparenchymal hemorrhage may be small (foci of petechiae) or large and often demonstrates a propensity to enlarge on follow-up studies.

In patients who present with post-traumatic coma upon initial assessment, CT scan may be unremarkable or present with any of the above findings. If patients fail to follow the expected clinical course with little improvement, diffuse axonal injury (DAI) should be considered. Due to CT's poor sensitivity for DAI, the imaging work-up of DAI should include MRI. Findings of DAI include small hemorrhages at the gray–white interface, corpus callosum, and dorsal midbrain. The most sensitive modality for the evaluation of DAI is unenhanced MRI, specifically susceptibility-weighted imaging (SWI), which may demonstrate areas of susceptibility artifact (Figure 2.9); diffusion-weighted imaging (DWI), which may demonstrate foci of

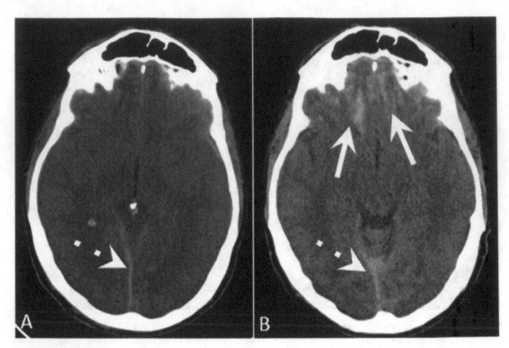

Figure 2.8 Axial CT performed on admission (a) and 12 hours later (b) demonstrating the enlargement of bilateral frontal lobe contusions (solid arrows). Subdural hematoma along the posterior falx is present (dashed arrow).

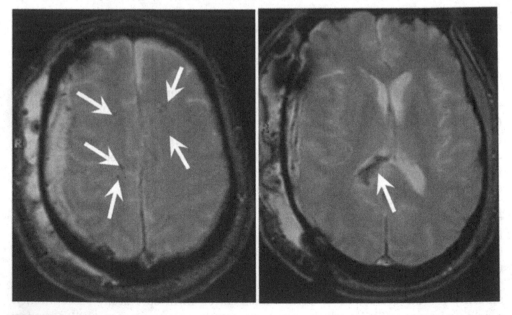

Figure 2.9 Axial MR gradient echo images of the brain demonstrating multiple foci of susceptibility artifact (arrows) representing areas of DAI. Incidental note is made of a right scalp hematoma and a right-sided subdural hematoma.

restricted diffusion; diffusion tensor imaging (DTI), which may demonstrate disruption of white matter fiber tracts; and FLAIR sequences, which may show increased T2/FLAIR signal in affected regions.

CT with bone algorithm is the best modality for the evaluation of calvarial and facial fractures. There is little role for MRI in the evaluation of fracture and CT is often adequate in the evaluation of abnormalities associated with facial fractures, such as entrapment of ocular muscles or retrobulbar hemorrhage.

2.5 Arterial Dissection

Arterial dissection can have a varied presentation and thus suspicion should be high for this entity, particularly when a young patient presents with symptoms of stroke. If positive, unenhanced CT most commonly demonstrates hypodensity in the MCA territory corresponding to ischemic infarction. Ischemia may also present in watershed territories (Figure 2.10) due to decreased perfusion. Subsequent evaluation with head and neck CTA will demonstrate a smooth intimal flap or area of thrombosis at the site of dissection (Figure 2.11), which may be long or short. If MRA is employed to evaluate for suspected dissection, T1-weighted fat-saturated or proton density sequences should be obtained as these sequences increase identification of methemoglobin within the vessel wall (Figure 2.12).

2.6 Dural Venous Sinus Thrombosis

In patients presenting with ischemic changes, occasionally with associated hemorrhage, that do not conform to an arterial vascular territory, dural venous sinus thrombosis should be considered. On unenhanced CT, hyperdensity within the dural venous sinuses (Figure 2.13), cortical veins, or deep veins may be suggestive of the diagnosis. Further evaluation with CTV

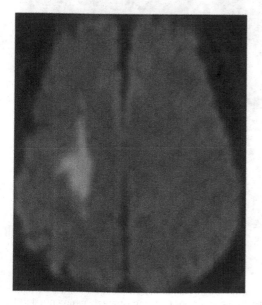

Figure 2.10 Diffusion-weighted MRI demonstrating restricted diffusion within the corona radiata representing a watershed territory infarction. ADC map (not shown) confirmed restricted diffusion.

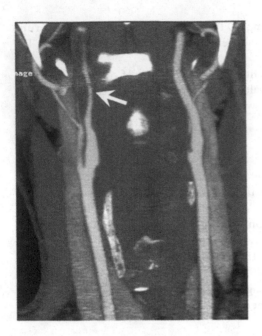

Figure 2.11 Neck CTA in the same patient as in Figure 2.10 demonstrating smooth tapering of the right internal carotid artery (arrow) consistent with arterial dissection.

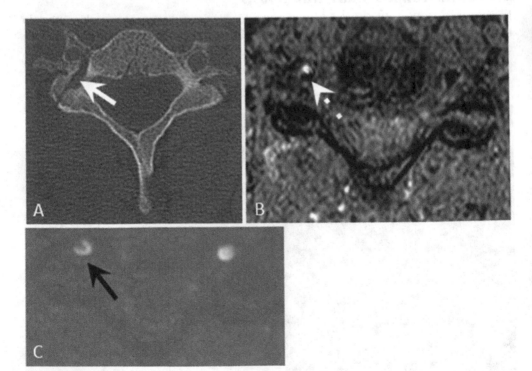

Figure 2.12 Axial CT image of the cervical spine (a) demonstrates a minimally displaced fracture involving the right transverse foramen (solid arrow). Axial T1 fat-saturated MRI of the cervical spine (b) demonstrates hyperintense signal within the right vertebral artery at the level of the fracture (dashed arrow). Axial 2D time-of-flight MRA image of the cervical spine (c) confirms a dissection flap within the right cervical artery (black arrow) at this location.

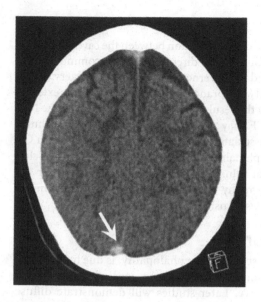

Figure 2.13 Unenhanced axial CT showing a hypertense superior sagittal sinus (arrow) demonstrating the "delta" sign of dural venous sinus thrombosis.

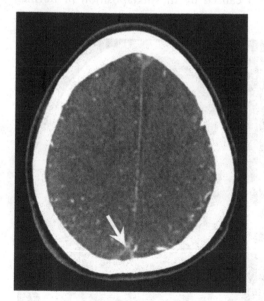

Figure 2.14 Axial CT venogram shows a filling defect within the superior sagittal sinus (arrow) in the same patient as in Figure 2.13, demonstrating the "empty delta" sign of dural venous sinus thrombosis.

will demonstrate a filling defect within affected structures, the so-called "empty delta sign" (Figure 2.14) when the superior sagittal sinus is involved. MR venography (MRV) will demonstrate increased signal (absence of the expected flow void) within affected dural venous sinuses on T1-weighted images due to methemoglobin within the thrombus.

2.7 Carotid–Cavernous Fistula

Carotid–cavernous fistula (CCF) is an abnormal communication between the cavernous sinus and the cavernous internal carotid artery. CCF may be direct, where the communication occurs directly between the cavernous sinus and the cavernous internal carotid artery (ICA), or indirect, where the communication exists between branches of the internal and/or external carotid arteries. Direct CCF is most commonly the result of trauma causing a tear in the ICA while indirect CCF is often spontaneous. CCF may present with pulsatile exophthalmos, pulsatile tinnitus, or progressive vision loss. Associated imaging findings found on both CT and MRI include proptosis, dilated superior ophthalmic vein, enlarged extraocular muscles, and rarely SAH (caused by rupture of cortical veins). Although the gold standard for the diagnosis for CCF is digital subtraction angiography (DSA), CTA has proven useful in the diagnosis of CCF. MRA has been found to be less sensitive and is not recommended.

2.8 Global Hypoxic-Ischemic Injury

Global hypoxic-ischemic injury, or hypoxic-ischemic encephalopathy, is due to interruption of normal brain perfusion, most commonly secondary to cardiac arrest. In the hyperacute state, the head CT will be negative. Later studies will demonstrate diffuse edema with diffuse loss of gray–white differentiation and effacement of the basal cisterns and other CSF-containing spaces. Diffuse edema often spares the cerebellum, giving rise to the "white cerebellum sign" (Figure 2.15) caused by the juxtaposition of normal

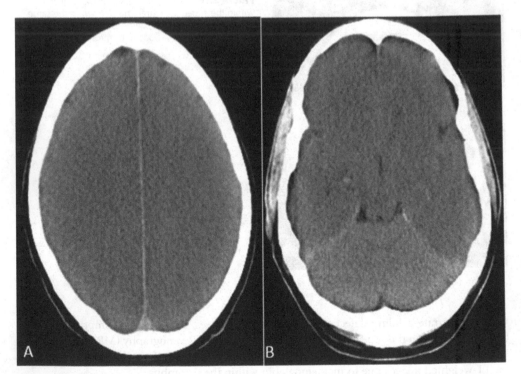

Figure 2.15 Unenhanced axial CT of the brain demonstrating diffuse loss of gray–white differentiation and sulcal effacement (a). Relative hyperdensity of normal cerebellar parenchyma relative to hypodense brain parenchyma (b). This patient had recently experienced prolonged cardiac arrest, and these findings are consistent with diffuse cytotoxic cerebral edema.

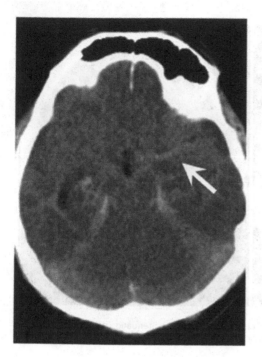

Figure 2.16 Unenhanced axial CT of the brain demonstrating hyperdensity within the left Sylvain fissure (arrow). In this patient with global hypoxic-ischemic injury this represents the "pseudosubarachnoid hemorrhage" sign.

cerebellar parenchyma and diffusely edematous cerebrum. Similarly, diffuse hypodensity of cerebral parenchyma gives the appearance of relative hyperdensity of intracranial vascular structures, which may be confused with hemorrhage, the "pseudo-SAH sign" (Figure 2.16). Another important sign in the evaluation of global hypoxic-ischemic injury is the "reversal sign," which is characterized by reversal of the normal attenuation pattern of gray and white matter in the cortex and basal ganglia (Figure 2.17). MRI imaging will demonstrate diffuse restricted diffusion involving the cerebral cortex and basal ganglia. Although T2/FLAIR sequences may appear normal early in the course of the injury, imaging performed 24 hours after the insult will demonstrate increased signal involving the cortex and basal ganglia.

2.9 Subarachnoid Hemorrhage

Acute SAH is best identified as hyperdense material within the subarachnoid space (Figure 2.18), which may be diffuse or focal. SAH may be traumatic or spontaneous in etiology with common nontraumatic causes, including ruptured aneurysm, nontraumatic perimesencephalic hemorrhage, cortical vein thrombosis, and arteriovenous malformation. Aneurysmal SAH tends to be most pronounced in the basilar cisterns, whereas traumatic SAH is usually seen in the sulci. However, due to the large number of potential etiologies, once SAH is identified, CT angiography (Figure 2.19) should be performed if a traumatic etiology is considered unlikely. Regardless of whether an etiology is identified, continued imaging monitoring of patients with SAH is recommended to evaluate for late complications such as hydrocephalus and vasospasm.

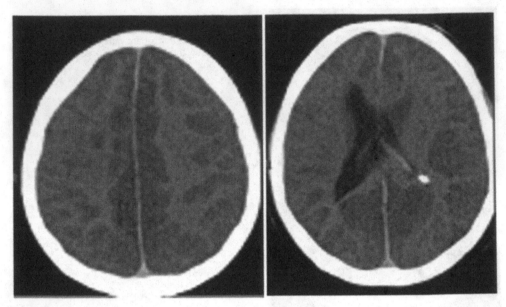

Figure 2.17 CT images demonstrating the "reversal sign" characterized by hypoattenuation of gray matter relative to white matter in this patient with diffuse hypoxic-ischemic injury.

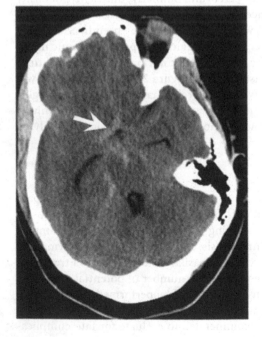

Figure 2.18 Unenhanced axial CT demonstrating hyperdense material within the suprasellar cistern (arrow) consistent with SAH.

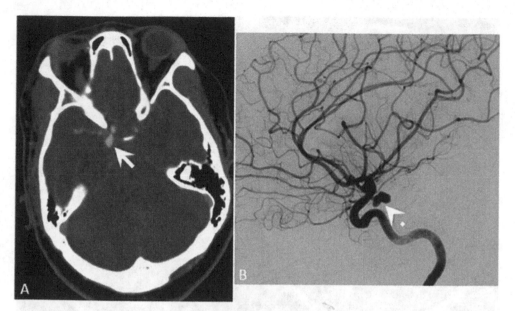

Figure 2.19 Axial CTA performed in the same patient as in Figure 2.18, demonstrating a right posterior communicating artery aneurysm (solid arrow) (a). Digital subtraction angiography in the same patient confirming presence of the aneurysm (dashed arrow) (b).

2.10 CNS Infection

Findings of intracranial infection are often occult on unenhanced CT imaging. Occasionally, hyperdense purulent material may be present within the subarachnoid space, suggestive of meningitis. Hypodensity within brain parenchyma may be indicative of cerebritis in the correct clinical setting, particularly if the location of the hypodensity does not follow known vascular territories and appears vasogenic, rather than cytotoxic. Regardless of the sensitivity, a head CT is still a critical component of the work-up of the CNS infection patient in order to exclude contraindications to lumbar puncture. The most sensitive imaging modality for the evaluation of CNS infection is enhanced MRI.

MRI findings in meningitis may present as hyperintense signal within the subarachnoid space on FLAIR imaging with associated leptomeningeal enhancement (Figure 2.20). Enhanced MRI may also evaluate for intracranial abscess formation (Figure 2.21) and intracranial empyema (Figure 2.22). Of note, certain causative agents demonstrate relatively specific patterns of infection. For example, preferential involvement of the temporal lobes in herpes simplex encephalitis (Figure 2.23) and subcortical vesicle formation in neurocysticercosis (Figure 2.24).

2.11 Toxic Exposures

Imaging findings in toxic exposures may be nonspecific and head CT may appear normal for the first 24 hours. When positive, unenhanced CT may demonstrate symmetric hypodensity involving the basal ganglia or cortex. Further evaluation may be performed with MRI, which may demonstrate areas of restricted diffusion and T2/FLAIR hyperintensity that can

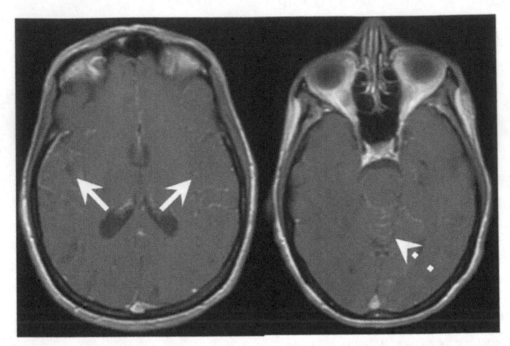

Figure 2.20 Enhanced axial T1-weighted fat-saturated MRI of the brain demonstrating bilateral temporal (solid arrows) and cerebellar (dashed arrow) meningeal enhancement in a patient with coccidioidomycosis meningitis.

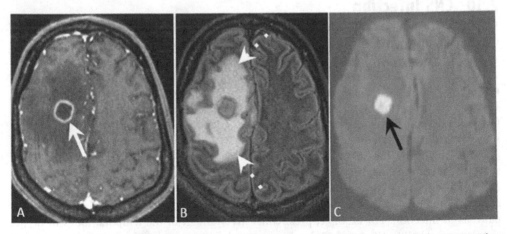

Figure 2.21 Axial T1 post-contrast (a), FLAIR (b), and diffusion-weighted (c) MRI of the brain demonstrate rim-enhancing mass (solid arrow) within the right centrum semiovale. The presence of restricted diffusion (black arrow) and surrounding edema (dashed arrows) are consistent with pyogenic abscess.

correspond to hypodensities seen on the CT scan. Patterns of involvement may be suggestive of the underlying metabolic derangement or exposure, such as involvement of the globi pallidi in carbon monoxide poisoning (Figure 2.25), but history is often essential in determining the underlying etiology.

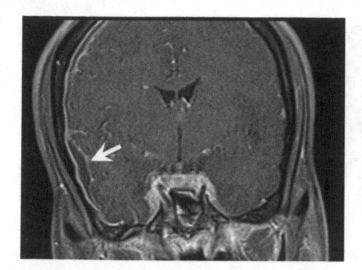

Figure 2.22 Coronal enhanced T1-weighted fat-saturated MRI of the brain demonstrates a rim-enhancing subdural fluid collection adjacent to the right temporal lobe (arrow), consistent with a subdural empyema.

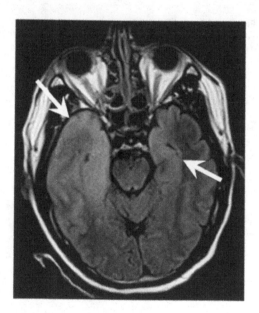

Figure 2.23 Axial FLAIR MRI image of the brain demonstrating increased T2 signal in the bilateral temporal lobes (arrows) in a patient with herpes simplex encephalitis.

2.12 Spinal Trauma

CT has become the standard for imaging of the spine in the setting of trauma, and cervical spine CT should always be considered in multiple trauma cases. CT is very sensitive for the detection of acute fractures (Figure 2.26) and malalignment

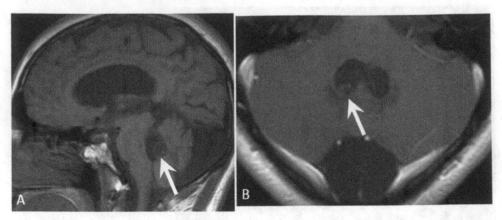

Figure 2.24 Sagittal T1-weighted unenhanced (a) and axial T1-weighted enhanced (b) images demonstrating a T1 hypointense nonenhancing cystic lesion (arrows) with a central dot, representing a scolex and the vesicular stage of neurocysticercosis.

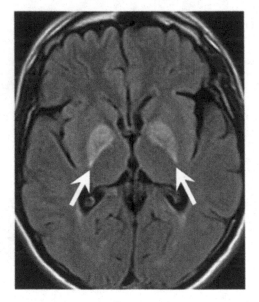

Figure 2.25 Axial FLAIR MRI demonstrating increased T2 signal within the bilateral putamen (arrows) in a patient with carbon monoxide exposure.

(Figure 2.27), but insensitive for acute ligamentous injury, EDH, and spinal cord injury. In patients with clinical findings of myelopathy in the setting of trauma, unenhanced MRI of the spine should be performed in conjunction with CT as these modalities are complementary in the evaluation of osseous and soft tissue abnormalities. Potential soft tissue abnormalities that are readily evident on MRI include traumatic disc herniation, ligamentous injury, EDH, and acute spinal cord injury.

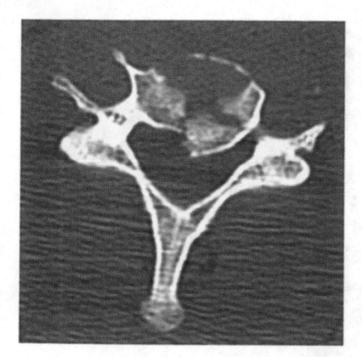

Figure 2.26 Axial CT image demonstrating a burst fracture of the C7 vertebral body.

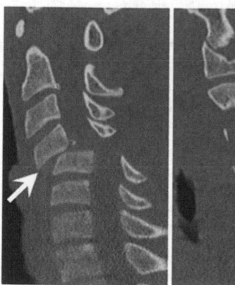
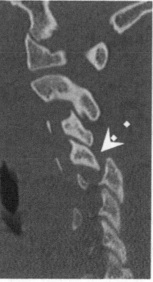

Figure 2.27 Sagittal CT images in the same patient demonstrate anterolisthesis of C4 on C5 (solid arrow) with associated facet fracture dislocation (dashed arrow).

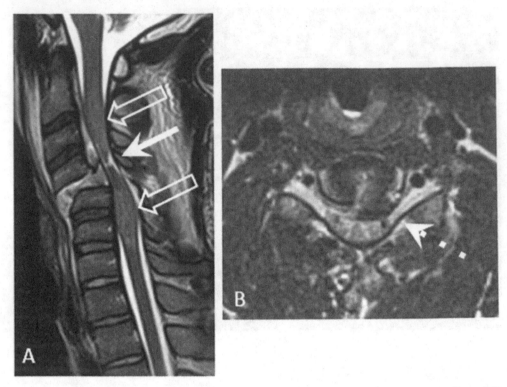

Figure 2.28 Sagittal STIR (a) and axial T2-weighted (b) MRI of the cervical spine, in the same patient as Figure 2.27, demonstrate hematoma and retropulsion of fracture fragments causing compression of the spinal cord (dashed arrow). Edema (open arrow) within and transection of the spinal cord (solid arrow) is also present.

Fluid-sensitive sequences are particularly useful for identifying edema or hematoma that may be causing mass effect upon the spinal cord (Figure 2.28). Susceptibility weighted or gradient echo images should also be acquired as these may demonstrate hemorrhage within the spinal cord, an indicator of poor clinical prognosis. MRI may also be used in the determination of fracture acuity as edema within a fracture denotes an acute process. If malignancy is suspected, MRI may also aid in the differentiation between benign and pathologic fractures.

2.13 Spine Infection

Spinal infections are predominantly centered at the vertebral body–intervertebral disc space. Risk factors for spine infection include recent surgery, intravenous drug users, bacteremia, or patients with chronic conditions (e.g., diabetes mellitus). Evaluation is best performed with enhanced MRI, with little role for spine CT (with the exception of patients who are unable to undergo MRI). Imaging findings include vertebral body and end-plate destruction with edema, loss of disc height, and enhancement within the intervertebral disc (Figure 2.29). Extension of infection into the spinal canal in the form of an epidural abscess (Figure 2.30) can cause significant spinal canal stenosis and may be the cause of neurologic deficits.

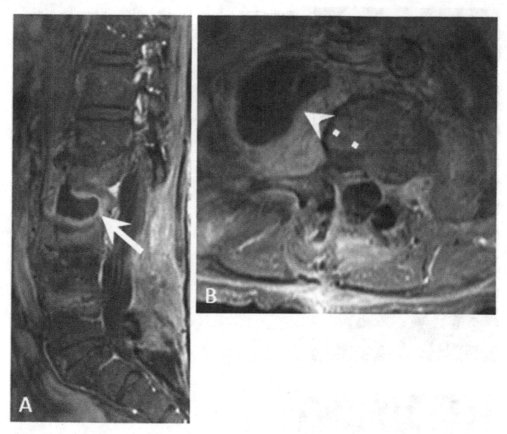

Figure 2.29 Sagittal (a) and axial T1-weighted contrast-enhanced (b) MRI of the lumbar spine demonstrating a rim-enhancing fluid collection at the L2–L3 disc space (solid arrow) with enhancement of the vertebral bodies, consistent with discitis/osteomyelitis with abscess formation. A psoas abscess is also present (dashed arrow).

2.14 Degenerative Disease of the Spine

Back pain is a common complaint of patients presenting to the ED. The ACR recommends imaging evaluation of back pain only in the setting of suspected cancer, suspected infection, focal neurologic deficit, prolonged symptom duration, or immunosuppression, as most cases of simple radicular pain are self-limited or can be treated without advanced imaging. In these instances, primary evaluation should be with enhanced MRI. Without a recent history of trauma, CT is not recommended. Spine radiographs are of little benefit and are not recommended.

MRI evaluation of the spine in the setting of degenerative disease may demonstrate spinal canal or foraminal stenosis secondary to disc herniation (Figure 2.31), facet hypertrophy, and/or ligamentous hypertrophy. In patients presenting with acute onset of foot drop, saddle anesthesia, or bladder/bowel dysfunction, the most pressing etiology to exclude is cauda equina syndrome where a lesion within the spinal canal causes severe compression of the spinal cord and/or cauda equina. In patients who cannot undergo MRI, CT myelography may be employed to evaluate for cord compression.

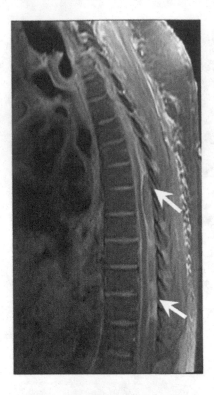

Figure 2.30 Enhanced T1-weighted fat-saturated MRI of the thoracic spine demonstrating a rim-enhancing epidural fluid collection (arrows) causing anterior displacement of the spinal cord, consistent with epidural abscess.

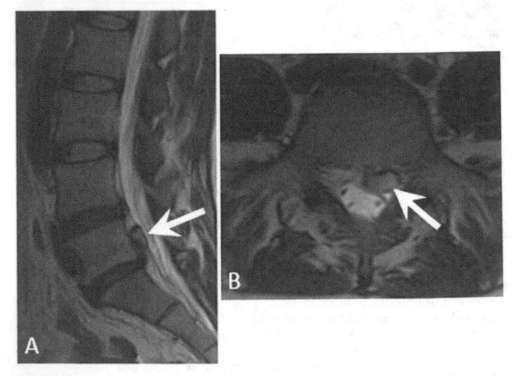

Figure 2.31 Sagittal (a) and T2-weighted (b) MRI of the lumbar spine demonstrate a left paracentral disc extrusion (arrows) at L4–L5. There is superior migration of the extrusion, without sequestration.

2.15 CT and MRI Safety Considerations in Neurologic Imaging

2.15.1 Computed Tomography Safety

Ionizing radiation exposure is associated with a potential increased risk of developing cancer after a latent period of typically 10–20 years, although the reported range is 4–60 years. These risks are considered greater for children. CT scans are the single largest source of radiation exposure to the US population and have recently received increased attention from medical professional organizations, the media, and patients. There have also been serious overexposures to patients in recent years, including almost 400 patients who had brain perfusion CT scans performed for evaluation of stroke, due to use of an inappropriate scanning protocol. These patients experienced erythema and hair loss, resulting in a FDA investigation and intervention followed by substantial increased regulatory requirements. Physicians must be aware of these potential risks and have the necessary information for informed discussions with patients and families.

Although the risk from one CT scan to an individual patient is very low, it is not zero. Thus, the exposure of patients to imaging studies utilizing ionizing radiation should always be a benefit–risk decision. CT exams should be ordered only after a physical examination, review of recent imaging exams, and a determination that the results of the CT imaging will impact the clinical decision-making and subsequent treatment. Patients should be queried about recent imaging performed at other locations.

In response to increased concerns about medical radiation exposures, there have been several consortia of medical specialties that have developed guidelines, education, and other resources to address radiation risks of imaging, appropriateness criteria, and dose reduction strategies. Emergency physicians should be familiar with these websites:

- Image Gently® is focused on pediatric dose reduction.
- Image Wisely® is aimed at adult radiation protection.
- Choosing Wisely® provides advice to patients and physicians regarding the reduction of unnecessary tests and procedures, including CT and other imaging studies, with specific recommendations from the American College of Emergency Physicians.
- RadiologyInfo.org provides information to patients about imaging exams, including typical radiation exposures.
- ACR Appropriateness Criteria® includes guidelines intended to assist physicians in making accurate imaging decisions for a variety of clinical conditions. These guidelines rate the appropriateness of different radiologic procedures with detailed comments and relative radiation levels (RRL) noted.

There are various radiation metrics used in describing radiation exposures from different imaging modalities. In CT, the metrics are $CTDI_v$ (CT dose index-volume), DLP (dose-length product), and effective dose. All CT scanners provide $CTDI_v$ and DLP values, but these metrics are based on standard phantom measurements and do not directly represent patient exposure.

Effective dose is the most common dose metric used, as it can be used to compare various imaging modalities. It is used to estimate radiation risk from an imaging study to the population, not an individual patient, as there are wide ranges in radiation exposures from various modalities. Effective dose is expressed in millisieverts (mSv) and accounts for the radiosensitivity of the exposed organs, not just the absorbed dose. The ACR Appropriateness

Table 2.1 Effective doses and relative risk levels by imaging study

Imaging procedure	Effective dose (mSv)	RRL (adult)
CT head (single-pass w/o contrast)	2	Low
CT head (with and without contrast)	4	Low
CT angiography	1	Very low
CT brain perfusion for acute ischemic stroke (AIS)	20	Moderate
CT multiphase angiography for AIS	0.8	Very low
CT spine	6–10	Low

Criteria[a] categorize the RRL and radiation risk by imaging study, from no risk to moderate risk. Radiation exposure from most diagnostic imaging studies does not normally exceed 100 mSv, which is considered to be high risk. Everyone is exposed to natural background radiation, which varies by location and elevation, but is generally considered to be approximately 3 mSv/year. Typical effective doses and relative risk levels by neurologic imaging study are shown in Table 2.1.

Radiation exposure to pregnant or potentially pregnant patients receiving CT scans is considered to be of negligible risk, unless the abdomen or pelvis is being imaged. The CT radiation beam is very well collimated and there is minimal scatter radiation to the fetus. Single-pass scans of the abdomen and pelvis are considered to be low risk and can be performed when necessary. The administration of iodinated contrast is not contraindicated in pregnant or lactating patients, as there are no data suggesting any harm to the fetus or baby. It is important, however, to be aware of organizational policy regarding imaging pregnant and lactating patients, as policies can vary substantially.

CT scanning of pediatric patients should be performed judiciously to reduce radiation exposure and the need for repeated studies. Alternative imaging studies using nonionizing modalities should be performed before CT (e.g., ultrasound or MRI). When CT evaluation is needed, single-pass, limited scan area, and low-dose CT scans will often provide sufficient information for diagnosis.

2.15.2 Magnetic Resonance Imaging Safety

MRI generates images using strong magnetic fields and radiofrequency waves, with no ionizing radiation exposure to patients. However, awareness of other very serious safety concerns is essential to ensure patient and personnel safety in MRI. There have been deaths and serious injuries to patients, staff, and others as a result of failure to understand these risks and follow recommended MR safety guidelines primarily established by the ACR, FDA, the Joint Commission, and the MR industry.

MRI scanners generally operate at 1.5 or 3 Tesla, with some medical research MRI units having much greater field strengths. These are very strong magnetic fields; the earth's magnetic field, in comparison, is 0.3–0.6 microTesla. These large superconducting magnets generate a static magnetic field which is *always on*, requiring MR safety precautions to be strictly followed at *all* times. "Quenching" the magnet, or releasing the liquid helium surrounding the magnet core into the atmosphere, is the only way the magnetic field can be turned off quickly. A quench subjects the magnet to potentially serious damage, however, and should only be initiated if a person is pinned to the magnet by a large ferromagnetic object and in immediate life-threatening, physical distress.

It is because of the risks of the static magnetic field, which is always on, that no ferromagnetic materials or any large metallic, nonferrous objects should be brought into the MRI scan room. Ferrous objects (e.g., non-MR-safe oxygen tanks, ventilators, or patient beds/transport carts) can become a projectile hazard and be pulled into the bore of the magnet. Nonferrous metallic objects (e.g., a metallic infusion pump) may experience forces that cause these objects to twist and pull.

MRI scanners also generate time-varying gradient and radiofrequency magnetic fields during scanning sequences. These fields can also affect ferrous and nonferrous implantable devices in patients (e.g., pacemakers, vascular clips, and nerve stimulators). The risks of these fields include auditory concerns, requiring hearing protection; induced voltages in implanted electrodes or retained wires in sensitive areas; thermal effects that can cause injuries to human tissues (e.g., burns); and permanent neurologic impairment.

It is because of the multitude of potential risks that comprehensive MRI screening must be performed on patients, staff, and family who will be entering the MRI room. All MRI facilities have four zones identified to ensure that MRI safety is maintained. Zones I and II are generally unrestricted areas prior to the areas under strict access control, Zones III and IV. Zone IV is the MRI room and Zone III is the area adjacent to the MRI room that accesses Zone IV. Screening of all patients, staff, and others accompanying the patient into Zones III and/or IV should occur in Zone II, but may also be performed in Zone III. This screening process must be comprehensive and performed each time, regardless of previous screenings and exams.

MR technologists, in conjunction with the radiologist, have final responsibility for ensuring that the patient has been adequately screened prior to being scanned. A major challenge in screening emergent patients is that they may not be conscious or able to participate in the screening process. Querying family members can be part of the screening process for these patients. Other imaging exams (e.g., CT scans or radiographs) that have been performed during the current visit should be reviewed as part of the screening for implants, leads, or other devices. Ferromagnetic detectors add another level of confidence to screening, but cannot generally identify ferromagnetic items in the patient. Shortcuts to comprehensive patient screening or insistence upon scanning patients who have not been adequately screened places patients, staff, and equipment in jeopardy of serious harm. It is also important to closely monitor unresponsive patients during MR scans to identify potential hazardous events that cannot be communicated to staff (e.g., thermal effects).

Pregnant patients may be scanned as there has been no evidence of harm to the fetus from MRI. Gadolinium-based MR contrast is not routinely given to pregnant patients, with the exception of cases where the benefit of using gadolinium outweighs the risks. The administration of MR contrast is not contraindicated in lactating patients, as there are no data suggesting any harm to the baby.

Pediatric patients present special challenges both from the screening requirements and because they often require sedation for MRI exams. It is common for a family member to accompany a child during the scan, and the child may bring comfort items into the MR room. Again, comprehensive screening of everyone and everything entering the MR room is mandatory. Special attention to monitoring of body temperature during MR exams is necessary, particularly in the neonatal and young pediatric population as hypo- and hyperthermia can occur.

It is essential to be aware of specific organizational policies and procedures regarding MRI scanning, screening, and safety requirements.

2.16 Summary

Neurologic complaints are a common source of ED presentations, and imaging plays a critical role in the initial work-up of these patients. Although initial imaging evaluation is commonly performed with CT, some complaints, particularly those involving the spine, are better assessed with MRI. This use of more advanced imaging in the emergent setting should be guided by a combination of clinical presentation, CT findings, and results of other testing.

Pearls and Pitfalls
• Spinal cord compression and cauda equine syndrome suspicion require stat MRI.
• The interventional treatment window of AIS has expanded to 24 hours and beyond.
• Rehemorrhage within 36 hours of injury can happen in epidural hematoma.
• CT scans are often unremarkable in diffuse axonal injury patients.
• CTV may be required to diagnose dural venous thrombosis.
• CT scans of pregnant patients have negligible risk unless to the abdomen or pelvis.

Bibliography

ACR. ACR Appropriateness Criteria® low back pain. Available at www.acr.org/~/media/ACR/Documents/AppCriteria/Diagnostic/LowBackPain.pdf. Accessed 25 July 2015.

Albers GW, Marks MP, Kemp S, et al. Thrombectomy for stroke at 6 to 16 hours with selection by perfusion imaging. *N Engl J Med* 378(8):708–718.

American College of Radiology. ACR Appropriateness Criteria®. Available at www.acr.org/ac.

American College of Radiology. ACR-SPR practice parameter for imaging pregnant or potentially pregnant adolescents and women with ionizing radiation. 2014. Web.

American College of Radiology. Manual on contrast media V10. 2015. Web.

Aviv RI, Mandelcorn J, Chakraborty S, et al. Alberta Stroke Program early CT scoring of CT perfusion in early stroke visualization and assessment. *AJNR Am J Neuroradiol* 2007; 28(10):1975–1980.

Goyal M. Randomized assessment of rapid endovascular treatment of ischemic stroke. *N Engl J Med* 2015;372(11):1019–1030.

Image Gently. Image Gently® and CT scans. Web.

Joint Commission. Sentinel Event Alert 38: Preventing accidents and injuries in the MRI suite. 2008.

Kanal E, Barkovich J, Bell C, et al. ACR guidance document on MR safe practices: 2013. An MRI accreditation safety review tool. *J Magn Reson* 2013; 37:501–531.

Menon BK, d'Esterre D, Qazi EM, et al. Multiphase CT angiography: a new tool for the imaging triage of patients with acute ischemic stroke. *Radiology* 2015;275 (2):510–520.

Miller NR. Diagnosis and management of dural carotid-cavernous sinus fistulas. *Neurosurg Focus* 2007;23(5):E13.

National Academies. *Health Risks from Exposure to Low Levels of Ionizing Radiation BEIR VII, Phase 2.* National Academies, 2006.

National Council on Radiation Protection and Measurements. *Ionizing Radiation Exposure of the Population of the United States: Recommendations of the National Council on Radiation Protection and Measurements, March 3, 2009.* National Council on Radiation Protection and Measurements, 2009.

National Institute of Neurological Disorders and Stroke rt-PA Stroke Study Group. Tissue plasminogen activator for acute ischemic stroke. *N Engl J Med* 1995;**333**(24):1581–1587.

Nishijima DK, Offerman SR, Ballard DW, et al. Immediate and delayed traumatic intracranial hemorrhage in patients with head trauma and preinjury warfarin or clopidogrel use. *Ann Emerg Med* 2012;**59**(6):460–468.

Nogueira RG, Jadhav AP, Haussen DC, et al. Thrombectomy 6 to 24 hours after stroke with a mismatch between deficit and infarct. *N Engl J Med* 2018;**378**(1):11–21.

Powers WJ, Rabinstein AA, Ackerson T, et al. 2018 guidelines for the early management of patients with acute ischemic stroke: a guideline for healthcare professionals from the American Heart Association/American Stroke Association. *Stroke* 2018;**49**(3):e46–e110.

Sullivan TP, Jarvik JG, Cohen WA. Follow-up of conservatively managed epidural hematomas: implications for timing of repeat CT. *AJNR Am J Neuroradiol* 1999;**20**(1):107–113.

US Food and Drug Administration. MRI (Magnetic resonance imaging). 2015.

Wong HJ, Sistrom CL, Benzer TI, et al. Use of imaging in the emergency department: physicians have limited effect on variation. *Radiology* 2013;**268**(3):779–789.

Electroencephalography

Timothy Quezada, Andrea Synowiec, and Kevin M. Kelly

3.1 Introduction

The electroencephalogram (EEG) is created by differential amplification of cortical postsynaptic excitatory and inhibitory potentials. As a neurophysiologic monitor, it can be used as a bedside tool to assess an unresponsive patient in an emergency setting, particularly in the case of a patient with a history of epilepsy or an unexplained coma. Use of EEG in the emergency department (ED) can be technically challenging; both obtaining and interpreting the study may pose difficulty in small community hospitals or remote settings.

3.2 Technical Setup

A minimum of 16 electrodes placed on the scalp utilizing the International 10–20 System of Placement is recommended for a thorough and accurate evaluation of cortical rhythms. Therefore, an EEG technician is typically necessary to set up the study; however, EEG headcaps and other "rapid" EEG substitutes are now being marketed for use in EDs. Electrodes are referenced to each other in various combinations and create a read-out called a "montage." While any montage can be used, an anterior–posterior longitudinal bipolar montage (AP bipolar or "double banana" montage) can be learned and utilized most easily; most EEG atlases are based in the AP bipolar montage. Note that Fz/Cz/Pz (midline) and A1/A2 ("ear") electrodes are omitted in the AP bipolar montage. For EEG, even-numbered electrodes are on the right and odd-numbered electrodes are on the left (Figure 3.1).

Differential amplification is used to minimize environmental artifacts. However, in the electrically contaminated environment of an ED setting, artifacts are common. Recognizing common artifacts is essential for the correct interpretation of the EEG in the ED. A 25–30-minute EEG recording is a typically adequate duration and a video component is ideal when available.

3.3 The Normal EEG

The appearance of the normal EEG changes with the age and arousal state of the patient. In the awake adult with eyes closed, a sinusoidal rhythm is expected from posterior head regions, typically ranging across 8–11 Hz (cycles/s). This rhythm typically suppresses with eye opening. Slower waves are seen in drowsiness. Sleep may show both slowing and some occasional high-amplitude sharp waves (vertex waves) from the central (C3, C4) and parietal (P3, P4) electrodes.

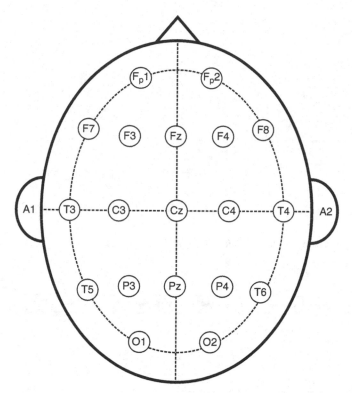

Figure 3.1 Electrode placement according to the International 10–20 System. Fp (frontopolar), F (frontal), C (central), P (parietal), O (occipital), A (auricular).

3.4 The Abnormal EEG

3.4.1 Abnormalities of Slowing, Voltage, and Reactivity

Slowing may be seen intermittently or persistently on the EEG and localized on the EEG as generalized (diffuse) or focal. A diffusely slow EEG is characterized by ≤7 Hz activity, frequently with high-voltage (amplitude) waveforms (Figure 3.2). It is characteristic of an encephalopathic patient, nonspecific for the type of encephalopathy, and may lack reactivity (i.e., EEG changes in response to patient stimulation). Focal slowing can be seen independent of or in combination with diffuse slowing and may indicate a focal area of cerebral dysfunction; imaging may be considered in these patients, especially if a focal CNS process is not part of the patient's clinical history. Diffuse or focal slowing may be seen in a postictal state. Excessively low-voltage recordings without frank electrocerebral activities typically portend a poor or grave prognosis unless an underlying potentially reversible cause can be identified (e.g., medication overdose, hypothermia, or near-drowning).

3.4.2 Interictal Epileptiform Abnormalities

Interictal (between seizures) epileptiform abnormalities are by definition nonictal; however, their presence implies a decreased seizure threshold. Interictal epileptiform abnormalities

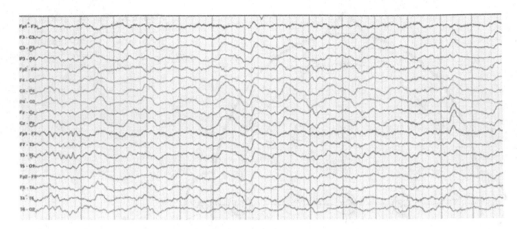

Figure 3.2 EEG with diffuse slowing and high-amplitude waveforms.

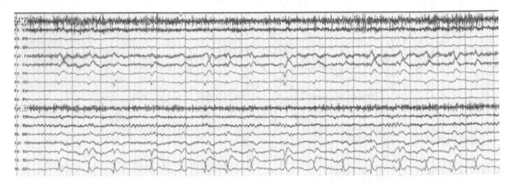

Figure 3.3 Lateralized periodic discharges with spike-and-wave complex associated with right hemispheric infarcts.

may be generalized, as in the classic 3 Hz spike-and-wave complexes associated with genetic absence epilepsy, or focal, as in spikes or sharp waves seen in the temporal region in a patient with temporal lobe epilepsy.

3.4.3 Seizures and Nonconvulsive Status Epilepticus

Seizure discharges in patients with genetic epilepsies are the easiest to identify, with well-formed spike/polyspike-and-slow wave complexes seen either diffusely or with bifrontal maximal voltages. However, most patients who present to the ED with an altered level of consciousness due to nonconvulsive status epilepticus (NCSE) do not have these findings. In these cases, recurrent spike and/or sharp wave discharges are often seen, but may be irregular-appearing or may wax and wane. Rhythmic or periodic patterns of discharges may be seen (Figure 3.3), which in certain circumstances may indicate electrographic (EEG alone) or electroclinical (EEG and clinically apparent) seizures.

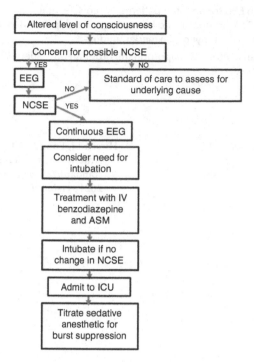

Figure 3.4 EEG use and diagnostic and treatment decisions for NCSE.

Rhythmic activity that starts focally and spreads across the EEG may also represent generalized seizure activity. For patients who have EEG findings that are suspicious for, but not clearly diagnostic of, status epilepticus, use of an IV antiseizure medication (ASM), including benzodiazepines, can be considered (Figure 3.4).

A diagnosis of NCSE is made based on history, neurologic examination, and EEG findings. When the EEG is strongly supportive or diagnostic of NCSE, continuous EEG monitoring is recommended if available. Based on the patient's presentation and a corresponding potential need to protect their airway, intubation should be considered. Treatment with a benzodiazepine or an ASM, such as phenytoin, valproate sodium, or levetiracetam, is initiated. Note that ASMs have less sedative potential than a benzodiazepine but a slower onset of action. If NCSE is not aborted with a benzodiazepine and an ASM, the patient requires intubation prior to treatment with a sedative anesthetic, typically midazolam or propofol, admission to an intensive care unit, and titration of the anesthetic to an EEG burst suppression pattern.

Pearls and Pitfalls

- Know when to order an EEG in the ED and when to insist on an emergent EEG. If uncertain, consult the neurology service.
- Treating an encephalopathic patient without an EEG can be harmful (e.g., administering a benzodiazepine to a postictal patient when presumed to be in NCSE).
- Know when to transfer rather than admit a patient when EEG services are not available.

- When ordering an EEG for agitated patients, when safe, hold sedating medications that will affect the EEG (i.e., propofol and benzodiazepine drips), and instead consider use of medications such as fentanyl or dexmedetomidine.
- When deferring an acute EEG is appropriate, order an outpatient EEG following discharge from the ED.

Bibliography

Fisch BJ. *Fisch & Spehlmann's EEG Primer: Basic Principles of Digital and Analog EEG.* Elsevier, 1999.

Hirsch LJ, Fong MWK, Leitinger M, et al. American Clinical Neurophysiology Society's standardized critical care EEG terminology: 2021 version. *J Clin Neurophysiol* 2021;38(1).

Lumbar Puncture

Troy Desai, Dan Geary, Chris Troianos, and Richard Feduska

4.1 Lumbar Puncture

Lumbar puncture (LP) is a diagnostic procedure that can be performed successfully in most patients with minimal discomfort. The key factors to a successful LP are an understanding of the anatomy of the lumbar spine, careful positioning of the patient, and a thorough palpation of the bony landmarks to identify the lumbar interspaces.

4.2 Anatomy of the Lumbar Spine

The spinal cord terminates at the conus medullaris. Ultrasound studies have demonstrated that 84.3% of neonates between the 40th gestational week (term) and 23 weeks post-term have a conus medullaris more cephalad than the L1–L2 interspace and 98% have a conus medullaris more cephalad than the L3 vertebra. Since the level of the conus medullaris is more variable in children, LPs should be attempted at or below the L3–L4 space in children (Figure 4.1).

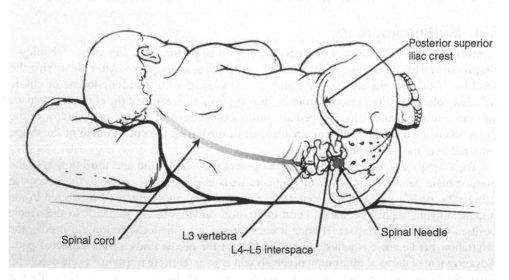

Figure 4.1 Lumbar puncture in an infant – left lateral decubitus fetal position.

The conus medullaris is at or more cephalad to the L2 vertebral body in most adults. In rare instances it may be at the level of the L3 body. An LP should not be performed routinely above the level of the L2–L3 space. An imaginary line connecting the posterior iliac crests crosses at the level of the L4 vertebral body. This is an important landmark for identifying the L3–L4 and L4–L5 interspaces.

The spinous processes of the lumbar vertebrae are angled downward at approximately 10–15 degrees from the vertical plane of the spine. Flexion of the lumbar spine will open the space between the spinous process and allow easier access to the subarachnoid space.

In the midline approach, the spinal needle will pass through three layers of ligament: the supraspinal ligament, the interspinal ligament, and finally the ligamentum flavum. After piercing the ligamentum flavum, the needle crosses the dura mater and the adherent arachnoid mater to enter the CSF-filled intrathecal space.

A descriptive video tutorial of lumbar spine anatomy is available at: www.usra.ca/VirtualSpine/LumbarAnatomy.htm.

4.3 Positioning for the Lumbar Puncture

The patient may be placed either in the lateral decubitus position or the sitting position. Each position has advantages and disadvantages. The sitting position allows for better estimation of the midline, which is particularly useful for obese patients. Similarly, the spinous processes can be palpated beginning in the thoracic (or cervical) region and then palpated downward toward the lumbar region using the gluteal folds as a visual guide (Figure 4.2). CSF pressure must be measured in the lateral decubitus position as measurements in the sitting position. The lateral position allows for better positioning of the patient by drawing the knees toward the abdomen. However, the soft tissue overlying the paraspinous muscles tends to sag toward the midline in the lateral position and may give a false impression of the true midline. Careful palpation of the spinous processes is needed to ensure that the midline is correctly identified while in the lateral position (Figure 4.3).

4.4 Midline Approach

Lumbar puncture is an invasive procedure that must be performed using aseptic technique. Preprocedural hand washing, mask, hat, and sterile gloves are required. After identifying the L3–L4 or L4–L5 interspace, the overlying skin is washed with povidone-iodine or chlorhexidine solution using a circular motion, moving from the region of the chosen interspace and extending outward. The prepped area must extend beyond the cut-out window of the drape to ensure a sterile field. The area is then draped, with the cut-out area of the drape centered over the chosen interspace.

The interspace is straddled on its lateral borders with the second and third fingers of the nondominant hand. A skin wheal of 1% lidocaine is injected in the center of the interspace using a 25- or 26-gauge needle. Deeper infiltration of local anesthetic is then injected in the midline, angling slightly cephalad. Local infiltration provides tactile feedback to the needle position within the interspace. If bone is encountered with the local infiltration needle, the infiltration needle angle is adjusted until passage of the needle finds an unobstructed path. Advancement of the local infiltration needle should encounter more resistance as the needle tip enters the supraspinal and interspinal ligaments. This is valuable tactile feedback that indicates the center of the interspace, passing through the ligaments between the spinous processes.

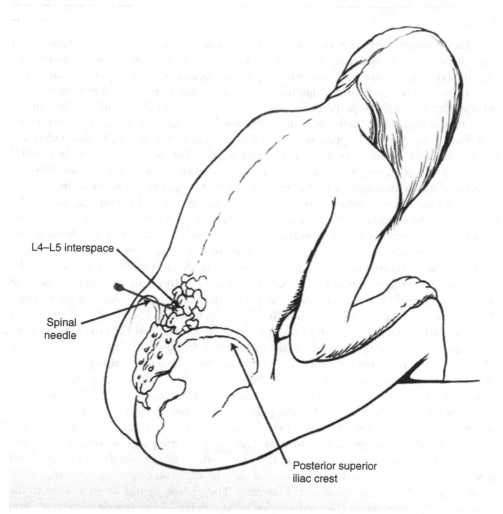

L4–L5 interspace

Spinal needle

Posterior superior iliac crest

Figure 4.2 Lumbar puncture in an adult.

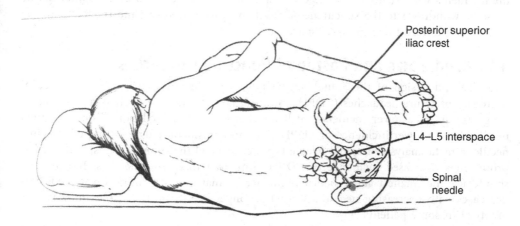

Posterior superior iliac crest

L4–L5 interspace

Spinal needle

Figure 4.3 Lumbar puncture in an adult – left lateral decubitus fetal position.

Prior to insertion of the spinal needle, the local anesthetic wheal can be massaged to allow palpation of the interspace and to ensure an accurate starting point for the insertion of the spinal needle. Spinal needles are of two types: cutting edge needles and conical-tipped or "pencil point" needles. Cutting edge needles do not require an introducer because their cutting edge passes through the skin easily. Conical-tipped needles require a short introducer needle to facilitate insertion of the spinal needle through the skin. It is important to note that using a conical-tipped spinal needle requires repositioning of the introducer needle direction before reinserting the spinal needle. The benefit of reduced post-LP headaches with conical-type spinal needles makes use of an introducer needle worthwhile.

Straddling the interspace with the second and third digits of the nondominant hand, the spinal needle is held between the thumb and index finger of the dominant hand. The bevel of cutting needles should be directed laterally to pass through the dural fibers in a longitudinal direction rather than transecting the longitudinally oriented dural fibers. Conical-type needles do not require this attention to needle tip orientation. As the spinal needle is advanced through the skin and adipose tissue, the firm midline ligaments will be encountered. The ligamentum flavum is the final layer of ligament and may provide the tactile sensation of "leathery" resistance as the needle is advanced. With passage through the dura mater, a "popping" sensation is often encountered. The stylette of the spinal needle is withdrawn and the hub of the spinal needle is examined for flow of CSF. If no CSF flows, the stylet is replaced in the spinal needle hub and the needle is slowly advanced again, repeating the process of removing the stylette and waiting a few seconds for CSF flow. A paresthesia may occur if the needle is within the intrathecal space or it may be lateral and encountering a nerve root. In either case, the needle should be withdrawn a few millimeters and if the paresthesia abates, the stylet can be withdrawn and the hub examined for CSF flow. If steady CSF flow occurs and the patient no longer has the paresthesia, the procedure may proceed by measuring an opening pressure and collecting CSF. Conversely, if there is CSF flow after slightly withdrawing the spinal needle, the paresthesia may have occurred due to encountering a nerve root, which usually means the needle was directed laterally. The patient should be queried as to the location of the paresthesia (i.e., left side or right side), and the needle withdrawn and redirected for the next needle pass. Spinal needles are flexible and the spinous ligaments are quite firm. Bending the needle at the hub after the spinal needle is positioned within the ligaments will usually not change the direction of the needle tip. The spinal needle must be withdrawn to the subcutaneous level in order to redirect the trajectory of the needle path toward the intrathecal space.

4.5 Needle Size and Postdural Puncture Headaches

The size and design of the spinal needle play a significant role in the incidence of postdural puncture headaches (PDPH). Studies have shown that decreasing the needle gauge results in a lower incidence of headache. Conical "pencil point" design spinal needles have a lower incidence of PDPH than an equivalent gauge cutting edge spinal needle; a meta-analysis of spinal needle types concluded that noncutting spinal needles produced a decreased incidence of PDPH compared to cutting needles. Ideally, one should use the smallest gauge pencil point needle that is practical; however, CSF flow decreases with decreasing needle size so the longer CSF collection times may not be practical in some patients.

4.6 Obtaining an Opening Pressure and Fluid Collection

An opening pressure is measured when CSF is encountered. A manometer tube with a three-way stopcock at its base is attached to flexible tubing. The flexible tubing is carefully connected to the hub of the spinal needle, with attention paid not to alter the position of the spinal needle. The patient should relax the neck and hips from the flexed position so that an accurate opening pressure can be obtained. The stopcock is turned to allow CSF flow into the manometer while the manometer is held in an upright position. The opening pressure is the level at which the CSF column stops rising in the manometer. The normal range of CSF pressure in adults is 10–20 cmH$_2$O. The fluid in the manometer is then drained into the collection tubes by turning the stopcock at the base of the manometer. Approximately 3–4 mL of fluid are collected in each of the four tubes. Additional CSF fluid can then be collected directly from the spinal needle hub. After sufficient CSF has been collected, the spinal needle is withdrawn from the patient. Some advocate reinsertion of the stylet before withdrawing the spinal needle to minimize the possibility of aspirating a nerve root into the needle tip.

4.7 Lumbar Puncture Video Resource

The *New England Journal of Medicine* has an excellent online video demonstrating the technique of LP: www.nejm.org/doi/full/10.1056/NEJMvcm054952. The video also discusses the role of LP in the diagnosis of neurological conditions.

4.8 Epidural Blood Patch

The epidural blood patch is considered the definitive treatment of the PDPH. Epidural blood patches are most effective when performed greater than 24 hours following a dural puncture. The incidence of complete relief of headache after the first epidural blood patch is ≥75%. If the PDPH is not resolved within 24 hours after the first epidural blood patch, a repeat blood patch also has a success rate of ≥75%. Persistent headaches after two blood patches should prompt an investigation of an alternative cause of the headache.

The epidural blood patch consists of injecting 20 mL of the patient's blood into the epidural space at the site of the dural puncture. The general theory of epidural blood patch treatment is that the injected blood forms a clot over the CSF leak site and prevents further CSF leakage as the hole in the dura heals. The injected blood volume may work to relieve the headache by increasing pressure within the CSF space, thereby relieving the traction on cranial structures caused by CSF loss. Contraindications for the procedure are the same as those for LP. In addition, fever and bacteremia increase the risk of infection in the epidural space. This procedure is most often performed by anesthesia personnel and rarely by emergency medicine physicians. Conservative treatments should be discussed when obtaining informed consent from the patient. PDPHs usually resolve within 7 days. Conservative treatments, including bed rest, hydration, analgesics, caffeine, and abdominal binders, may be tried before utilizing an epidural blood patch. Severe headaches or limited patient function may make conservative treatments an impractical choice. Risks of the procedure include dural puncture, infection, backache, and partial or complete failure to resolve the headache.

4.9 Contraindications to Lumbar Puncture

1. Increased intracranial pressure.
2. infection overlying the area of the LP site.
3. thrombocytopenia or other coagulopathy.

Patients at risk for development of bleeding complications must be monitored for signs of sensory change, motor weakness, and symptoms of cauda equina syndrome. Epidural hematoma development must be diagnosed early and treated by neurosurgical decompression to reduce the incidence of permanent neurologic dysfunction. Experienced practitioners consider a platelet count of 80,000 to be the lower limit when performing LP. When a low platelet count is present, an experienced practitioner should attempt the LP so that the number of needle passes is kept to a minimum. The American Society of Regional Anesthesia and Pain Medicine developed evidence-based guidelines for patients who are receiving anticoagulant therapy. The most current guidelines can be accessed at the ASRA website: www.asra.com/advisory-guidelines. The ASRA recommendations for neuraxial blocks (spinal or epidural anesthesia) are applicable to diagnostic LPs since the approach to all of these procedures is identical. A summary of the ASRA recommendations is outlined below.

4.10 Thrombolytic Therapy

Patients receiving thrombolytic drugs are at an increased risk for developing spontaneous epidural hematomas. Patients who had an LP and subsequent thrombolytic therapy should be closely monitored for neurologic changes. Lumbar puncture should be avoided for 10 days following thrombolytic drugs.

4.11 Heparin Unfractionated (UFH)

4.11.1 Intravenous UFH

1. Delay heparin administration for one hour after LP.
2. Patients receiving IV UFH should have the infusion stopped 2–4 hours before the LP and coagulation assessed prior to LP. Patients who have been on IV heparin for several days are at risk for heparin-induced thrombocytopenia and should be checked for a normal platelet count before attempting LP.

SQ heparin: Patients receiving twice-daily dosing of 5000 units have no contraindications to LP.

4.11.2 Low Molecular Weight Heparin (LMWH)

Patients receiving LMWH treatment should have an LP delayed until 24 hours after the last dose of LMWH. LMWH treatment should be delayed for 24 hours following an LP.

4.12 Warfarin

Warfarin should be stopped for 4–5 days before performing an LP and the INR should be normal at the time of LP. In emergencies, vitamin K or fresh frozen plasma can be given and the INR checked for normalization.

4.13 Antiplatelet Medications

Aspirin and NSAIDS. These drugs by themselves seem to pose no additional risk for spinal hematoma. When used in the presence of other medications altering coagulation, extra concern should be exercised due to the increased risk for bleeding.

4.14 Thienopyridine Derivatives

Clopidogrel should be discontinued for 7 days prior to LP.

4.15 Platelet GP IIb/IIIa Antagonists

Abciximab should be discontinued for 24–48 hours.

Eptifibatide and tirifiban should be discontinued for 4–8 hours.

4.16 Thrombin Inhibitors

This includes desirudin, lepirudin, bivalirudin, argatroban.

The thrombin inhibitor effect is monitored by the aPTT (activated partial thromboplastin clotting time) and is present for 1–3 hours following intravenous delivery. aPTT should be obtained if the patient recently received a thrombin inhibitor.

4.17 Fondaparinux

Fondaparinux causes factor Xa inhibition. The FDA issued a black box warning for spinal/ epidural hematomas. The safe time period for LP following fondaparinux administration has not been established.

4.18 Direct Thrombin and Activated Xa Inhibitors

Draft recommendations by ASRA are given in Table 4.1.

4.19 Herbal Therapy

This includes garlic, ginkgo and ginseng.

Herbal medications used alone do not pose a significant risk concern for spinal/epidural hematoma following LP.

Table 4.1 Draft recommendations by ASRA for direct thrombin and activated Xa Inhibitors

Drug	Time before LP	Time after LP
Dabigatran	5 days	6 hours
Apixaban	3 days	6 hours
Rivaroxaban	3 days	6 hours
Prasugrel	7–10 days	6 hours
Ticagrelor	5–7 days	6 hours

4.20 Ultrasound Guidance When Performing an LP

Palpation of bony landmarks in the obese patient is challenging. Ultrasound imaging allows for identification of the bony landmarks in the lumbar spine and imaging of deeper soft tissue structures. The sacrum can be identified and the level of each lumbar spinous process can be marked. Using transverse and paramedian sagittal oblique images, spinous interspaces can be accurately marked to allow accurate skin surface starting points for LP. The paramedian sagittal oblique view also provides information regarding the angulation between adjacent spinous processes. Ultrasound imaging can be combined with the use of the surface anatomy to confirm correct location of the L3–L4 interspace. Imaging of soft tissue structures such as the dura mater and intrathecal space provides valuable information as to the needle depth needed to reach the intrathecal space. Almost all studies using ultrasound for epidural placement, spinal anesthesia, and LP have used ultrasound preprocedurally to obtain landmarks and mark the skin. Very few studies have used real-time ultrasound to guide the needle placement.

Ultrasound acquisition of spinal images allows for rapid imaging of spinous structures and has proven useful in the ED for LPs. In spinal anesthesia with patient BMIs >35, ultrasound-guided first attempt success rates were twice as high as landmark-guided first attempt success rates. Ultrasound image acquisition has a learning curve and may require 40 cases before the operator develops competency. A tutorial for ultrasound-guided techniques for LP is available at: http://viewer.zmags.com/publication/70ed5a23#/70ed5a23/1.

Pearls and Pitfalls

- LP at or below the L3–L4 space in children due to variable conus medullaris levels.
- Opening pressures must be measured with the patient in the lateral decubitus position.
- The spinal needle must be withdrawn to the subcutaneous level to redirect the trajectory adequately.
- Reinserting the spinal needle stylet before withdrawing the needle may minimize any potential nerve root damage.
- When an emergent LP is required on a patient that is anticoagulated, have the most experienced provider perform the LP and use ultrasound assistance to minimize the number of insertions.

Bibliography

Carson D, Serpell M. Choosing the best needle for diagnostic lumbar puncture. *Neurology* 1996;**47**:33–37.

Chin KJ, Karmakar MK, Peng P. Ultrasonography of the adult thoracic and lumbar spine for central neuraxial blockade. *Anesthesiology* 2011;**114**:1459–1485.

Chin KJ, Perlas A, Chan V, et al. Ultrasound imaging facilitates spinal anesthesia in adults with difficult surface anatomic landmarks. *Anesthesiology* 2011;**115**:94–101.

Ferre RM, Sweeney TW. Emergency physicians can easily obtain ultrasound images of anatomic landmarks relative to lumbar puncture. *Am J Emerg Med* 2007;**25**:291–296.

Halpern S. Postdural puncture headache and spinal needle design: metanalysis. *Anesthesiology* 1994;**81**:1376–1383.

Horlocker TT, Wedel DJ, Rowlingson JC, et al. Regional anesthesia in the patient receiving antithrombotic or thrombolytic therapy. *Reg Anesth Pain Med* 2010;**35**:64–101.

Paech MJ, Doherty DA, Christmas T, et al. The volume of blood for epidural blood patch in obstetrics: a randomized, blinded clinical trial. *Anesth Analg* 2011;**113**:126–133.

Safa-Tissront V, Thormann F, Malassine P, et al. Effectiveness of epidural blood patch in the management of post-dural puncture headache. *Anesthesiology* 2001;**95**(2):334–339.

Stachan A, Train J. Aspirating cerebrospinal fluid speeds up procedure. *BMJ* 1998;**316**:1018.

Wolf S, Schneble F, Troger J. The conus medullaris: time of ascendence to normal level. *Pediatr Radiol* 1992;**22**:590–592.

Chadd E. Nesbit and Deeksha Agrawal

Coma, Delirium, and Dementia

Chapter

5

5.1 Introduction

Alterations in mental status are a frequently encountered chief complaint that the emergency physician is asked to evaluate. These changes vary from marked depression of mental status to extreme over-activation. The differential diagnosis of altered mental status (AMS) is perhaps one of the broadest encountered in medicine. Here we will discuss alterations in mental status, and a diagnostic approach to these types of patients.

A normal level of consciousness is the result of two functions of the brain, arousal and cognition. Each of these functions resides in a different area of the brain. Arousal is a function of the reticular activating system (RAS), which is composed of neurons located in the pons, medulla, and midbrain, while cognition is dependent on properly functioning cortical hemispheres. Disruption of either of these components will lead to alterations in mental status. Improper functioning of the RAS will manifest as an alteration in the level of arousal, with either depressed or excited states possible. Alterations in cognition may be more subtle. Forgetfulness, confusion, and hallucinations are all possible presentations.

In the broadest terms, coma is depression of mental status due to disruption of the RAS. Delirium is also due to dysfunction of the RAS, but unlike coma it manifests as a periodically excited state of arousal and altered cognition. Dementia is the result of dysfunction of the cerebral cortex. In this disease state the level of arousal is typically normal, but cognition is altered.

In this chapter we will discuss each one of these problems: coma, delirium, and dementia. These may all initially be classified as being alterations in mental status, but they have different etiologies, treatments, disposition from the ED, and eventual outcomes.

5.2 Coma

The comatose patient is manifested by a markedly depressed level of consciousness. This is due to dysfunction of the RAS. The brainstem or both cerebral hemispheres may be disrupted by either a structural or metabolic insult. Notice that *both* cerebral hemispheres must be affected for depression in the level of consciousness to occur. In general, disruption of one hemisphere by itself does not cause depressed consciousness, but this may occur when the disruption also causes a mass effect that alters the function of the brainstem.

Coma presents a diagnostic conundrum as patients in this state, by definition, are unable to provide a history as to what has taken place. If the patient has arrived by EMS, speak with the pre-hospital personnel. They often have critical information about the patient and can relay what was found at the scene. They may have spoken to family or bystanders who are not present in the ED. They may have seen pill bottles at the scene that could provide clues to underlying medical issues such as hypertension, cardiac problems, or diabetes. EMS personnel can also provide the ED physician with a description of the scene, such as where the patient was found, which may help provide clues to the presentation. Similarly, the same information may be available from an accompanying relative or friend and should be immediately sought out as part of the initial evaluation.

5.2.1 Initial Approach to the Comatose Patient

The initial evaluation of these patients is aimed at identifying immediately life-threatening conditions. A number of common, reversible causes of coma can be identified with an "ABCDE" approach. If any problems are identified during this brief exam they should be immediately addressed as many of these problems may prove to be rapidly fatal. A paper by Moore and Wijdicks (2013) lists the three most common out-of-hospital causes of coma as intoxication (both illicit and legal drugs), diabetic emergencies, and traumatic head injuries.

A = Airway. An inadequate supply of oxygen to the brain will lead to coma, and ultimately death. Ensure that the airway is patent, check pulse oximetry or an ABG, and immediately provide oxygen by nonrebreather mask.

B = Breathing. Just because the patient is breathing does not necessarily mean that they are adequately ventilating. Pulse oximetry and end tidal CO_2 detectors are readily available technologies and should be applied as a part of the routine acquisition of vital signs of critically ill patients. Hypoxia and hypercarbia will both cause AMS. The causes of hypoxia and hypercarbia are myriad, but the correction of these states is often relatively simple. A dose of naloxone of 0.4–2 mg IV may be diagnostic and therapeutic in this setting. Naloxone may also be given either IM or intranasal if IV access is not immediately available. Manual ventilation by bag valve mask may be needed while preparations are made to intubate the patient if they do not improve quickly.

C = Circulation. The brain is dependent on glucose as well as oxygen for normal function. Hypoperfusion limits the amount of blood going to the brain, which may result from cardiac arrest or arrhythmia and may lead to coma. Standard ACLS protocols should be employed in this case. Septic, distributive, and cardiogenic shock may also be the cause of hypoperfusion. The patient should have IV access established, be fluid-resuscitated, and, if needed, be started on vasoactive medications appropriate to the type of shock being treated.

D = Dextrose and disability. All patients with coma/AMS should have a bedside blood glucose level checked. Given that glucometers are readily available, 50% dextrose should only be given for documented hypoglycemia, instead of empirically as part of a "coma cocktail" as has been done before point-of-care testing was readily available. The level of disability should also be ascertained here. The Glasgow Coma Score (GCS), AVPU (alert, voice, pain, unresponsive), or FOUR (full outline of unresponsiveness) score may be used here to measure the level of consciousness (LOC). Any obvious lateralizing neurological signs should be noted. Are the pupils deviated to one side? Tonically deviated pupils looking toward the side of unilateral twitching suggest seizure, while tonically deviated pupils looking away from the hemiplegic side suggests a hemispheric lesion such as stroke. Unequal pupils may be indicative of intracranial hemorrhage with impending herniation.

E =Exposure. The patient should be undressed rapidly. They should be examined for signs of trauma such as bruising, deformities, or bleeding. If there is any indication of trauma, or uncertainty about the circumstances under which the patient was found, cervical spine precautions should be taken and a rigid c-collar should be applied. The presence of rashes, petechiae, or cellulitis may indicate an infectious source. Urinary catheters, dialysis fistulae, or chemotherapy ports may also suggest causes of the presentation.

5.2.2 Differential Diagnosis of Coma

Once the patient has been assessed and treated for any immediately life-threatening causes of coma, the physician must begin to determine the underlying cause of the coma if not already identified in the initial rapid assessment. The differential diagnosis of coma is broad and it is helpful to think of general categories of causes rather than trying to remember exhaustive lists of diagnoses.

The first step in the decision tree is to determine whether the coma is due to structural or nonstructural causes. As noted above, the three most common out-of-hospital causes of coma are intoxication (both illicit and legal drugs), diabetic emergencies, and traumatic head injuries. A recent published report determined the most common etiologies of nontraumatic coma as derived from a comprehensive literature review. Tables 5.1 and 5.2 list the structural and nonstructural/metabolic etiologies that were found in the review. The included studies were noted to be heterogeneous in nature, but the most common causes of nontraumatic coma found were stroke, postanoxic injury, poisonings, and metabolic

Table 5.1 Structural causes of coma

Acute CVA
CNS infections
Malignancy
Other neurological causes

Table 5.2 Nonstructural causes of coma

Poisoning – drug/alcohol
Epilepsy
Postanoxic encephalopathy
Respiratory hypercarbia
Infection
Metabolic
Hepatic encephalopathy
Eclampsia
Unclassified/miscellaneous

derangements. The best outcomes were noted for poisonings and epilepsy, whereas the worst outcomes were seen with stroke and postanoxic encephalopathy patients. It is important to note that although some of these categories list a single class of cause of coma, there may be many different etiologies within that given class. For instance, the metabolic class of nonstructural coma contains hypoglycemia, hyperglycemia, hypercalcemia, hyponatremia, uremia, hepatic encephalopathy, and many other causes of global neuronal dysfunction. Figure 5.1 outlines a general approach to the initial management and work-up of coma.

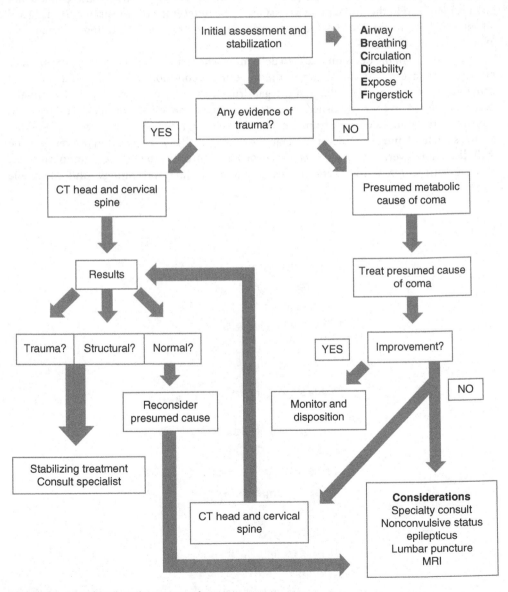

Figure 5.1 An approach to the work-up of coma.

5.2.3 Physical Examination

When presented with a situation in which the patient cannot provide a history, the physical examination should enable a narrowing of the differential diagnosis. A complete set of vital signs should also be a part of the routine physical examination. Abnormalities in the vital signs may help guide the formation of the differential diagnosis. Hypertension may suggest intracranial hemorrhagic encephalopathy. Hypotension may be due to shock secondary to infection. Variations in respiratory rate and pattern suggest possible causes of coma. Extremes of temperature may also lead to alterations in the LOC.

Once the initial brief assessment has been completed, a detailed examination of the patient should be undertaken. A significant amount of information may be gained simply by looking at the patient briefly before beginning a detailed physical examination. Note any movement that the patient is making, especially if they are moving only one side of the body. Twitching or jerking movements may indicate seizure or encephalopathic states. Abnormal odors, such as the fruity breath of the diabetic patient in ketoacidosis, may provide clues to you.

A head-to-toe physical examination should be performed to assess for any evidence of trauma. Careful note should be made of any evidence of head injury, such as bleeding, scalp deformity, or the presence of hematoma. Any such finding should immediately lead to placement of a cervical collar as there is the possibility of spinal cord injury in these patients. If there is any doubt about trauma, place the cervical collar. It is easily cleared once the patient is awake and cooperative. Missing a spinal injury can be catastrophic.

The level of responsiveness of the patient is an important part of the physical examination. A simple method, such as the AVPU scale, may be used initially. In this system, the patient is either alert, or responds to verbal or painful stimuli, or is unresponsive, providing a gross assessment of the level of responsiveness. The GCS (Table 5.3) was initially developed to aid in the assessment of head-injured patients. Its use has been expanded and it is now used for assessment of essentially all types of patients with decreased levels of responsiveness. The GCS is broken down into three scales for eye, motor, and verbal responsiveness; the eye component is a four-point scale, motor is five, and verbal is six, for a total of 15 possible points. The lowest score is 3. A score of less than 8 is generally used by emergency physicians as an indicator for intubation.

Table 5.3 Glasgow Coma Score

Eyes	Verbal	Motor
4 = spontaneous	5 = normal	6 = follows commands
3 = verbal stimulus	4 = disoriented	5 = localizes pain
2 = painful stimulus	3 = incoherent	4 = withdraws
1 = no response	2 = incomprehensible	3 = decorticate
	1 = no speech	2 = decerebrate
		1 = no movement

Although the GCS has been used for more than 40 years, it is not without critics. There are inconsistencies in its application. Some practitioners simply assign the lowest possible score if a value is not obtainable, as is often the case in intubated coma patients. A study by Balestreri et al. (2004) showed a lack of correlation between GCS and outcomes in traumatic brain injury. The GCS fails to account for hemiplegia and does not have a scale for brainstem reflexes or abnormal respiratory patterns.

The FOUR score (Table 5.4) was developed in response to some of the perceived shortcomings of the GCS. This score has four components: eye, motor, brainstem, and respirations. Each of these is scored on a four-point scale. It will detect a locked-in syndrome, a condition in which the patient is awake and aware but unable to move anything except their eyes vertically. It will also accurately reflect a vegetative state where the eyes will open but do not track the examiner.

Table 5.4 The FOUR score

Eye response

Eyelids open or opened, tracking or blinking to command = 4

Eyelids open but not tracking = 3

Eyelids closed but open to loud voice = 2

Eyelids closed but open to pain = 1

Eyelids remain closed with pain = 0

Motor response

Thumbs up, fist, or peace sign = 4

Localizes pain = 3

Flexion response to pain = 2

Extension response to pain = 1

No response to pain, or generalized myoclonic status = 0

Brainstem reflexes

Pupil and corneal reflexes present = 4

One pupil wide and fixed = 3

Pupil **or** corneal reflexes absent = 2

Pupil **and** corneal reflexes absent = 1

Absent pupil, corneal, and cough reflexes = 0

Respiration

Not intubated, regular breathing pattern = 4

Not intubated, Cheyne–Stokes breathing pattern = 3

Not intubated, irregular breathing = 2

Intubated, breathing above ventilator rate = 1

Intubated, apnea, or breathing at ventilator rate = 0

Modified from Wijdicks et al., 2005.

5.2.4 Respiratory Pattern

As outlined above, an initial assessment of the comatose patient must start with management of the airway. If there is doubt as to the patient's ability to protect their own airway, or if there is evidence of hypoventilation or a failure to oxygenate, then the ED physician must take control of the airway, secure it, and provide the patient with appropriate ventilation and oxygenation. Further discussion of airway management is beyond the scope of this chapter and a standard text of emergency medicine will provide a thorough discussion of this subject. While preparing to manage the airway, observation of the respiratory pattern and rate may provide some clue as to the etiology of the coma.

- Decreased respiratory rate, especially accompanied by small pupils, is highly suggestive of narcotic overdose. Naloxone may be both diagnostic and therapeutic. It is not unreasonable to attempt a dose of naloxone in the appropriate clinical setting while preparing to intubate. For patients with significantly decreased respiratory drive, it may be reasonable to administer 2 mg of naloxone IV or intranasal naloxone 1 mg in each nostril.
- Conversely, an increased respiratory rate may be seen in cases of metabolic acidosis. The respiratory rate increases in an attempt to "blow off" excess CO_2 and normalize the blood pH.
- Cheyne–Stokes respirations is a breathing pattern in which periods of hyperventilation are followed by periods of apnea. This can be seen in various metabolic derangements, head injury, and stroke.
- Ataxic breathing is simply a pattern of highly irregular breathing. This may be a sign of dysfunction of the respiratory centers located in the medulla. Presence of this highly disordered breathing pattern may be an indicator for intubation.
- There are also various types of pre-apneic breathing that are usually harbingers of impending respiratory arrest. These include gasping respiration and patterns where the patient opens their mouth with each breath. This is sometimes called "guppy" or "fish-mouth breathing."

5.2.5 Pupillary Response

Close examination of the pupils can provide a significant amount of information about the etiology of coma. Care should be taken to make note of the size, reactivity, and symmetry of the pupils. This should be done prior to the administration of any drugs for management of the airway as this will change the pupillary exam. The administration of paralytics by either EMS or ED physicians will obviously confound the pupillary exam. Eye surgery and prosthetics may also prove confounding. There are some specific pupillary findings that may be of help in determining the etiology of coma.

- The presence of small, pinpoint pupils, especially when coupled with respiratory depression, may be indicative of narcotic overdose.
- Reactive pinpoint pupils are the classic finding in pontine hemorrhage.
- Unequal pupils are seen in uncal herniation as the innermost portion of the cerebrum is forced over the tentorium, into the brainstem, and causes compression of the oculomotor nerve. The parasympathetic fibers are often affected, leading to dilation of the ipsilateral pupil.
- Metabolic insults usually leave the pupils reactive.

Tokuda et al. (2003) used pupillary evaluation for assessment of the etiology of coma. They evaluated 115 patients presenting to the ED with coma; 60% had coma of metabolic origin (overdose, sepsis, alcohol) and 40% were due to structural lesions (hemorrhage, infarct, mass). They found that loss of the pupillary light reflex or the presence of anisocoria was predictive of structural lesions with odds ratios of 11.02 and 7.5, respectively. This finding may allow the ED physician to rapidly narrow the differential diagnosis simply by examining the pupils. Greer et al. (2012) also demonstrated that the pupillary light reflex was associated with prognosis in their series of 500 consecutive patients in coma without evidence of trauma with a mean odds ratio of 12.51, range [6.01, 22.56] for a modified Rankin scale less than or equal to 3, which they defined as independent.

Other elements of the physical exam may help to narrow the differential diagnosis. Abnormal vital signs, skin color, abnormal odors, presence of medical alert bracelets, and the general appearance of the patient may help to narrow the differential diagnosis. For an exhaustive listing of potentially relevant physical exam findings, please refer to Moore and Wijdicks (2013).

5.2.6 Laboratory Testing

Laboratory testing should be performed in a logical fashion to narrow the differential diagnosis. In addition to the finger stick glucose obtained as part of the rapid initial assessment, additional laboratory tests should be ordered as appropriate. A "shotgun" approach to ordering tests may prove to be less than helpful and, at times, proves to be confounding. A more focused approach, with the goal of addressing specific probable etiologies, is likely to be a more rewarding approach. A complete blood count (CBC) with platelets, PT/INR, metabolic panel, liver and thyroid function tests, and an ammonia level is a reasonable starting point. If there is concern for an infectious etiology, a chest x-ray, urinalysis, blood cultures and lumbar puncture may also be considered. Although invasive, the lumbar puncture may provide crucial information when other laboratory and imaging studies have not provided an explanation. Serum and urine osmolality, salicylate and acetaminophen levels, and calculation of the osmolar gap should be obtained and calculated if there is thought of ingestion or intoxication.

The utility of the urine drug screen is of question in this setting. Positive results may be misleading. A positive test simply indicates the presence of the substance or one of its metabolites, depending on what the particular drug screen is actually measuring. It may also be a false positive. For instance, bupropion, labetalol, and ofloxacin have been shown to cause false positives in urine drug screens. In addition, many illicit synthetic or semi-synthetic compounds simply do not show up on standard urine drug screens.

5.2.7 Neuroimaging

Any comatose patient presenting to the ED with evidence of trauma or lateralizing neuro-logical findings should have a noncontrast CT scan of the brain. Lack of an immediately clear diagnosis, such as hypoglycemia or alcohol intoxication, should also prompt brain imaging while the laboratory work-up is being undertaken. Consideration should be given to continuing the scan through the cervical spine when there is any indication of trauma above the level of the clavicles.

CT scanning is typically the first imaging modality to be employed as it is readily available in most EDs and scanning of the head and cervical spine takes less than a minute. CT scanning is excellent for detecting acute intracranial hemorrhage, hydrocephalus, edema, and hyperdense basilar and middle cerebral arteries. It is also excellent for detection of bony trauma. CT scanning, however, does lose sensitivity in detection of abnormality in the posterior fossa due to bony artifact. Detection of abnormality such as intracranial hemorrhage, mass, edema, or hydrocephalus necessitates consultation of a neurologist or neurosurgeon, or may be a reason for transfer to a higher level of care.

MRI may have a role in the ED when it is readily obtainable. MRI shows great detail of the cerebral vessels and should be obtained when there is concern for basilar or cerebellar artery occlusion without clear evidence on CT scan. MRI also provides a clearer picture of the posterior fossa and shows cortical and subcortical detail not seen on CT scans. Venous sinus thrombosis and posterior reversible encephalopathy syndrome (PRES) may also be missed on CT scan and only seen on MRI. Availability and time to complete a scan are the largest drawbacks to MRI, often relegating this imaging modality to a role employed by specialist consultants.

Not every comatose patient presenting to the ED needs to have a CT scan of the brain. The hypoglycemic patient who rapidly recovers after administration of D50 does not need a CT scan, nor does the elderly patient with a fever and infected urine or pneumonia. These patients should be closely monitored and, if they do not progressively improve with proper treatment of the suspected etiology, then the diagnosis needs to be rethought and neuroimaging may be appropriate. When there is any doubt as to a traumatic vs a nontraumatic etiology, the CT scan of the brain should be obtained emergently.

5.2.8 Coma Mimics

There are a few coma-like states that deserve special mention as these may require expert consultation to accurately diagnose and may be easily mistaken for true coma. Detection of the so-called "locked-in" state may now be accomplished by use of the FOUR score, as outlined above. In this condition, sometimes seen after a basilar artery stroke or central pontine myelinolysis, the patient is awake and completely aware of their surroundings, but is unable to move anything except their eyes and eyelids, frequently communicating by blinking or moving the eyes vertically. Akinetic mutism is a condition caused by bilateral frontal lobe or midbrain lesions in which the patient is alert but unable to move or speak. They may move their eyes, do not have spontaneous motor movement, but are not paralyzed. EEG is often needed to make the diagnosis and typically shows severe generalized slowing. Survivors of severe head injury or hypoxic/ischemic injury may present in a vegetative state. Usually the history, obtained from a caretaker, is sufficient to separate this state from that of acute coma. Depending on the specific injury, the patient may show various neurological responses, including normal sleep–wake cycles, but they will have no awareness of their surroundings. EEG, if obtained, will show some intermittent periods of alphawave activity instead of the generalized slowing or "burst suppression" pattern often seen in coma patients. Finally, catatonic patients are akinetic and mute. They may display "waxy flexibility" in that the limbs will remain in the position placed by the examiner. These patients may have a history of severe depressive illness or schizophrenia, but a number of organic causes, such as drug reaction, metabolic abnormality, and encephalitis, may lead to this condition.

5.3 Delirium

Delirium, an acute, generalized brain dysfunction, has been called by a number of names – acute confusional state, brain failure, and encephalopathy to name a few. Previous definitions of delirium have included alterations in the LOC of the patient. The *Diagnostic and Statistical Manual of Mental Disorders* (DSM-5) has removed mention of consciousness from the definition and now defines delirium by its cognitive features. Table 5.5 lists the new DSM-5 criteria for the diagnosis of delirium.

Delirium is very commonly seen in hospital and ED settings; in some case series an estimated 10–30% of the patients over the age of 65 seen in the ED have delirium. It is also commonly seen in the inpatient setting, particularly in the intensive care unit. A recent review notes that 30–50% of cases of delirium are preventable. However, despite the prevalence of delirium, it is often misdiagnosed and may go undetected in the acute clinical setting. A number of bedside clinical tools have been developed to aid in the diagnosis of delirium. The Confusion Assessment Method (CAM) is probably the most widely used tool employed to assist in the diagnosis of delirium. This tool has been validated in a number of studies and has a sensitivity of 94%, a specificity of 89%, and very good inter-rater reliability.

Delirium is also associated with significant mortality. Delirium in the ED has been shown to be an independent predictor of morality at 6 months. In one series, mortality in delirious patients was 37% vs 14.3% in nondelirious patients. This observed increased mortality was independent of whether the patient came from a nursing facility or another location.

5.3.1 Assessment

Unlike some presentations of coma, the delirious patient usually isn't experiencing an immediate, potentially life-threatening emergency. However, these patients are often very complex medically, and their current presentation may be a manifestation of a significant underlying illness. Similar to the initial assessment of the comatose patient, obtaining a history of the present illness from a family member or caregiver is critically important as many delirious patients may not be able to provide a complete and/or accurate history or medication list.

It may be useful to ask relatively closed questions of the patient, if possible, and any accompanying family or caregivers. Specific questions about how the patient's behavior has

Table 5.5 DSM-5 criteria for diagnosis of delirium

- Disturbance in attention and awareness.
- Disturbance develops over a short time, is an acute change from baseline, and tends to fluctuate.
- There is an additional disturbance in cognition (e.g., memory deficit, disorientation).
- The disturbances in Criteria 1 and 3 are not better accounted for by a pre-existing neurocognitive disorder and do not occur in the context of coma.
- There is evidence of history, physical exam, or lab findings that the disturbance is a direct physiological consequence of another medical condition, substance intoxication or withdrawal, exposure to a toxin, or due to multiple etiologies.

changed, when the change was noticed, and any new medication or dosage changes may help to point to a cause of the delirium.

Delirium, like coma, has a multitude of potential etiologies (Table 5.6). Age may help to determine the cause of the presentation of the patient. Younger patients in their twenties and thirties may be more likely to be experiencing delirium from drug or alcohol use/abuse or withdrawal syndromes from these substances. The very young and elderly may have delirium caused by illnesses such as pneumonia, urinary tract infection, or other febrile illness. Delirium due to medications is often seen in the elderly. In general, the causes of delirium can be grouped into a few classes of causes, namely toxic, metabolic, and infectious etiologies.

There are a number of factors that predispose a patient to the development of delirium. Inouye et al. (2014) used validated models to list a number of factors that predispose to the development of delirium. These predisposing factors are shown in Table 5.7. Similarly, precipitating factors from validated predictive models of delirium are shown in Table 5.8.

Medications have been identified as the cause of a high percentage of cases of delirium. In particular, anticholinergic medications, such as antihistamines, muscle relaxants, and antipsychotics, have been noted to be "high risk" for precipitating delirium. Benzodiazepines, dopamine agonists, and meperidine also have significant potential to precipitate delirium (Kalish et al., 2014).

5.3.2 Physical Examination

The physical examination in the delirious patient, as in the comatose patient, may suggest a cause. Many of the same physical signs seen in coma may be seen in the delirious patient when the precipitating factor is a medical condition. Fever, tachycardia, tachypnea, respiratory depression, and hyper- or hypotension may all point to potential causes. Hypoxia,

Table 5.6 Differential diagnosis of delirium

Hypoxia/hypercarbia
Hypo or hyperglycemia
Decreased perfusion: Cardiac? Blood loss?
Dehydration – decreased intake, increased output?
Electrolyte disturbance – K^+, Ca^{++}, Mg^{++}
Infection – UTI, pneumonia
Alcohol and drug intoxication or withdrawal
Medications
Vitamin deficiency
Thyroid storm
Adrenal insufficiency
Hypo- or hyperthermia
Primary CNS cause – bleed, mass, infection
Hypertensive emergency (PRES syndrome)

Table 5.7 Predisposing factors for delirium

Dementia or pre-existing cognitive impairment
History of delirium
Functional impairment
Sensory impairment
Severe illness
Depression
History of CVA or TIA
Alcohol abuse
Older age

Table 5.8 Precipitating factors for delirium

Polypharmacy
Use of physical restraints
Bladder catheters
Physiological and metabolic abnormalities
Infection
Major surgery
Trauma or unplanned hospital admission
Coma

hypercarbic respiratory failure, and hypoglycemia may all present as delirium. A simple bedside blood glucose measurement and a pulse oximetry reading help to address many of these issues.

The physical examination in the delirious patient must also include an assessment of the patient's cognitive function. In the ED setting, quick assessment of the patient's orientation and the ability to complete an attention-type task, such as naming the days of the week, months of the year, or serial sevens, may be sufficiently informative when time is limited.

5.3.3 Laboratory Testing and Imaging

Testing ideally should be performed in a manner guided by the history and findings on the physical examination. Consideration should be given to ordering a CBC, a metabolic panel, urinalysis, ammonia levels, liver function tests, and thyroid studies. A chest x-ray may reveal pneumonia or mass while the EKG may show cardiac ischemia or an acute myocardial infarction. An arterial blood gas may also be indicated. When there is concern for carbon monoxide toxicity, pulse oximetry will be normal and CO-oximetry will need to be obtained.

Lumbar puncture should be considered in the febrile patient with headache or signs of meningeal irritation.

Neuroimaging also may be indicated for the delirious patient. However, it is frequently normal and should target specific populations with a high pretest probability of abnormality on the imaging. Patients with focal neurological findings, any history of trauma, or the presence of a fever may require a CT of the head or an MRI. A seemingly minor head injury in a patient taking any of the many available anticoagulants should be assessed with a noncontrast scan of the head to evaluate for any kind of intracranial hemorrhage. MRI as a primary imaging modality is rarely indicated for the initial evaluation of the delirious patient, but may be indicated as part of a more complete work-up in the setting of continued delirium without identification of an etiology.

5.3.4 Disposition of the Patient with Coma or Delirium

The patient presenting to the ED with an acute coma state is often discharged from the ED when hypoglycemia or intoxication is diagnosed, two of the most common reasons for acute coma. Although the treatment may be quite simple in many of these cases, such as administration of dextrose, the ED physician must address any underlying cause of the presentation such as inadvertent insulin overdose. Causes other than the most simple intoxication or case of hypoglycemia will likely require admission.

The delirious patient is somewhat more complicated with regard to disposition. When a cause of the delirium is identified, such as a new medication, and the patient improves after a period of observation and there is good follow-up, it may be reasonable to discharge them to home with another responsible party. However, the vast majority of cases of delirium will not be so clear-cut, or are the result of significant metabolic abnormalities, and will likely require in-hospital observation or admission to delineate the problem and initiate treatment.

5.4 Dementia

When a cognitively impaired patient presents to the ED, it is important to differentiate between delirium and dementia. As described above, delirium typically has an acute onset with fluctuating course and impaired attention. Dementia, on the other hand, is characterized by multiple cognitive complaints along with global deterioration of functioning, progressive over several months to years. Attention and consciousness are generally preserved.

In older ED patients the prevalence of cognitive impairment is 23–40%. Alzheimer's disease is the most common type of dementia and accounts for about 70% of cases. In the United States this accounts for a healthcare cost of $148 billion per year, in part due to longer lengths of stay, more diagnostic testing, and more frequent admissions. Alzheimer's disease is characterized by cognitive impairments in addition to at least one of the following: aphasia (language disturbance), apraxia (impaired motor ability), agnosia (failure to recognize objects), or impaired executive functioning (disturbance in planning and organizing).

Other forms of dementia include frontotemporal dementia, dementia with Lewy bodies, vascular dementia, and prion diseases. Frontotemporal dementia involves an insidious onset of cognitive deficits, gradual progression, and behavioral abnormalities, such as disinhibition, apathy, loss of sympathy, perseveration, and hyperorality. Dementia with Lewy bodies is characterized by fluctuating cognition, followed by parkinsonian symptoms and signs, psychiatric abnormalities, such as REM behavior disorder, autonomic instability, and falls. Vascular dementia is associated with onset of cognitive deficits that are temporally related to one or more cerebrovascular events. Patients typically have focal neurological deficits due to stroke. Finally, prion disease is characterized by rapidly progressive cognitive decline and is associated with myoclonus and ataxia.

All dementias have prominent neuropsychiatric symptoms, including depression, apathy, agitation, aggression, hallucinations, delusions, misidentification, pacing, wandering, hoarding, and sleep–wake cycle disturbance. The most common cause of death in patients with dementia is pneumonia.

5.4.1 Diagnosis

It is important to identify cognitive dysfunction when evaluating geriatric patients in the ED. However, time constraints and the sheer volume of patients in the EDs limit the emergency physician's ability to administer lengthy screening examinations, such as the Mini Mental Status Examination (MMSE). The MMSE has also been noted to be suboptimal in identifying mild cognitive impairment and is a copyrighted tool. Numerous brief screening tools have been developed to aid ED physicians in their evaluation, but none has proven to be a sufficiently sensitive and reasonably specific instrument.

Recent data have suggested that the Six-Item Screener may be of some benefit. The Six-Item Screener consists of three questions on temporal orientation (day, month, and year) and three-item recall – immediate and after 3 minutes. A score of ≤4 is used as the cutoff for impairment. An abnormal score would warrant further testing, such as a more detailed MMSE testing.

Initial assessment for dementia should include a noncontrast CT or MRI scan to rule-out structural abnormalities. Other comorbidities and reversible causes of dementia include depression, B12 deficiency, and hypothyroidism; therefore, B12 level and TSH should be part of routine testing for dementia. Finally, syphilis serology (RPR) as a routine test is discouraged unless the patient has some specific risk factor, history of syphilitic infection, or resides in a high-risk area.

5.4.2 Management

Management of patients with dementia involves pharmacologic and nonpharmacologic approaches. Agitation and psychosis are commonly encountered psychological symptoms of dementia and should be treated with atypical antipsychotics, while being cognizant of their tolerability and side effects, including mortality. Recent studies have suggested better efficacy of olanzapine and risperidone with increased side effects, but better tolerability of quetiapine with reduced efficacy. Antidepressants have shown limited benefit for depression in dementia, but may be due to the exclusion of severely demented patients in these studies.

Specifically, when frontotemporal dementia is suspected, the physician should be cognizant that dopamine agonists can worsen psychiatric symptoms by increasing hallucinations and delusions. Conversely, dopamine antagonists used for hallucinations can worsen parkinsonian symptoms.

Nonpharmacologic interventions are typically not feasible in the ED setting but are important to discuss with the patient and the caregiver. These usually involve educating the caregiver about stress-reducing techniques, enhancing communication with the patient, and simplifying the environment and tasks for the patient.

All patients should be evaluated for falls, suicidal ideation, wandering, abuse, and neglect. Many patients have other comorbid conditions that may require hospital admission and treatment by multidisciplinary teams, including internal medicine, psychiatry, neurology, case management, and social work.

5.4.3 Disposition of the Dementia Patient

A new diagnosis of dementia is generally not going to be made in the ED based on a single visit. This diagnosis will likely be made by the primary care provider or a consultant to whom the patient has been referred. The goal of the ED physician is to ensure that there is no acute, reversible cause of the patient's presentation to the ED at that time. A basic metabolic and infectious work-up searching for possible reversible causes of worsening dementia leading to the presentation is good practice. Infection, electrolyte abnormalities, and new or altered doses of medications may all precipitate a change in the mental status of the patient with dementia. Head CT may be warranted if there is concern for trauma. Fever and an acutely AMS should prompt consideration of the possibility of CNS infection and possible lumbar puncture. The patient with a negative work-up, good support, and close follow-up is likely safe for discharge to home after discussion with caregivers regarding the results and plan for outpatient follow-up.

5.5 The Neuropsychiatric Patient

Neuropsychiatry is the branch of psychiatry concerned with mental disorders resulting from diseases of the central nervous system. These patients may present for evaluation of changes in mood, behavior, or cognition. They may also present as being frankly psychotic. These patients fall into two broad classes: those who present with neuropsychiatric symptoms but no known CNS disorder, or those with a known CNS disorder who present with changes of mood or behavior. Regardless of the etiology of the symptoms, the general approach involves stabilization of the patient, determination of the cause of the presentation, and determination of an appropriate disposition for the patient.

5.5.1 Assessment

Due to the nature of their presentation, these patients are often not able to provide a reliable history and this often must be obtained from an accompanying family member or friend. Specific attention should be paid to the exact nature of the patient's symptoms, any exacerbating or palliating factors, any medication use and/or changes in medications or dosages, and any recent changes in the patient's overall medical condition. Patients presenting without an already established diagnosis of a CNS disorder require an extensive work-up to determine if there is an underlying disorder such as dementia, Huntington's disease, Parkinson's disease, multiple sclerosis, or a brain tumor. In patients with a known diagnosis, the presence of an exacerbating medical condition must be investigated as a possible cause of an acute deterioration from baseline.

A detailed assessment of the patient's mental status is critically important. In addition to detecting disorders of cognition or acute confusion, the mental status exam also serves as a baseline for comparison in future exams. Examination of this type is generally beyond the scope of that necessary or practical in the setting of the ED.

5.5.2 Treatment

Neuropsychiatric patients may present in extremely agitated or violent states. The primary goal in the acute setting must be to stabilize the patient such that they do not present a danger to themselves or the treating staff. Treatment of aggression and agitation will also serve to facilitate examination of the patient. Patients should be moved to quiet rooms to minimize stimulation. Ideally they would be placed in a seclusion room devoid of any objects that could potentially be used as weapons. Lorazepam given intravenously or intramuscularly is often used as a sedative due to a good safety profile. Up to 2 mg IV or IM may be given. Respiratory depression is rare, but can occur. Haloperidol is another option; 1–10 mg IM or IV may be used. There is a risk of QT prolongation with this medication. Ziprasidone 10–20 mg IM may also be used for control of the violent patient. A combination of haloperidol and lorazepam, typically 5 mg and 2 mg, either IV or IM, may be used for severely agitated patients. Patients should be monitored closely for any signs of respiratory depression.

5.5.3 Disposition

Ultimately, the patient must either be admitted to the hospital or discharged. The change in the patient's behavior may be due to a new medical condition or worsening of a chronic condition that may be medical or neurological in nature. If the patient is to regain their baseline status, the underlying disorder must be treated and the patient should be admitted to the appropriate inpatient service, likely either a medical service or neurology. Admission to a psychiatric service is indicated if the patient's behavior remains deranged in the absence of a medical condition, a nonworsening underlying neurological condition, or when there is no obvious cause for the deterioration. If the patient can be treated in the ED and shows improvement, they may be appropriate for discharge from the ED with close follow-up.

5.6 Transient Global Amnesia

Transient global amnesia (TGA) is a clinical syndrome that typically presents between 50 and 70 years of age. It is characterized by sudden onset of anterograde amnesia and repetitive questioning without any focal neurological deficits. Patients can have some degree of retrograde amnesia, especially surrounding events that occurred in recent years. They repeatedly ask the same questions and are unable to form new memories. However, they are able to perform previously learned activities, such as driving, without any difficulty. Patients have a profound lack of insight into their condition and thus appear restless or nervous. They do not have any loss of awareness or personal identity. They are attentive, can follow complex commands, and generally do not tend to confabulate. Deficits may last up to 24 hours. Triggers include activities associated with the Valsalva maneuver, emotional stress, immersion in cold or hot water, intense physical activity, sexual intercourse, or pain.

Diagnosis is based on a clinical history obtained from a capable observer and patient's physical examination. Presence of focal neurological deficits should prompt the clinician to consider other diagnoses (Table 5.9), such as stroke/TIA. Currently, there are no specific diagnostic studies that can confirm the diagnosis of TGA. Additional diagnostic studies are

Table 5.9 Differential diagnosis of TGA

Stroke/TIA
Focal onset seizure
Transient epileptic amnesia Postictal state
Post-traumatic amnesia
Metabolic abnormalities
Dissociative disorders Psychogenic amnesia

based on the need to exclude other diagnoses. CT of the head is typically normal. MRI of the brain, performed at 48 hours of symptom onset, can frequently show hyperintensity in unilateral or bilateral hippocampi on diffusion-weighted imaging (DWI), T2-weighted sequences, and fluid-attenuated inversion recovery (FLAIR) sequences. These changes are typically reversible. EEG is usually normal but can be considered to rule-out an epileptic etiology and not to confirm the diagnosis of TGA. Other testing may include a urine drug screen (UDS), serum ethanol level, comprehensive metabolic panel (CMP), and CBC.

The pathophysiology of TGA is currently unknown but has centered around three main mechanisms: vascular (due to venous flow disturbances or focal arterial ischemia), epileptic, or migraine. The episodes are typically self-limiting and resolve without any interventions within 24 hours. There is no specific treatment for TGA. Memory usually recovers completely within days, but mild impairment can occasionally persist for weeks. Long-term outcomes are unknown. Studies have suggested an approximate recurrence rate of 2–23%. There does not seem to be an increased risk of ischemic stroke, but more studies are required to adequately assess the risk of epilepsy and cognitive decline.

5.7 Conclusion

The patient who presents to the ED with AMS may do so for any number of reasons, ranging from the acute onset, immediately life-threatening presentation caused by intracranial hemorrhage to the slow, progressive decline of Alzheimer's dementia. The ED physician must quickly evaluate this spectrum of patients, address immediately life-threatening or reversible causes of the presentation, and then initiate laboratory testing and imaging as needed in an attempt to determine the etiology of the other presentations. History and physical examination should guide laboratory testing and imaging, focusing on including or excluding likely causes. Expert consultation may be necessary in some cases to arrange for definitive treatment or specialized diagnostic testing. Ultimately the ED physician must make the decision regarding disposition of the patient. If the patient is to be discharged, the ED physician must ensure that the patient is stable and has appropriate follow-up for the problem that brought them to the ED.

Pearls and Pitfalls

- An "ABCDE" approach to the comatose patient may reveal a reversible cause.
- Coma can be considered broadly as due to either structural or nonstructural causes.
- Pupillary responses in the comatose patient provide an important part of neurologic evaluation.
- Urine drug screen in the comatose patient may yield false positive results.
- Delirium in the elderly is often caused by polypharmacy.
- Delirium is often misdiagnosed in the acute clinical setting.
- Delirium is often superimposed in elderly demented patients presenting to the ED with a change in their level of consciousness.

Bibliography

ACEP, AGS, ENA, SAEM, Geriatric Emergency Department Guidelines Task Force. Geriatric emergency department guidelines. *Ann Emerg Med* 2014;**63**(5):e7–25.

American Psychiatric Association. *Diagnostic and Statistical Manual of Mental Disorders*, 5th ed. APA Press, 2013.

Arena JE, Rabinstein AA. Transient global amnesia. *Mayo Clin Proc* 2015;**90** (2):264–272.

Balestreri M, Szonskya M, Chatfield DA, et al. Predictive value of the Glasgow Coma Scale after brain trauma: change in trend over the past ten years. *J Neurol Neurosurg Psych* 2004;**75**:161–162.

Bartsch T, Butler, C. Transient amnesic syndromes. *Nature Rev Neur* 2013;**9**: 86–97.

Brown J. ED Evaluation of transient global amnesia. *Ann Emerg Med* 1997;**30** (4):522–526.

Carpenter CR, DesPain B, Keeling TN, et al., The Six-Item Screener and AD8 for the detection of cognitive impairment in geriatric emergency department patients. *Ann Emerg Med* 2011;**57** (6):653–661.

Doebbeling CC. Behavioral emergencies. In *Merck Manuals Professional Edition*. 2008. Available at www.merckmanuals.com/professional/ psychiatric-disorders/approach-to-the-patient-with-mental-symptoms/behavioral-emergencies. Accessed June 5, 2018.

Edlow JA, Rabinstein A, Traub SJ, Wijdicks EF. Diagnosis of reversible causes of coma. *Lancet* 2014;**384**:2064–2076.

Fong T, Davis D, Growdon MA, et al. The interface between delirium and dementia in elderly adults. *Lancet* 2015. http://dx.doi.org/ 10/1016/S1474-4411(15)00101-5.

Greer DM, Yang J, Scripko PD, et al., Clinical examination for outcome prediction in nontraumatic coma. *Crit Care Med* 2012;**40**:1150–1156.

Horsting MWB, Franken MD, Meulenbelt J, et al. The etiology and outcome of non-traumatic coma in critical care: a systematic review. *BMC Anesthesiol* 2015;**15**:65–72.

Inouye SK, Westendrop RG, Saczynski JS. Delirium in elderly people. *Lancet* 2014;**383**:911–922.

Kales HC, Gitlin LN, Lyketsos CG. Assessment and management of behavioral and psychological symptoms of dementia. *BMJ* 2015;**350**:h369.

Kalish VB, Gillham JE, Unwin BK. Delirium in older persons: evaluation and management. *Am Fam Phys* 2014;**90**(3):150–158.

Knopman DS, DeKosky ST, Cummings JL, et al. Practice parameter: diagnosis of dementia. An evidence based review. *Neurology* 2001;**56**:1143–1153.

Moore SA, Wijdicks EF. The acutely comatose patient: clinical approach and diagnosis. *Sem Neurol* 2013;**33**:110–120.

Saitman A, Park H-D, Fitzgerald RL. False-positive interferences of common urine drug screen immunoassays: a review. *J Anal Toxicol* 2014;**38**(7):387–396.

Samaras N, Chevalley T, Samaras D. et al. Older patients in the emergency department: a review. *Ann Emerg Med* 2010;**56**(3):261–269.

Scheel M, Malkowsky C, Klingebiel et al. Magnetic resonance imaging in transient global amnesia. *Clin Neurorad* 2012;**22**:335–340.

Tokuda Y, Nakazato N, Stein GH. Pupillary evaluation for differential diagnosis of coma. *Postgrad Med J* 2003;**79**:49–51.

Weisberg LA, Garcia C, Strub R. Stupor and coma. In *Essentials of Clinical Neurology*.

2015. Available at: http://tulane.edu/som/departments/neurology/programs/clerkship/essentials-clinical-neurology.cfm. Accessed August 15, 2015.

Wijdicks EFM, Bamlet WR, Maramattom BV et al. Validation of a new coma scale: the FOUR score. *Ann Neurol* 2005;**58**(4):585–593.

Wilber ST, Lofgren SD, Mager TG et al. An evaluation of two screening tools for cognitive impairment in older emergency department patients. *Acad Emerg Med* 2005;**12**:612–616.

Wong CL, Holroyd-Leduc J, Simel DL, Straus SE. Does this patient have delirium? *JAMA* 2010;**304**:779–786.

Headache

Sandeep Rana, Ye Vivian Liang, Paul S. Porter, Charles Q. Li, Dolores Santamaria, and Andrea Synowiec

6.1 Introduction

Headache as a presenting symptom is commonly encountered by the emergency department (ED) physician. The differential diagnosis of headaches is extensive and the etiologies can range from benign to life-threatening. These patients can pose a diagnostic and therapeutic challenge to the treating clinician. This chapter encapsulates the clinical approach, appropriate evaluation, and treatment options in patients presenting with the complaint of headache.

6.2 Evaluation

6.2.1 History

Patients typically present to the ED for headaches that are new and/or particularly severe; alternatively, they may present due to recurrent headaches that are not responding to treatment. Taking a detailed history (Table 6.1) can help elucidate whether the headache represents symptoms of a primary headache syndrome or symptoms that are secondary to another underlying medical or organic condition.

6.2.2 Physical Examination

Assessment of vital signs, particularly blood pressure and temperature, is important in patients with headaches, as uncontrolled hypertension can present with headache as an initial symptom. Headaches in the setting of fever may herald intracranial infection such as meningitis, cerebral abscess, etc. Palpation of temporal arteries, paranasal sinuses, and temporomandibular joints is also relevant in assessing patients with headaches. Neurological examination should include assessment of mental status, speech, cranial nerves, visual field testing, fundoscopy, motor, sensory, and cerebellar function. Assessment should include evaluation for neck rigidity and asymmetry of deep tendon reflexes.

6.2.3 Diagnostic Tests

When a patient presents with severe headaches, the clinician's chief goal is to accurately differentiate between primary and secondary causes of headache (Table 6.2). Obtaining a detailed history is the foundation for correct diagnosis. Life-threatening etiologies must be quickly differentiated from other, more benign causes of headache. Testing should be planned to maximize the likelihood of detecting acute intracranial pathology while minimizing exposure to unnecessary radiation or invasive testing (Table 6.3).

Table 6.1 Aspects of history that should be elicited

How long the patient has had headaches, the course of headaches, including the severity and frequency

Provoking or alleviating factors

Any warning symptoms that precede the headaches (i.e., prodromes or auras)

Typical duration of headaches: minutes, hours, or days

Location of pain: hemicranial, holocephalic, retroorbital, etc.

Quality of pain: throbbing, constant, stabbing, etc.

Onset and tempo of pain: thunderclap with pain most severe at its onset, or a slow increase in intensity of pain

Associated symptoms, including nausea, emesis, photophobia, neck stiffness, lacrimation, etc.

Recent changes in medications

Medical comorbidities: hypertension, immunocompromised status, etc.

Table 6.2 Differential diagnosis of headaches

Primary headaches	Secondary headaches
• Migraine	• Concussion
• Tension-type headaches	• Cerebrovascular disease
• Trigeminal autonomic cephalgias (TACs)	1. Stroke 2. Intracranial hematomas – parenchymal bleed, subdural, epidural hematomas
• Other primary headache disorders	3. Intracranial aneurysms/arteriovenous malformation (AVM) 4. Arterial dissection 5. Arteritis
	• Intracranial tumors
	1. Parenchymal – primary/metastatic
	2. Meningeal carcinomatosis
	• Intracranial infection
	1. Meningitis
	2. Encephalitis
	3. Intracranial abscess
	• CSF abnormalities
	1. Hydrocephalus
	2. Idiopathic intracranial hypertension (IIH)
	3. Low-pressure syndromes

Table 6.2 (cont.)

Primary headaches	Secondary headaches
	• Medication overuse headaches
	• Systemic diseases
	1. Hypoxia
	2. Dialysis
	3. Hypoglycemia
	4. Hypothyroidism
	• Diseases of extracranial structures
	1. Cervicogenic headaches (e.g., secondary to cervical spondylosis)
	2. TMJ
	3. Sinus diseases
	4. Glaucoma
	• Cranial neuralgias
	1. Trigeminal neuralgia
	2. Occipital neuralgia

Table 6.3 Red flags that should prompt a diagnostic evaluation in patients presenting with headaches (SNOOP5)

- **S**ystemic symptoms (fever, weight loss) or secondary risk factors (immunocompromised state, cancer)
- **N**eurological symptoms or signs (confusion)
- **O**nset: abrupt, peak <1 min (thunderclap)
- **O**lder: >50 (giant cell arteritis)
- **P**revious headache history (new or change in frequency, severity, pattern)
- **P**ostural
- **P**recipitated by Valsalva, exertion
- **P**ulsatile tinnitus (diplopia, transient visual changes: IIH)
- **P**regnancy

6.3 Imaging Studies

6.3.1 Noncontrast CT of Head

If a patient presents with a severe headache without a prior diagnosis of a primary headache, or an abrupt change of previous headache patterns, a noncontrast CT of the head is typically necessary. CT scanners are available in almost all hospital EDs and scans can be performed quickly. This testing provides useful information about bone integrity and allows for basic assessment of intracranial structures, which is especially useful for detecting intracranial hemorrhage, mass lesions, and assessment of abnormal fluid or air collections

6.3.2 MRI of the Brain

MRI of the brain can be added for better visualization of the sinuses, skull base, and posterior fossa. MRI with contrast will provide more detail if a tumor or abscess or diffuse/meningeal conditions such as meningitis, encephalitis, carcinomatosis, or low-pressure headaches is suspected.

An **MR or CT angiogram** is needed if brain aneurysm or vessel dissection is suspected. An **MR or CT venogram** may be needed to assess for cerebral sinus thrombosis if raised intracranial pressure (ICP) is suspected or in patients with a suspected or known hypercoagulable state.

6.4 Lumbar Puncture

If a patient presents with headache, confusion, and fever without a clear etiology, CSF examination is mandatory. Prior to lumbar puncture (LP), CT or MR brain imaging must be done in order to rule-out space-occupying lesions and to avoid life-threating brain herniation. The evaluation of CSF includes cell counts, assays for protein, glucose, culture, and bacterial antigens with PCR testing for infectious processes. When carcinomatous meningitis is suspected, cytology should also be ordered.

Assessment of opening pressure should be done routinely during LP, especially if there is concern for IIH. Ensure proper patient positioning to avoid falsely elevated opening pressures. This includes positioning the patient in the left lateral decubitus position with legs extended and relaxed and ensuring that the patient is not performing a Valsalva maneuver.

LP is also helpful to increase sensitivity of detection of subarachnoid hemorrhage (SAH), which may be too subtle to be seen on CT of the head. However, recent studies suggest that for patients evaluated with CT of the head <6 hours after onset of headache, LP does not add to the diagnosis. For atypical presentations or patients who present after 6 hours from the onset of headache, LP is needed to rule-out SAH in a small percentage of patients (typically less than 5%). CSF should be centrifuged to detect the presence of xanthochromia in these cases.

6.5 Serum Tests

If a patient >50 years old presents with new headaches or a change in headache pattern, serum ESR should be checked for evaluation of temporal arteritis. A peripheral white blood cell count with a differential will facilitate diagnosing most headaches with an infectious etiology. Carboxyhemoglobin levels or toxicology screening may be indicated if a patient has a potential toxic exposure. A serum Lyme titer should also be considered if a patient presents with severe headaches accompanied by a history of a bull's eye skin rash or tick bites, with or without cranial nerve palsies.

6.6 Primary Headache Syndromes

Migraine headaches: Every 10 seconds a patient in the United States will present to the ED complaining of head pain; 1.2 million of these visits will be due to acute migraine exacerbation. Migraine headaches are moderate-to-severe disabling headaches with pulsatile or steady unilateral or holocranial pain often associated with nausea, vomiting, and photophobia. Per the International Headache Society's diagnostic criteria, migraines typically last 4–24 hours without treatment. Migraines are often exacerbated by exertion or routine physical activity and patients typically prefer to lie down in a quiet, dark room. Approximately 32% of migraines will present with auras that are most often in the form of visual symptoms such as seeing bright flickering spots or lines surrounding a dark scotoma that slowly moves across the visual field. Less frequently, migraine can mimic stroke, presenting as slurred speech, confusion, or hemiparesis. These auras can vary in duration from 5 to 60 minutes.

Well established patients with migraine presenting with acute exacerbation usually do not need additional testing. Clinical history is essential to make this determination (Table 6.1). These patients should be treated with migraine-specific treatment and testing should be minimized.

Many patients who have been diagnosed with migraine may have used their acute medication or multiple acute medications prior to presentation to the ED. A careful history of therapies given at home will prevent dangerous drug interactions when formulating an acute treatment plan.

6.7 Acute Therapy for Migraine

6.7.1 Migraine-Specific Treatments

Many patients presenting with an acute migraine have become volume-depleted due to vomiting. Even in the absence of vomiting, migraine-associated nausea and/or anorexia can cause clinically significant dehydration. IV hydration is typically indicated and may independently reduce the severity of symptoms.

Triptans are selective serotonin receptor agonists (5HT-1B/1D receptor subtypes) that block the release of vasoactive and inflammatory peptides that are responsible for the pathogenesis of migraine. Currently there are seven triptans commercially available and all are efficacious in reversing the symptom complex of migraine. The onset of action and half-life varies with each product. All triptans are available for oral administration, although sumatriptan and zolmitriptan are also available as nasal sprays, and sumatriptan is also available as a subcutaneous injection in 3 mg and 6 mg doses. Due to the risk of coronary vasoconstriction, these medications should be limited to patients without significant cardiovascular risk factors (Table 6.4). Triptans are most effective in abolishing the attack when administered early in the evolution of the headache before the development of central sensitization or allodynia. Although a patient

Table 6.4 Contraindications for the use of a triptan or DHE

Coronary artery disease or Prinzmetal angina
Cerebrovascular disease
Peripheral arterial disease
Significant risk factors for vascular disease
Uncontrolled hypertension
Pregnancy
Prior serious adverse reaction with the drug
Use of a triptan or DHE within the preceding 24 hours

seen in an acute care setting for migraine has typically passed the early phase of their migraine attack, triptans may still be a very effective treatment. A careful history of timing and doses already administered at home is needed; more than two doses of any triptan in one 24-hour period is not advised.

Dihydroergotamine, marketed as DHE-45, is another very useful option for specific migraine treatment and is often more effective than triptans when used in the ED setting. DHE can be administered by nasal spray or subcutaneous injection, but intravenous administration is exceptionally effective. In IV administration, a PICC (peripherally inserted central catheter) line is preferred due to a potent vasoconstrictive effect on the peripheral vasculature. Due to this issue, DHE is contraindicated in patients with vascular disease in any form (Table 6.4). Pretreatment with an antiemetic 15–30 minutes before DHE will reduce the severe nausea associated with administration; additional side effects can include abdominal cramps and diarrhea. Typically, 1 mg DHE is given IV, although some patients may receive benefit from 0.5 mg instead, with an option to administer a second 0.5 mg dose 30 minutes later if significant improvement is not seen.

6.7.2 Nonspecific Treatments: The "Migraine Cocktail"

While migraine-specific treatments may abort the migraine entirely, nonspecific treatments consisting of anti-inflammatory, antiemetic, anticonvulsant, antipsychotic, and various other medications with centrally active properties are frequently used in combination to abort migraine (Table 6.5). Typical combinations given for migraine include an anti-inflammatory

Table 6.5 American Headache Society treatment recommendations for an adult patient with acute migraine in the ED

Treatment option	First-line treatment (% response)	Second-line treatment (% response)
Dopamine antagonist	**58.7**	21.2
NSAIDs	**49.0**	**26.0**
IV hydration	**48.1**	16.3
DHE	33.7	**28.8**
SC sumatriptan	21.1	5.8
Corticosteroids	15.4	22.1
IV magnesium	15.4	14.4
IV valproic acid	7.7	**31.7**
Ondansetron	7.7	2.9
Oral triptan	5.8	3.8
NS triptan	3.8	1.0
Peripheral nerve block	1.9	8.7
Opioids	1.0	1.8
IV levetiracetam	0	4.8
Barbiturate-containing combination medications	0	0

medication in conjunction with an antiemetic. Patients often have a personal knowledge of a particular combination of medications that has been helpful for them in the past. It is not unreasonable to consider this information in choosing an appropriate acute treatment.

Anti-inflammatory medications can include both steroidal and nonsteroidal options. Intravenous ketorolac, methylprednisolone, and dexamethasone have been used effectively to treat acute migraine. Note that recurrent doses of NSAIDs can raise the risk of renal toxicity; screening for a history of excessive outpatient NSAID use is important. Antiemetics have been proven in several retrospective studies to be helpful not only to control nausea and vomiting, but also to have efficacy in controlling the entire symptom complex of migraine. Dopamine antagonists such as chlorpromazine, prochlorperazine, metoclopramide, and serotonin antagonists such as ondansetron, as well as antihistaminics such as diphenhydramine are widely used in the ED setting to abort severe migraine status. Note that promethazine, once commonly used in migraine cocktails, should be avoided due to serious tissue injury associated with IV infusion.

Magnesium sulfate 1–2 g IV has also shown significant benefit as an abortive agent in treatment of an acute migraine attack in the ED setting.

Valproic acid 500 mg, rapidly infused via peripheral line over 15–20 minutes, is very safe and effective to abort acute migraine attacks and does not require cardiac monitoring.

Greater occipital nerve blocks can be performed bilaterally to acutely abort both acute migraine and status migrainosus.

Narcotics are not indicated for treatment of migraine in the ED.

6.8 Cluster Headaches

Cluster headache (CH) is one of the most distinctive and painful primary headache disorders in clinical practice. Most headache disorders evaluated in EDs are of a benign etiology, with migraine being responsible for 60% of all headache presentations. In contrast, CH accounts for only 2%. It is more common in males, with a male to female ratio of 3:1. CH is characterized by a series of sudden attacks of severe, side-locked temporal and retroorbital pain, lasting from 30 minutes to 2 hours. The pain is of terrible intensity and is typically described as boring or tearing and may be likened to a "hot poker in the eye" or as if "the eye is being pushed out." Patients often develop unilateral autonomic symptoms: redness, lacrimation, miosis, and partial ptosis of the ipsilateral eye. In contrast to those with migraine, patients experiencing CH are restless and often will be seen pacing in their room as opposed to lying quietly in the dark. Cluster headaches are relatively short-lasting, the pain intensifies rapidly, peaking in 5–10 minutes and may stay at maximal intensity for 45–90 minutes. After the attack the patient is pain-free but exhausted. In many patients there is a striking circadian pattern wherein the headaches tend to occur at a certain time of the day for several days or weeks in a row. The attacks commonly occur 1–3 times daily, although the inter-headache interval may vary from 3 to 48 hours. The daily attacks usually last for 1–2 months (the cluster period). The headaches then remit spontaneously only to recur again in a cluster of daily headaches months to years later. Alcohol and vasodilators such as nitroglycerine tend to precipitate attacks and patients often learn to avoid these agents.

Because of the rapid onset and short time to peak intensity of the pain of CH, a fast-acting symptomatic therapy is imperative. Oxygen inhalation has been the standard of care for the symptomatic relief of CH since it was introduced as an effective therapy by Horton.

If delivered at the onset of an attack via a nonrebreathing facial mask at 100% at a flow rate of at least 10–15 L/min for 15 minutes, approximately 70% of patients will obtain relief within 15 minutes.

Triptans: Subcutaneous sumatriptan is the most effective medication for the symptomatic relief of CH. In a placebo-controlled study, 6 mg of sumatriptan delivered subcutaneously was significantly more effective than placebo, with 74% of patients having complete relief by 15 minutes compared with 26% of patients treated with placebo. Sumatriptan 20 mg intranasally and zolmitriptan 5 mg intranasally also appear to be effective in the acute treatment of CH. Three doses of zolmitriptan in 24 hours are acceptable. There is no evidence to support the use of oral triptans in CH.

Dihydroergotamine: 1 mg IM is effective in the relief of acute attacks of CH. The intranasal form seems less effective, although some patients benefit from its use.

6.9 Secondary Headache Syndromes

6.9.1 Vascular Diseases

6.9.1.1 Subarachnoid Hemorrhage

When a patient presents with a "thunderclap" headache, characterized by abrupt, intense pain at the very onset of symptoms, it is important to rule-out SAH, often due to rupture of an intracranial aneurysm or an AVM. SAHs most commonly occur between the ages of 40 and 60 years; the mortality and morbidity are very high in these patients. The patients will typically complain of "the worst headache of my life" or "the pain knocked me to my knees." They may also have nuchal rigidity, nausea, vomiting, and seizures, with an altered level of sensorium, which can progress to coma. CT of the head without contrast is sensitive to detect more than 90% of SAHs. Posterior circulation aneurysms have a higher annual bleed rate compared to the anterior circulation; however, posterior circulation aneurysms are less common (30%) compared with the anterior circulation. A typical SAH due to a ruptured aneurysm is either located at the base of the skull (posterior circulation) or in the anterior circulation. Anterior communicating artery aneurysm rupture will have a typical "starfish" hyperdensity pattern on CT of the head (Figure 6.1).

Less than 10% of SAH patients have negative findings on CT of the head, therefore if clinical suspicion is high LP should be performed, with the CSF evaluated for xanthochromia, which can reflect even small amounts of hemorrhage. In the case of a traumatic LP, RBC counts should be compared in sequential tubes to confirm clearing of CSF and progression toward normal findings by the final tube. Some patients may have warning signs weeks prior to the rupture, including recurrent generalized headaches and cranial nerve palsies, due to a "sentinel bleed."

The on-call neurosurgery team should be alerted emergently when aneurysm rupture is confirmed in order to proceed with emergent aneurysm clipping or coiling. In the interim before surgery, nimodipine 60 mg orally should be started for prevention of vasospasm. Table 6.6 lists the differential diagnosis of a thunderclap headache.

6.9.1.2 Vascular Causes Other than SAH

Spontaneous intraventricular or parenchymal hemorrhage may present with new onset severe headache (Table 6.6). Parenchymal hemorrhage often has focal neurological signs accompanying the severe headache. The patient with posterior fossa hemorrhage such as

Table 6.6 Differential diagnosis of thunderclap headaches

Aneurysm/SAH or vasospasm

Sagittal sinus thrombosis

Pituitary apoplexy

Vertebral or ICA dissection

Reversible cerebral vasoconstriction syndrome

Sphenoid sinusitis

Intracranial hypotension

Pseudotumor cerebri

Colloid cyst

Tumor

Migraine

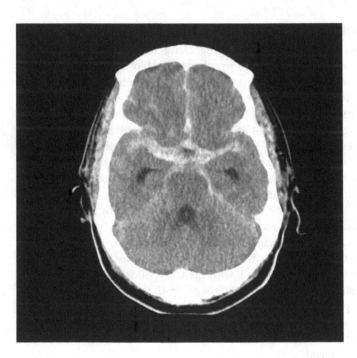

Figure 6.1 "Starfish" appearance of blood in the subarachnoid space. Courtesy of Dr. Charles Q. Li, Neuroradiology, Allegheny Health Network.

a hypertensive cerebellar bleed may quickly become comatose. CT of the head will show hyperdense hemorrhage in the affected area (Figure 6.2).

Carotid artery dissection typically presents with headache and neck pain with or without focal neurological signs. These patients may have an ipsilateral Horner's sign or ipsilateral blindness due to occlusion of the first branch of the carotid artery (i.e., the ophthalmic artery).

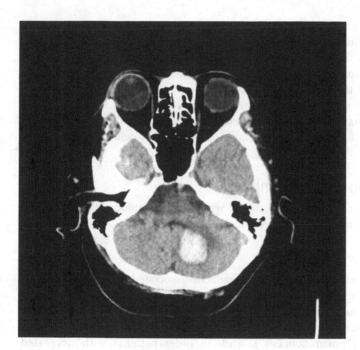

Figure 6.2 Intraparenchymal hemorrhage of the left cerebellar hemisphere. Courtesy of Dr. Charles Q. Li, Neuroradiology, Allegheny Health Network.

The patient often has a history of trauma such as whiplash injury. Similar to carotid dissection, the patients with vertebral artery dissection often have headache and neck pain, as well as brainstem symptoms such as vertigo, diplopia, dysarthria, or lateralized weakness. The diagnosis of dissection can be confirmed with neuroimaging such as CTA, MRA, conventional angiography, or duplex Doppler studies. In the appropriate clinical setting these patients may be treated with anticoagulation vs an antiplatelet agent.

Intracranial dural sinus thrombosis may present with varied symptoms ranging from dull headache to focal neurological symptoms to coma. Lateral sinus thrombosis may present with headache and an IIH Cavernous sinus thrombosis presents with acute onset of headache, unilateral proptosis, and ophthalmoplegia. The diagnosis of sinus thrombosis warrants further evaluation for parameningeal infections or a systemic hypercoagulable state. Cerebral venous infarcts with hemorrhage may be seen on imaging studies of the head and confirmed by venous imaging. Treatment of dural sinus thrombosis includes anticoagulation, which prevents further propagation of the clot. Anticoagulation is warranted even if the imaging studies reveal hemorrhagic infarcts. Broad-spectrum antibiotics also need to be administered in patients with cavernous sinus thrombosis associated with infection.

6.9.2 Vasculitis

Giant cell arteritis (temporal arteritis, TA) typically occurs in patients over 50 years of age and presents with unilateral headaches often associated with systemic symptoms of fever, malaise, weight loss, and polymyalgia rheumatica. Other clinical features include visual symptoms such as visual obscurations, with blindness as a dreaded complication, or rarely stroke. Laboratory findings reveal a raised ESR (usually in the range of 50–100 or higher) and C-reactive protein (CRP) levels. Definitive diagnosis of TA requires temporal artery biopsy and the pathologic demonstration of a vasculitis with mononucleated cell infiltration of all mural layers and the presence of giant cells. It is imperative that patients suspected to have TA receive empirical steroids, preferably prednisone at 1 mg/kg dose. Preparations for diagnostic arterial biopsy must not delay treatment with steroids.

6.9.3 Headache Due to Traumatic Injury

Simple closed head injury or complex head injury with subdural/epidural/subarachnoid blood can cause headaches with associated neurological deficits.

6.9.4 CNS Infection

CNS infections often present with acute onset headache associated with fever, nausea, and emesis. Bacterial meningitis is extremely serious; delayed diagnosis and treatment can lead to permanent neurological deficits or even death. The common bacteria causing meningitis in the United States are *Neisseria meningitidis* ("meningococcus"), *Streptococcus pneumoniae* ("pneumococcus"), and, in older patients with decreased immunity, *Listeria monocytogenes*. The diagnosis of CNS infection can be made by CSF study in suspected patients. Viral infections typically have lymphocytic pleocytosis with normal glucose and mildly elevated protein. Bacterial infections have pleocytosis with predominance of polymorphic cells, low glucose, and elevated proteins. Viral meningitis is more common than the bacterial form and is less serious in most cases. These cases typically cluster in the spring and fall seasons and improve with conservative management. One notable exception is caused by herpes simplex virus, which can cause both meningitis and encephalitis, which can be severe, often presenting with headaches, seizures, and focal neurological deficits. Patients often have a focal temporal lobe hypodensity or evidence of temporal hemorrhage on CT imaging. Admission is typically needed in these cases, including emergent neurologic and ID consultation. In patients suspected to have intracranial sepsis, broad-spectrum antibiotics including antiviral medicine should be started empirically.

6.9.5 Space-Occupying Lesion

Brain tumors and intracranial abscesses present with signs of raised ICP, namely headache, nausea, and vomiting. Many of these patients will have focal neurological deficits. Other causes of intracranial space-occupying lesions include subdural or epidural hematomas, which may present following a history of trauma or in the context of chronic anticoagulation. Fundoscopy in some patients with chronic space-occupying lesions will reveal papilledema. Change in mental status in these patients in association with anisocoria may be an ominous sign that heralds impending herniation. A colloid cyst in the third ventricle can cause periodic hydrocephalus, which at times can present as periodic headaches. The diagnosis can be made by CT or MRI of the brain, which will confirm the presence of space-occupying lesions that may or may not be accompanied by ventriculomegaly. Once mass lesions are confirmed, neurosurgery should be notified, and in the interim temporizing treatment of raised ICP with dexamethasone 10 mg IV or alternatives such as IV mannitol or IV hypertonic saline are warranted.

6.9.6 Idiopathic Intracranial Hypertension

IIH may present with headaches, blurry vision, nausea, and pulsatile tinnitus (sounds perceived occurring in the same rhythm as the pulse). Most commonly these patients are overweight women of childbearing age. Fundoscopic examination reveals papilledema (for example of bilateral papilledema seen on fundoscopic examination; see: http://eyelight photo.blogspot.com/2012/02/stereo-images-optic-disk-papilledema.html).

Physical examination may occasionally include meningismus and a sixth nerve palsy. Patients with IIH usually have normal imaging studies of the head, although careful review of MRI scans in some of these patients may reveal features of an empty sella turcica. The diagnosis of IIH is made by measuring the CSF opening pressure. The accurate measurement is best done with the patient in a lateral decubitus position with legs in an extended and relaxed posture. If the opening pressure is elevated, computed tomography venography (CTV) or magnetic resonance venography (MRV) are usually needed to rule-out cerebral sinus thrombosis. LP may provide temporary therapeutic relief, although most patients will require treatment with acetazolamide. If untreated, chronic papilledema will progress to optic nerve head atrophy and permanent vision loss. Educating the patient about potential risks and establishing a plan for follow-up care are essential prior to discharge from the ED.

6.9.7 Intracranial Hypotension (Spontaneous or Post-LP)

The cardinal clinical feature of a low-pressure headache is its distinctive positional nature, with significant or complete improvement in the supine position. Common causes are postdural puncture CSF leaks, spinal anesthesia, and following back surgery or trauma, although spontaneous cases are also reported. Brain MRI will typically show diffuse smooth dural thickening and enhancement, potentially accompanied by subdural effusions (Figure 6.3). Treatment for intracranial hypotension includes bedrest, hydration, and analgesics combined with caffeine intake. Most cases will spontaneously resolve over a few days. If headaches persist, treatment options include an epidural blood patch or surgical repair of the CSF leak.

Pearls and Pitfalls

- All patients with thunderclap headache should undergo CT scan of the head to rule-out SAH. If the scan is negative and the history is suggestive of a subarachnoid bleed, LP should be performed.
- Presence of xanthochromia in CSF is strongly indicative of a subarachnoid bleed.
- New onset of headache in individuals over 50 years of age should prompt evaluation for temporal arteritis.
- Do not use opioids or barbiturates for migraine patients due to the strong potential for headache recurrence, chronic nature of headache disorders, and potential for addiction.

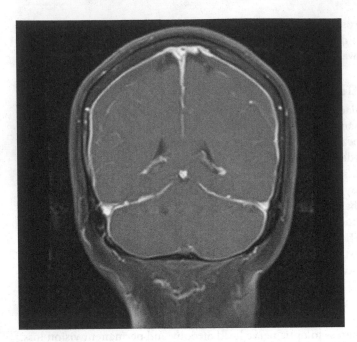

Figure 6.3 Coronal T1 image with contrast shows diffuse smooth pachymeningeal thickening; more subtle are bilateral subdural collections. Courtesy of Dr. Charles Q. Li, Neuroradiology, Allegheny Health Network.

Bibliography

Anthony M, Daher BN. Mechanism of action of steroids in cluster headache. In Clifford RF (ed.) *New Advances in Headache Research 2.* Smith Gordon, 1992.

Backes D, Rinkel GJ, Kemperman H, Linn FH, Vergouwen MD. Time-dependent test characteristics of head computed tomography in patients suspected of nontraumatic subarachnoid hemorrhage. *Stroke* 2012;**43**(8):2115–2119.

Barton CW Evaluation and treatment of headache patients in the emergency department: a survey. *Headache* 1994;**34**:91–94.

Bigal ME, Bordini CA, Tepper SJ, Speciali JG. Intravenous magnesium sulphate in the acute treatment of migraine without aura and migraine with aura: a randomized double-blind placebo-controlled study. *Cephalalgia* 2002;**22**(5):345–353.

Bigal ME, Bordini CA, Speciali JG. Intravenous chlorpromazine in the emergency department treatment of migraines: a randomized controlled trial. *J Emerg Med* 2002;**23**(2):141–148.

Bigal ME, Lipton RB. Excessive opioid use and the development of chronic migraine. *Pain* 2009;**142**(3):179–182.

Cete Y, Dora B, Ertan C, Ozdemir C, Oktay C. A randomized prospective placebo-controlled study of intravenous magnesium sulphate vs. metoclopramide in the management of acute migraine attacks in the Emergency Department. *Cephalalgia* 2005;**25**(3):199–204.

Demirkaya S, Vural O, Dora B, Topcuoglu MA. Efficacy of intravenous magnesium sulfate in the treatment of acute migraine attacks. *Headache* 2001;**41**(2):171–177.

Dodick DW, Capobianco DJ. Treatment and management of cluster headache. *Curr Pain Headache Rep* 2001;5:83–91.

Dougherty CO, Marmura MJ, Ergonul Z, Charleston LC, Szperka CL. Emergency and inpatient treatment of migraine: an American Headache Society survey. *Brit J Med Med Res* 2014;4(20):3800–3813.

Ekbom K Treatment of acute cluster headache with sumatriptan. *N Engl J Med* 1991;325:322–326.

Fogan L Treatment of cluster headache: a double-blind comparison of oxygen vs air inhalation. *Arch Neurol* 1985;42:362–363.

Frank LR, Olson CM, Shuler KB, Gharib SF. Intravenous magnesium for acute benign headache in the emergency department: a randomized double-blind placebo-controlled trial. *CJEM* 2004;6(5):327–332.

Ginder S, Oatman B, Pollack M. A prospective study of i.v. magnesium and i.v. prochlorperazine in the treatment of headaches. *J Emerg Med* 2000;18(3):311–315.

Grosberg BM, Solomon S Recognition and treatment of cluster headache in the emergency department. *Curr Pain Headache Rep* 2004;8:140–146.

Kostic MA, Gutierrez FJ, Rieg TS, Moore TS, Gendron RT. A prospective, randomized trial of intravenous prochlorperazine versus subcutaneous sumatriptan in acute migraine therapy in the emergency department. *Ann Emerg Med* 2010;56(1):1–6.

Orr SL, Aube M, Becker WJ, et al. Canadian Headache Society systematic review and recommendations on the treatment of migraine pain in emergency settings. *Cephalalgia* 2014;35(3):271–284.

Raskin NH. Repetitive intravenous dihydroergotamine as therapy for intractable migraine. *Neurology.* 1986;36:995–997.

Saper JR, Silberstein SD, Gordon CD, Hamel RL (eds.). *Handbook of Headache Management.* Williams & Wilkins, 1993.

Saper JR, Lake III AE. Continuous opioid therapy (COT) is rarely advisable for refractory chronic daily headache: limited efficacy, risks, and proposed guidelines. *Headache* 2008;48(6):838–849.

Schwartz TH, Karpitskiy VV, Sohn RS. Intravenous valproate sodium in the treatment of daily headache. *Headache* 2002;42(6):519–522.

Somerville BW. Treatment of migraine attacks with an analgesic combination (Mersyndol). *Med J Aust* 1976;1(23):865–866.

Swidan SZ, Lake III AE, Saper JR. Efficacy of intravenous diphenhydramine versus intravenous DHE-45 in the treatment of severe migraine headache. *Curr Pain Headache Rep* 2005;9(1):65–70.

Weakness

George A. Small and Melody Milliron

7.1 Introduction

Weakness is often a very complicated ED presenting complaint. A detailed history and physical examination, and diligent search for etiology are required. First, the clinician must elucidate true weakness vs fatigue. Fatigue is best defined as a decrease in the ability to perform motor functions. Fatigue may be the complaint for a broad differential diagnosis, including acute coronary syndrome, anemia, chronic inflammatory diseases, dehydration, hypoglycemia or other electrolyte derangements, adrenal insufficiency, a variety of infections, pulmonary disorders, medication side effects, and depression. These disorders are characterized by a lack of true muscular weakness on examination. True muscular weakness is not painful, and pain should guide the examiner to other etiologies such as fibromyalgia or polymyalgia rheumatica. True muscular weakness is graded 0 (no movement) to 5 (normal) (Table 7.1) and characterized by weakness with specific tasks. Proximal muscle weakness is suggested by difficulties in raising arms over the head or combing hair. Distal muscle weakness is characterized by tripping, issues with dexterity while buttoning clothes, or difficulty with fine motor tasks such as writing. Bulbar causes of weakness present with complaints of diplopia, choking, or ocular or speech issues. The patient's history is essential for appropriate differential diagnosis.

7.2 ABCs

As is true with any other ED patient, the ABCs trump any further detailed history or exam. If the patient has any signs of impending airway issues or unstable vital signs, emergent intervention is required. The presence of upper or lower motor neuron signs generally results in an appropriate (Table 7.2), expeditious differential diagnosis. Abrupt onset of weakness due to acute CNS or spinal cord pathology requires acute intervention. Neuromuscular junction, peripheral nerve, and myopathic causes of weakness tend to present more insidiously. Tachypnea, shallow breathing, inability to handle secretions, a weak voice, inability to lift the head, or a very low forced vital capacity (normal is 65 cc/kg) may suggest impending respiratory failure (Table 7.3). The three most common primary neurological causes of acute ED respiratory failure are previously unrecognized amyotrophic lateral sclerosis (ALS), myasthenia gravis, and Guillain–Barré syndrome. Respiratory failure due to neuromuscular cause presents differently than COPD, which presents with air trapping and an increased pCO_2. However, an ABG may be normal in patients with diaphragmatic and intercostal muscle weakness. Patients with a neuromuscular cause of respiratory failure typically have a decrease in tidal volume and compensatory tachypnea to maintain normal minute ventilation. As a result, pCO_2 may remain normal even in a decompensating patient. The judicious use of

Table 7.1 Muscle strength grading: British Medical Research Council staging of weakness

5	Normal motor strength against full resistance
4	Movement against some, but less than full resistance
3	Movement against gravity, but not against resistance
2	Not able to move against gravity
1	Trace contraction, muscle twitch
0	No contraction of movement

Table 7.2 Upper vs lower motor neuron signs

Upper motor neuron	Lower motor neuron
Spasticity	Decreased muscle tone
Hyperreflexia	Hyporeflexia
Positive Babinski	Negative Babinski
Likely diagnosis:	Likely diagnosis:
Acute CVA	Neuropathy
CNS mass	Myopathy
Spinal cord pathology	Neuromuscular junction disease

Table 7.3 Signs of impending respiratory failure in the weak patient

Tachypnea, shallow breathing
Inability to handle secretions
Weak voice
Inability to lift head
Low forced vital capacity – under 15 cc/kg (normal is 65 cc/kg), or rapidly declining
PaO_2 less than 70 on room air
Negative inspiratory force less than –30 cmH_2O or rapidly worsening

BiPAP allows the ED physician time to stabilize the patient and allows further investigation of the underlying etiology. If intubation is acutely indicated, avoid depolarizing agents (succinylcholine) due to the risk of an exaggerated hyperkalemic response. This response is typically more significant in patients with ALS, Guillain–Barré, and inherited myopathies (e.g., Duchenne's muscular dystrophy). Maintenance of respiratory function through assisted ventilation is critical while ED evaluation continues. If any vital sign abnormalities exist, they must be addressed before a detailed history and physical exam proceeds.

7.3 History

7.3.1 Onset

If no acute airway issue or vital sign abnormalities exist, further history and physical examination may continue. The onset of weakness may narrow the differential diagnosis (Table 7.4). Symptom duration may be difficult to establish in ED patients who cannot communicate, are elderly, or have a language barrier. Acute onset of weakness is typically within minutes to hours. This may suggest a vascular, metabolic, or toxic etiology. Subacute weakness (progressing over a week) is more common with disorders involving nerves, the neuromuscular junction, or muscles. Subacute fluctuating weakness may occur with toxic or metabolic disorders, neuromuscular junction disorders such as botulism, rarely periodic paralysis, or more commonly myasthenia gravis. Slowly progressive weakness over weeks or months is more likely associated with nonemergent conditions. Slowly progressive weakness in inflammatory myopathy such as dermatomyositis and polymyositis, and steroid-resistant inflammatory myopathy, a common cause of weakness in the elderly, result in a more subacute to chronic process. Patients with muscular dystrophies or primary disorders of the motor nerve, such as ALS, also experience gradual worsening weakness. These patients typically present to the ED with a complicating event, such as a fall.

7.3.2 Additional History

Additional history helps to narrow the differential diagnosis, allowing appropriate ED disposition. A history of risk factors including smoking, hypertension, hypercholesterolemia, diabetes, or heart disease, as well as unilateral symptoms, may lead to early diagnosis of stroke. Significant psychiatric history, such as somatoform disorder, leads to an evaluation for organic and nonorganic causes of weakness. A history of collagen vascular type syndromes or prior endocrinopathy may also be important in an accurate final diagnosis. A detailed review of systems informs the differential diagnosis.

In addition to past medical history, medication history is important. Diuretic use may result in electrolyte disturbances and generalized fatigue, not true weakness. Amiodarone, cisplatin, dapsone, INH, disulfiram, metronidazole, and vincristine may also cause weakness from polyneuropathy. Statin drugs may result in patients presenting with significant

Table 7.4 Weakness by onset

Acute	Subacute progressive	Subacute fluctuating	Slowly progressive
Vascular	Nerve disorder	Toxic	Inflammatory myopathies
Metabolic	Neuromuscular junction	Metabolic	
Toxic	Muscles	Neuromuscular junction	
		Muscles	

muscle fatigue with or without cramping. Drugs of abuse may also result in presentations to the ED. Nitrous oxide abuse with or without associated vitamin B12 deficiency may cause an acute myelopathy. Cocaine and amphetamine ingestion may result in cerebral infarction or bleeding, and present as unilateral weakness.

Obtaining an accurate social and travel history is also important. Insect envenomation, such as tick exposure, may result in acute neuromuscular junction disorders with areflexia. Botulinum toxin is increasingly used for cosmetic and neurological causes, and frequently causes cranial weakness. Naturally occurring botulism is much less common than iatrogenic botulinum-induced weakness. A history of travel in areas with known toxins from sea life also can result in an accurate diagnosis of weakness resulting from envenomation.

Family medical history may determine an inherited cause of weakness. These diseases include autosomal dominantly inherited myotonic muscular dystrophy, the most common muscular dystrophy of adults. Other rare problems such as Charcot–Marie–Tooth disease, which causes distal weakness, do not result in ED presentations unless a complicating event, such as a fall, exists. Metabolic disorders of muscle, including glycogen storage diseases and lipid storage diseases, are autosomal recessive and also are generally not ED presenting complaints.

7.4 Physical Examination: Symmetric vs Asymmetric Weakness

An attentive physical examination in the ED can further differentiate weakness into symmetric (bilateral) and asymmetric (unilateral) weakness. When weakness is unilateral, brain dysfunction is often the cause. Patients with primary intracerebral hemorrhage, ischemic stroke, or expanding neoplasms most commonly present with unilateral weakness of the face, arm, or leg, or some combination of the above. Abrupt onset likely signifies CNS ischemia or hemorrhage as determined by CT and/or MRI. Although hyporeflexia may occasionally occur acutely, hyperreflexia and pathological reflexes such as a Babinski sign are typically seen with acute CNS etiologies. Patients with glioblastoma multiforme and other CNS neoplasms typically present with focal seizures and/or headache, and altered mental status with or without unilateral weakness. Headache, nausea, and vomiting are typical indicators of intracerebral hemorrhage with abrupt onset of weakness. In HIV-positive patients, slowly progressive unilateral weakness with hyperreflexia requires CNS imaging to assess a vast differential diagnosis of infectious and neoplastic causes. Patients with slowly evolving brainstem lesions may present with combinations of cranial nerve weakness and bilateral lower extremity weakness. These presentations may mimic spinal cord, muscle, or nerve disease. However, CNS imaging helps the ED physician establish an accurate diagnosis. As mentioned, unilaterality of true weakness dramatically helps narrow the differential diagnosis of upper or lower motor neuron problems.

The hallmarks of a spinal cord process are: bilateral weakness without effect on cranial nerves or altered mental status, hyperreflexia, and urinary dysfunction. Sensory symptoms may accompany the weakness of cervical or thoracic myelopathy. Back pain typically occurs at the level of a lesion in epidural abscess, epidural hemorrhage, or transverse myelitis. Secondary causes of spinal cord problems are usually apparent from the patient's history: use of anticoagulants resulting in spontaneous hemorrhage, history of trauma such as gunshot wound or fall, or history of cancer with spinal metastases and cord compression. Primary intramedullary tumors such as astrocytomas, metastases, and ependymomas will be diagnosed by spinal imaging. Individuals with transverse myelitis after a viral illness often have weakness at a definable level, enhancement on MRI of the spine, and have CSF with elevated protein and cell counts. Multiple sclerosis can present as transverse myelitis as above, typically in a young female, but may occur at any age. Proper CNS and spinal imaging after physical examination, and CSF analysis when indicated, will aid in the differential diagnosis. In the last 15 years, particularly in spring and summer, an acute polio-like illness from West Nile virus (WNV) presents with pure unilateral or bilateral motor symptoms without sensory symptoms. WNV can present so abruptly as to cause respiratory failure or a combination of proximal and distal weakness, prompting ED evaluation. A high index of suspicion for WNV is required for inclusion in the accurate differential diagnosis.

7.5 Weakness Characterized as Proximal, Distal, Bulbar

The specific location of weakness can be divided generally into proximal, distal, and bulbar (cranial) (Table 7.5). In general, proximal weakness is typical of inherited diseases of motor neurons, acquired diseases of motor neurons, or particularly rare causes such as inherited spinal muscular atrophies. Inherited nerve problems and inherited muscle disorders such as muscular dystrophies generally do not present to the ED unless an acute complication, such as a fall, exists. Patients with acute onset symptoms with bilateral proximal weakness have difficulty arising from a seated position, raising their arms over their head, or even respiratory compromise. Toxins to nerve, muscle, and the neuromuscular junction may also present in this fashion. Patients reporting proximal muscle weakness will describe difficulty combing hair, rising from a chair, climbing stairs, or may present to the ED after a fall. Since all of these modalities require appropriate force generation from the hip girdle or periscapular muscles, the proximal nature of these problems is established. Continued physical examination reveals the presence or absence of reflexes, which further narrows the differential diagnosis to nerve, muscle disease, or spinal cord disease. The patient who "Gowers" essentially climbs up their own body to stand. This is pathognomonic of proximal weakness. Visual examination of the patient with proximal weakness may reveal scapular winging,

Table 7.5 Weakness: proximal, distal, bulbar

Proximal	Distal	Bulbar
Inherited diseases of motor neurons	Peripheral nerve	Myasthenia gravis neurons
Acquired diseases of motor neurons	Anterior horn cell disorders with botulism hypo- or areflexia (history of diabetes or alcoholism)	Botulism
Inherited spinal muscular atrophies		
Toxins to nerve and muscle		
Toxins to the neuromuscular junction		

noted as shoulder girdle weakness, or atrophy of proximal arm musculature, which further suggests a nerve or muscle process.

Distal weakness is generally found with patients who drop things frequently, have difficulty manipulating small objects, buttoning clothes, dragging feet, tripping over objects, or have difficulty ambulating on uneven ground. Diagnosis of slowly progressive distal weakness secondary to peripheral nerve or anterior horn cell disorders such as diabetic neuropathy, alcoholic polyneuropathy, or ALS depends on the ED physician's understanding of disease prevalence, and the presence of normal or pathological reflexes. In distal weakness with hypo- or areflexia, peripheral neuropathies are the most likely etiology; a history of diabetes or alcoholism is key to diagnosis. The presence or absence of sensory symptoms with weakness also helps to narrow the differential diagnosis. Sensory symptoms, defined as paresthesias or dysesthesias, never occur in motor neuron disorders, such as ALS or WNV, or in myopathies. Patients with frequent falls and stumbling with a marching gait, lifting knees up excessively while ambulating, suggest distal leg weakness. As the population ages and more patients are living with Parkinson's disease, rigidity may be misinterpreted as weakness as patients present with falls and fractures.

Bulbar weakness presents to the ED with alterations in muscles of the tongue, jaw, face and larynx. Symptoms are ocular (ptosis, diplopia), bulbar (dysphagia, dysarthria), and occasionally nasal speech. Myasthenia gravis is the most common neuromuscular junction disorder, and occasionally presents to the ED with fluctuating diplopia and/or swallowing issues. Myasthenia can be deadly if the patient is discharged with no diagnosis. As the problem worsens, the patient may experience severe complications, including acute respiratory compromise or obstruction of the oropharynx. A high index of suspicion is required by the ED physician in these cases. Patients who received botulinum toxin for neurological or cosmetic causes can also present with reversible bulbar weakness and acute problems in breathing and swallowing.

7.6 Weakness by Location: Anterior Horn, Peripheral Nerve, Neuromuscular Juncture, or at the Muscle Fiber

Diseases of the anterior horn are motor neuron diseases and include lead exposure, poliomyelitis, and WNV. Time of onset, age, family history, exposure, and occasional CSF evaluation lead to disease differentiation. Isolated pathology of motor nerves, distal to the nerve roots, can occur with heavy metal intoxication, such as lead, or iatrogenically with the use of dapsone or metronidazole. Historically, lead intoxication has been described in patients with bilateral wrist drop without trauma. Polio remains rare in the United States. Polio virus attacks anterior horn cells, resulting in hyporeflexia and asymmetric weakness, with proximal muscles affected more than distal. If bulbar involvement occurs, respiratory compromise follows. CSF evaluation shows pleocytosis with mononuclear cells, and normal to slightly high protein. WNV is now an endemic RNA virus in the United States with a *Culex* mosquito vector. Although most infections are asymptomatic, symptomatic patients present with fever, headache, nausea, and vomiting consistent with viral meningoencephalitis. Patients may also present with asymmetric weakness or facial involvement. Evaluation of these disorders is based on history and physical examination and may require CSF testing.

Peripheral nerve etiologies of weakness include diabetes and peripheral nerve compression. Diabetic neuropathy is typically bilateral, symmetrical, and in the lower extremities. History of diabetes often confirms the diagnosis. Mononeuropathy due to a peripheral nerve compression follows a classic anatomic pathway (e.g., carpal tunnel). This typically makes the diagnosis routine.

Diseases of the neuromuscular junction include myasthenia gravis, organophosphate exposure, botulism (see below), and tick envenomation. In all of these illnesses, reflexes are preserved. Myasthenia gravis typically presents with fluctuating bulbar symptoms. In an age of bioterrorism, organophosphate exposure from insecticides is of specific interest to the ED physician. Organophosphate poisoning presents with the often classic DUMBBELS (defecation, urination, miosis, bronchospasm, bradycardia, emesis, lacrimation, salivation) and possible respiratory paresis. The toxic effect of these agents lies in their inhibition of acetylcholinesterase, thus stimulating and then inhibiting at the neuromuscular junction by uncatabolized acetylcholine. Weakness of skeletal and bulbar muscles, marked fasciculations, and the constellation of the above findings will alert the ED physician to this diagnosis. Treatment with decontamination and high-dose atropine and 2-PAM (pralidoxime) is standard. Tick paralysis is caused by a neurotoxin released by the Rocky Mountain Wood tick (*Dermacentor andersoni*) or Eastern dog tick (*Dermacentor variabilis*). Ascending paralysis is caused by neurotoxin production that inhibits liberation of acetylcholine at the neuromuscular junction. Several days after female tick attachment, fatigue and paresthesias progress to weakness, ataxia, and walking difficulties. After diligent search, removal of the tick is curative within hours.

Diseases affecting the muscle fiber include neuropathies and myopathies. Neuropathies are a class of nerve disorders that cause distal muscle weakness, altered sensation, and hyporeflexia. Myopathies are inflammatory or congenital disorders of muscle that rarely present to the ED. Symptoms include muscle pain without sensory changes, preserved reflexes, and proximal upper and lower extremity weakness. The patient may have an associated collagen vascular syndrome. The presence of pain and an elevated CPK, with or without an elevated sedimentation rate, confirms the diagnosis. The chronic use of steroids in many patients may also present quite similarly to an inflammatory myopathy.

Another etiology of symmetric weakness is myelopathy. Nontraumatic myelopathy is a spinal cord disease that presents with bilateral motor weakness, sensory deficits, and bowel and bladder symptoms due to upper motor neuron interruption. Arm weakness localizes disease to the cervical cord, whereas leg weakness without arm weakness localizes to the thoracic cord. Reflexes typically start as hyporeflexic and then over days progress to hyperreflexia more typical of upper motor neuron pathology (Table 7.6).

Table 7.6 Weakness by location: anterior horn, peripheral nerve, neuromuscular junction, or at the muscle fiber

Anterior horn (motor neuron diseases)	Peripheral nerve	Diseases of the neuromuscular junction	Muscle fiber
Lead exposure	Diabetic neuropathy	Myasthenia gravis	Neuropathies
Poliomyelitis	Peripheral nerve compression	Organophosphate exposure	Myopathies
West Nile virus		Botulism	
		Tick envenomation	

7.7 Weakness: Ascending vs Descending

Classification of weakness as ascending or descending may also help narrow the differential diagnosis (Table 7.7). Ascending weakness causes include acute inflammatory demyelinating polyneuropathy (AIDP), also known as Guillain–Barré syndrome, and tick paralysis (as discussed above). AIDP is the most common primary acquired cause of ascending paralysis in the United States. It commonly presents to the ED with symmetrical weakness and decreased or absent reflexes 2–4 weeks after a febrile illness. The hallmarks of AIDP are rapid progression within 2–4 weeks, and an elevated CSF protein without cells. Approximately 70% of patients recall a prior febrile illness, and up to 30% require ventilator support. Prompt diagnosis and use of gamma globulin or plasma exchange greatly decreases the time course. AIDP generally occurs as a sensory–motor syndrome. AIDP may acutely worsen with respiratory compromise, requiring close monitoring in a critical care setting.

Descending weakness causes include botulism and polio (as discussed above). Botulism infection with *Clostridium botulinum* produces weakness from a toxin generated from bacterial spores. Clostridia are gram-positive, spore-forming bacteria found dormant in the soil, seawater, and air. The toxin produced results in inhibition of calcium-dependent release of acetylcholine at the presynaptic membrane of the neuromuscular junction, resulting in descending weakness, flaccid paralysis, and autonomic dysfunction, with intact sensation and cognition. Several varied clinical types of botulism exist: foodborne (8% of the 112 CDC-confirmed cases in 2010), infantile (76%), and wound botulism (15%). Contaminated canned goods account for approximately 65% of foodborne outbreaks of botulism. Foodborne botulism presents nonspecifically in the initial stages, with gastrointestinal symptoms such as nausea, vomiting, diarrhea, and abdominal pain developing 1–5 days after exposure. These symptoms would typically be mistaken for other forms of food poisoning. Later, bulbar symptoms (diplopia, dysarthria, and dysphagia) develop and clarify the diagnosis. The vast majority of wound botulism is seen in injection drug users, especially those who inject subcutaneously. Wound botulism does not cause significant gastrointestinal symptoms. Neurologic symptoms can develop as early as 12–24 hours after exposure and initially involve cranial nerve symptoms. Infantile botulism is due to spores, often in honey, that grow and produce toxin in the immature gut. Thus, the course is more indolent as it takes time for toxin production. Ninety-five percent of cases occur before the age of 6 months and are rare after 1 year. Infantile botulism also begins with bulbar symptoms, such as a poor suck and inability to hold the head up, as well as constipation. With disease progression more generalized weakness occurs, creating classic findings of a "floppy baby," with a weak cry and ptosis. Most patients do not progress to intubation but will require ICU monitoring

Table 7.7 Selected causes of ascending vs descending weakness

Ascending weakness	Descending weakness
Acute inflammatory demyelinating polyneuropathy (Guillain–Barré syndrome)	Botulism
Tick paralysis	Polio

for respiratory difficulties. Iatrogenic complications may also arise from injection of botulinum toxin for medical or cosmetic reasons.

A final common pathway in botulism occurs as a descending flaccid paralysis develops. Bulbar palsies present initially followed by arm and leg muscles being affected, proximally to distally. If disease progresses unrecognized and untreated, intercostal and diaphragm muscles may be affected and respiratory failure may occur. Once respiratory failure occurs, the patient requires ventilatory support until the motor end-plate recovers, which may take several months. Botulism does not alter mentation, sensation, or cause fever, so these symptoms should suggest investigations for other etiologies. Treatment includes supportive care, immune globulin, and possible wound debridement in wound botulism. If bulbar symptoms occur as a side effect of botulinum toxin use for medical or cosmetic reasons, supportive care is indicated. Testing, evaluation, and treatment with antitoxin for botulism are best performed after consultation with the local health department, and ultimately with the CDC.

7.8 Further ED Evaluation

As the differential for weakness is vast, a comprehensive list of all possible testing is not feasible in this text. In general, laboratory testing is useful only to exclude nonneuromuscular causes of weakness. An ED evaluation with EKG, hemoglobin, electrolytes, glucose, troponin, and urinalysis is standard. Further testing, including CNS or spinal imaging, is guided by the history and physical examination. Treatment of specific etiologies is dependent on the suspected diagnosis and disposition. Unless acute respiratory issues, risk for acute decompensation, or upper motor pathology is identified, the patient's disposition is typically to home.

In conclusion, the complaint of weakness in the ED should be evaluated for a serious etiology. A meticulous history with closed-ended questions regarding the patient's specific inability to perform certain tasks and a careful neurological examination are key. Documentation of the distribution of weakness, presence or absence of sensory symptoms, and possible involvement of cranial innervated musculature enables the ED physician to formulate an informed differential diagnosis, and diagnostic and treatment plans.

Pearls and Pitfalls

- Fatigue can be misdiagnosed as frank weakness.
- The three most common primary neurological causes of acute ED respiratory failure are previously unrecognized ALS, myasthenia gravis, and Guillain–Barré syndrome.
- If emergent intubation is required for respiratory failure due to a suspected neuromuscular cause, avoid depolarizing agents due to the risk of an exaggerated hyperkalemic response.
- pCO_2 may be normal in neuromuscular causes of respiratory failure.
- Differentiating upper vs lower motor neuron signs of weakness can narrow a differential diagnosis.
- Sudden respiratory compromise due to cosmetic use of botulinum toxin is rare but can go undiagnosed if relevant history is not obtained.
- Bulbar weakness due to myasthenia gravis can progress rapidly with severe consequences if untreated.

Bibliography

Andrus P Michael Guthrie J. Acute peripheral neurologic lesions. In Tintinalli JE, (ed.) *Tintinalli's Emergency Medicine*, 7th ed. McGraw-Hill, 2011.

Asimos AW. Evaluation of the adult with acute weakness in the emergency department. Available at: www.uptodate.com/home .index.html. 2015

Donaghy M. *Brain's Diseases of the Nervous System*, 10th ed. Oxford University Press, 2002.

Dyck P, Thomas P. K. (eds.). *Peripheral Neuropathy*, 3rd ed. W. B. Saunders, 1993.

Engel AG, Franzini-Armstrong C (eds.). *Myology*, 2nd ed. McGraw-Hill, 1994.

Fernández-Frackelton, M. Bacteria. In Marx J (ed.) *Rosen's Emergency Medicine*, 8th ed. W. B. Saunders, 2013.

Fuchs, S. Weakness. In Schafermeyer R (ed.) *Strange and Schafermeyer's Pediatric Emergency Medicine*, 4th ed. McGraw-Hill, 2014.

Handel, DA, Gaines SA. Chronic neurological disorders. In Tintinalli JE (ed.) *Tintinalli's Emergency Medicine*, 7th ed. McGraw Hill, 2011.

Lewis ED, Mayer SA, Noble JM (eds.). *Merritt's Neurology*, 10th ed. Lippincott Williams and Wilkins Publishers, 2000.

Miller ML Approach to the patient with muscle weakness. 2015. Available at: www .uptodate.com/home.index.html.

Sethi RK, Thompson LL. *The Electromyographer's Handbook*, 2nd ed. Little Brown and Company, 1989.

Stone KC. Neurologic emergencies. In Stone KC (ed.) *Current Diagnosis and Treatment Emergency Medicine*, 7th ed. McGraw Hill, 2011.

Swanson PD. *Signs and Symptoms in Neurology*. Lippincott, 1984.

Chapter

8

Musculoskeletal and Neurogenic Pain

Nestor Tomycz and Thomas P. Campbell

8.1 Introduction

Pain is one of the most common presenting complaints in the emergency department (ED), both acute pain and exacerbation of chronic pain syndromes. Acute pain is accompanied by anxiety and sympathetic hyperactivity, whereas chronic pain is often associated with affective symptoms of depression. *Nociceptive* (musculoskeletal, inflammatory, or somatic) pain involves activation of the peripheral receptors secondary to tissue damage from trauma or heat. *Neuropathic* pain involves direct activation of either sensory nerves or ganglia by nerve injury or disease. Differentiation between nociceptive and neuropathic pain in the ED can be difficult, but should be considered for successful management of the pain.

8.2 Facial Pain

8.2.1 Nociceptive Syndromes

Dental pain is the most common cause of orofacial pain in adults. Odontalgia is best treated with regional nerve blocks. This technique prevents reliance on opioids and the potential for abuse and dependence. When necessary for severe abscess, antibiotics and urgent dental referral are required.

Acute sinusitis is diagnosed by localized pain and tenderness, purulent rhinorrhea for greater than 2 weeks, and fever. Blood tests and radiographs are not needed in immunocompetent patients and treatment includes decongestants and oral antibiotics. Immunocompromised and toxic-appearing patients should have an emergent CT scan and consultation to prevent intracranial spread of infection.

Temporo-mandibular joint dysfunction presents with localized joint tenderness to palpation that is exacerbated with joint movement, decreased range of motion, and/or crepitus on joint movement. Treatment is usually with nonsteroidal anti-inflammatory drugs (NSAIDs) and dental referral.

Disorders of the eyes, ears, neck, and salivary glands can also be sources of facial pain, but are far less common.

8.2.2 Neuropathic Syndromes

Trigeminal neuralgia presents with sudden paroxysms of lancinating pain that lasts for seconds to minutes, often recurring many times per day. The pain can occur without provocation or provoked by sensory stimulation of facial trigger points. The diagnosis is

Table 8.1 Causes of facial pain in the ED

Nociceptive	Neuropathic
Odontalgia	Trigeminal neuralgia
Sinusitis	Herpetic neuralgia
TMJ syndrome	Glossopharyngeal neuralgia Occipital neuralgia
Disorders of the eyes, ears, neck and salivary glands	

usually made clinically without neuroimaging. However, if symptoms are bilateral, patient age is less than 40 years, or there is sensory loss on exam, consultation and imaging should be considered. The extremely short duration of the pain is usually not improved with anti-inflammatory medications or opioids. Carbamazepine or gabapentin are the initial drugs of choice for treatment, but baclofen and pimozide have also been used with limited success.

Other facial neuralgic conditions (Table 8.1) such as glossopharyngeal neuralgia are very rare and must be differentiated from mass lesions or vascular lesions with neuroimaging (MRI/MRA). Treatment is the same as trigeminal neuralgia and may include surgery for refractory severe cases.

Acute herpetic neuralgia most often involves the first division of the trigeminal nerve. Treatment with antiviral medications and steroids during the first 72 hours of rash has shown to reduce events of postherpetic neuralgia, and the acute episode may require a short course of opioids to help control the pain. If ophthalmologic involvement is considered, emergent consultation should be obtained. Pain beyond one month of the lesion resolution is considered postherpetic neuralgia and is more common in those over age 60 years. Treatment for postherpetic neuralgia can include tricyclic antidepressants and some success has been achieved with antiseizure medications such as gabapentin, pregabalin, and divalproex sodium. Severe cases may benefit from regional nerve block.

8.3 Neck and Upper Extremity Pain

This chapter deals with nociceptive and neurogenic pain, but clinicians must be careful to assess neck, upper extremity, and truncal pain to distinguish those pain syndromes from referred pain from ischemic processes of visceral organs that can be confounding on examination.

8.3.1 Nociceptive Syndromes

The most common cause of neck pain in the ED is cervical strain (Table 8.2), which is characterized by paracervical tenderness, muscle spasm, and discomfort on movement. Most cases are successfully treated with heat and anti-inflammatory medications.

Cervical osteoarthritis is the most common cause of neck pain in patients over age 40 years. Pain is usually generated from the apophyseal joints and isolated in the neck and shoulders. Radiation into the upper extremities suggests nerve root involvement.

Table 8.2 Causes of neck and upper extremity pain in the ED

Nociceptive	Neuropathic
Cervical strain	Cervical radiculopathy
Cervical osteoarthritis	Brachial plexus disorders
Rheumatoid	Erb–Duchenne palsy
Ankylosing spondylitis	Dejerine–Klumpke palsy
Inflammatory upper extremity causes	Radiation plexitis
Septic arthritis	Idiopathic brachial plexitis
Noninfectious arthritis	Thoracic outlet syndrome
Tendonitis	Complex regional pain syndrome (reflex sympathetic dystrophy)
Bursitis	Suprascapular nerve palsy
Tenosynovitis	Radial nerve neuropathies
Ischemic causes	Ulnar nerve neuropathies
Acute arterial dissection	Median nerve neuropathies
Subclavian steal syndrome	Carpal tunnel syndrome
Coronary artery ischemic referred pain	
Traumatic causes	

Compression fractures can also cause acute pain syndromes, but rarely involve the nerve root. Most arthritic symptoms can be managed with NSAIDs, but when severe may require referral or imaging to determine the type of arthritis, consideration of additional medications, and/or need for surgical intervention. It is not uncommon for patients with complicated arthritic conditions to require management from pain specialists.

Rheumatoid arthritis (RA) is a systemic erosive polyarthritis primarily involving small joints. Joints of the hand are the most commonly involved joints and the cervical spine is the second most common. Bony and ligamentous disruption from spinal involvement in RA can be life-threatening and should be considered in those patients with consistent histories. These patients are often treated with biologicals or immune modulators and may require urgent consultation.

Ankylosing spondylitis (AS) is a spondyloarthropathy with many similarities to the arthritis of Reiter's syndrome, psoriasis, and arthritis related to inflammatory bowel disease. These disorders are characterized by spondylitis, sacroiliitis, tendon insertion inflammation, asymmetrical oligoarthritis, and often extra-articular manifestations such as uveitis, urethritis, and mucocutaneous lesions. Dysfunction of the lower thoracic and lumbar sacral spine is most common in these syndromes, but it can involve the cervical and upper thoracic spine. Pain, limited range of motion, and radiologic abnormalities such as a "bamboo spine" in AS are common findings. Pain management is usually begun with NSAIDs and physical therapy, but often requires consultant-directed therapy with anti-TNF-alpha agents, sulfasalazine, methotrexate, and steroids.

Inflammatory upper extremity disorders are a frequent cause of upper extremity pain. Local infection of the joints is usually obvious with severe pain, redness, and warmth, and requires aspiration and joint fluid analysis to determine if the etiology is infectious. Nonbacterial arthritis from rubella, Epstein–Barr virus, or hepatitis is always associated with systemic findings and resolves spontaneously when the systemic infection resolves. Gout and pseudogout require anti-inflammatory treatment to shorten the course of inflammation and pain. Bacterial septic arthritides usually require surgical drainage and appropriate antibiotics and pain management. Tendonitis, bursitis, and tenosynovitis are most common in the shoulder, elbow, and thumb. The clinical exam usually reveals extreme pain on motion of these joints and tendon insertions and often is related to overuse syndromes such as tennis elbow and de Quervain's disease. These entities are self-limited and best treated with NSAIDs, subsequent physical therapy with range-of-motion exercises, and steroid injections for cases lasting greater than 4 months.

8.3.2 Neuropathic Syndromes

Lesions of the cervical spine (see Table 8.3) generally result in deep segmental pain, which is often not well localized. Segmental weakness, sensory loss, and hyporeflexia are present in the upper extremities. The lower extremities exhibit spasticity, weakness, sensory loss, hyperreflexia, and a positive Babinski sign. Urinary or fecal incontinence occur as later symptoms. Lesions of the cervical spine are best visualized by MRI or CTA.

Table 8.3 Cervical nerve root pathology localization on exam

Disc involved	Nerve root involved	Area of pain	Area of sensory change	Motor weakness	Altered reflex
C3–C4	C4	Shoulder	Variable	± Deltoid	None
C4–C5	C5	Shoulder, lateral upper arm	Shoulder	Deltoid ± biceps	Biceps
C5–C6	C6	Shoulder, upper arm, lateral forearm, thumb, and index finger	Lateral forearm and thumb	Biceps, triceps wrist extensors	Brachioradialis and biceps
C6–C7	C7	Posterolateral upper arm, shoulder, and neck	Index and middle fingers	Wrist flexors, finger extensors, and triceps	Triceps
C7–T1	C8	Ulnar forearm and hand	Medial forearm, fourth and fifth digits of hand	Hand intrinsics, finger flexors, and wrist extensors	None

Cervical radiculopathy is caused by cervical spondylosis and disc disease. Cervical herniated nucleus pulposus can occur either from trauma or from disc degeneration. Radiation of the pain to the neck and upper limb in a segmental fashion is common. Clinical findings include segmental sensory loss, motor weakness, and reflex changes (see Table 8.3). Herniated nucleus pulposus of the lower cervical roots of C6–C7 account for 70% of cases and C5–C6 for 20%. Neck pain on exam may reveal greater pain on lateral head movement toward the side of the radiculopathy. Significant sensory loss, weakness, and intractable pain require neuroimaging and consultation. Pain management can be difficult and often requires opioid medication for acute phases prior to surgery.

Thoracic outlet syndrome is a rare condition to diagnose in an ED but should be considered when shoulder and arm pain is accompanied by paresthesias of the median or ulnar nerve distribution. The syndrome is caused by compression of the lower trunk of the brachial plexus and subclavian artery from impingement due to abnormal first thoracic ribs, clavicle, fascia, or scalene muscles. Weakness, atrophy, and vascular changes in the distal forearm and hand are common. Diagnostic clinical maneuvers include the Wright maneuver to reproduce symptoms with the arm abducted and rotated 90 degrees while the elbow is flexed 90 degrees, or the Adson maneuver to extend and rotate the patient's head to the affected side with maximal inspiration to palpate a weakened pulse with the maneuver. Treatment for the pain includes NSAIDs, flexibility and stretching exercises, and postural and ergonomic adjustments. Surgery is occasionally required.

Complex regional pain syndrome causes neurologically mediated shoulder and arm pain characterized by vasomotor and dermal changes and premature osteoporosis. The syndrome is also known as reflex sympathetic dystrophy and defined as an unexplained syndrome of continual pain that is not limited to a single nerve distribution, disproportionate to an initial noxious event, and associated with abnormal vascular and sweat gland activity. Early referral of these patients to a pain specialist is important, as well as appropriate use of nerve blocks to allow the patient to tolerate physical therapy.

Palsies and neuropathies (see also Chapter 20). Suprascapular nerve palsy results from suprascapular nerve compression, resulting in pain at the glenohumeral or acromioclavicular joints and weakness in abduction and external rotation at the shoulder. Radial nerve palsy occurs at the level of the spiral groove of the humerus (also known as Saturday night palsy due to inebriated patients compressing the radial nerve for long periods of time), the radial tunnel, or the wrist. Ulnar neuropathy may be reflected as pain at the elbow when compressed in the cubital tunnel, or pain at the wrist when impingement occurs in Guyon's canal. Median nerve compression can become symptomatic, causing pronator teres syndrome, which results in proximal arm pain on pronation with weakness and sensory loss in the hand, or the anterior intraosseous syndrome, which results in similar weakness and is generally painless. Finally, carpal tunnel syndrome is the most common nerve entrapment in the upper extremity and is covered in other chapters of this book. Treatment of the pain includes splinting, NSAIDs, physical therapy, and surgical release.

8.4 Thoracic and Truncal Pain

8.4.1 Nociceptive Syndromes

Nociceptive pain in the truncal region (see Table 8.4) is often caused by metastatic tumors. Benign tumors rarely originate or cause pain in this region. Symptoms of

Table 8.4 Thoracic and truncal pain

Nociceptive	Neuropathic
Tumor of the spine	Tumors of the spine (spinal cord compression)
Diffuse idiopathic skeletal hyperostosis (DISH)	Thoracic disc disease (HNP)
Ischemia or inflammation of truncal organs (heart, pleura, esophagus)	Herpetic neuralgia
	Epidural abscess
	Transverse myelitis
	Spinal cord infarction

metastatic tumor pain include slowly progressive back pain that is often worse in the supine position, localized tenderness to percussion, and often accompanied by other symptoms of malignancy such as weight loss, malaise, fevers, and night sweats. Plain radiographs are often unremarkable, but urgent MRI is indicated when neurologic deficits are identified on examination. Diffuse idiopathic skeletal hyperostosis (DISH) is characterized by ossification of paravertebral ligaments, most commonly in the thoracic spine. Pain is usually relieved with physical therapy and NSAIDs.

8.4.2 Neuropathic Syndromes

The thoracic region is the most common spinal location for metastatic disease; nearly 70% of spinal cord compression cases arise from thoracic cord involvement. This is covered in other sections of this book.

Acute herpetic or postherpetic neuralgia is common in the thoracic region. Treatment is discussed in the facial pain syndrome portion of this chapter. Epidural abscess is rare but most common in the thoracic region and can cause back and abdominal pain. Signs and symptoms are discussed in other chapters of this book. Primary thoracic disc disease is not common and usually requires nonemergency MRI for diagnosis.

Spinal cord infarction is a rare event usually secondary to aortic dissection; however, it can also result from atheroembolic disease, vasculitis, sepsis, and iatrogenic complication of catheter placement. The pain is acute to the back, chest, or abdomen, and accompanied by acute partial anterior myelopathy, which spares vibratory and proprioceptive sensation.

8.5 Low Back and Lower Extremity Pain

8.5.1 Nociceptive Syndromes

Lumbar strain is the most common source of backache. The pain is usually acute or subacute with a pattern of recurrent episodes of the pain. The pain can radiate down the leg, but unlike radiculopathy, rarely goes below the knee. Physical examination reveals local tenderness with paraspinal muscle spasm and restricted range of motion. Plain radiographs are almost always unremarkable and are not indicated (Table 8.6). Avoidance of strenuous activity, application of cold and heat, and liberal use of NSAIDs usually manages the pain. If opioids are necessary acutely, short-acting agents should be chosen and they should be limited to a small number without refill. Children and adolescents are most likely to have congenital malformations, postural abnormalities, or osteochondritis. Young adults are the most common age group to diagnose strains or direct trauma, discogenic disease, or systemic disorders causing back pain, such as RA, AS, and Reiter's syndrome. Older adults are most likely to have osteoarthritis with spondylitic changes, spinal stenosis, and vertebral metastases (see Tables 8.5 and 8.6).

Table 8.5 Causes of low back and lower extremity pain

Nociceptive	Neuropathic
Disorders of the lumbar spine	Disorders of the lumbar spine
Lumbosacral strain	Conus medullaris syndrome
Trauma	Cauda equina syndrome
Discogenic disease	Spinal stenosis
Systemic arthritides (RS, AS)	Lumbar HNP
Congenital spinal diseases	Disorders of the lower extremities
Degenerative spinal disorders	Lateral femoral cutaneous neuropathy
Spinal stenosis	Peroneal neuropathy
Vertebral osteomyelitis	Joplin's neuroma
Sacroiliitis	Morton's neuroma
Tumors	
Abdominal aortic aneurysm	
Peptic ulcer disease	
Disorders of the kidneys Disorders of the female reproductive tract	
Prostatitis	
Diverticulitis	
Hemoglobinopathies	
Disorders of the lower extremities	
Vascular (ischemic): acute arterial occlusion	
Deep venous thrombosis	
Systemic and septic arthritides	
Acute gout	
Tendonitis, bursitis, and tenosynovitis	

Table 8.6 Indications for radiography in back pain

Neurological deficit

Significant trauma

Suspected pathological lesions (carcinoma) or metastasis

Suspected infection

Immunocompromised patients

Patients on dialysis

Patients with recent spine surgery

Intravenous drug users

Vertebral osteomyelitis presents as subacute pain progressing over weeks to months, worsening with activity and continuing at rest. It is associated with comorbid conditions such as diabetes, IV drug abuse, and recent infection of the skin, urinary tract, or lungs. Pathogens are most commonly *Staphylococcus* and *Pseudomonas* species. Signs and symptoms are discussed in other chapters in this book.

Sacroiliitis has a bimodal age distribution and in the young can be an early indication of AS. In older adults it is usually nonspecific inflammation or arthritis. Local tenderness and joint stress while prone or supine can be diagnostic. Plain radiographs are not helpful. Treatment is with NSAIDs and physical therapy.

Lumbar pain can have many intra-abdominal and systemic causes and a thorough examination is required to diagnose abdominal aortic aneurysm, peptic ulcer, pancreatitis, kidney disease, gynecologic disease, prostatitis, diverticulitis, sickle cell crisis, or thalassemia.

Nociceptive pain in the lower limb is most often due to vascular and inflammatory conditions. Deep venous thrombosis and acute arterial occlusion are more common in the lower limb than arms, and septic and systemic arthritis should be considered.

Tendonitis, tenosynovitis, and bursitis can involve the knee, hip, ankle joints, and foot. Trochanteric bursitis at the hip, prepatellar bursitis of the knee, and calcaneal bursitis of the heel are the most common sites for bursitis. Treatment involves joint rest, NSAIDs, and local injection with a steroid and lidocaine for severe cases.

Acute gouty arthritis presents with an acute single joint arthritis, usually in the foot or ankle. Initial diagnosis may require joint fluid analysis. Treatment includes NSAIDs, colchicine, or low-dose steroids. Allopurinol can prevent the attacks, but should not be used in the acute phase.

8.5.2 Neuropathic Syndromes

Conus medullaris syndrome is usually painless, with initial symptoms of bowel and bladder dysfunction, and bilateral sensory loss in a saddle distribution. Motor weakness is usually mild, but hyperreflexia and Babinski signs can be seen.

Cauda equina syndrome, by comparison, is subacute, painful, and involves unilateral sensory and motor dysfunction in the limb ipsilateral to the pain. Sphincter weakness occurs later in the course of the syndrome. Spinal compression from tumor, disc, hemorrhage, fracture, infection, or spondylolisthesis can cause this syndrome. Emergent MRI or CT myelogram is indicated, with an IV steroid bolus and emergent surgical consult.

Spinal stenosis results from narrowing of the spinal canal most commonly from osteoarthritis. Symptoms usually progress slowly with back pain that can radiate down one or both legs. Symptoms may mimic claudication of the legs or discogenic disease, but are usually relieved by flexion of the spine such as bending over to push a shopping cart. CT or MRI is used to confirm the diagnosis and is emergent if there are any acute neurologic changes. Treatment involves NSAIDs, adjuvant analgesics such as antidepressants, antiseizure medications, lidocaine patches, centrally acting muscle relaxants, physical therapy, and surgical repair.

Lumbar disc herniation presents as back, buttock, and leg pain (Table 8.7) with compression of the nerve root; pain radiates below the level of the knee. Pain is generally relieved when the patient is supine. Positional changes, coughing, sneezing, and defecation all increase the pain due to increasing intradiscal pressure. Numbness, paresthesias, and weakness follow or precede pain in the leg. Heel-to-toe walking and sensory, motor, and reflex testing allow diagnosis of disc and nerve root involvement. Straight leg raising stretches the L5 and S1 nerve roots and exacerbates pain on exam. Extending the hip while prone stretches the L2–L4 nerve roots and exacerbates pain originating at those locations. Management includes reduced strenuous activity, NSAIDs, and muscle relaxants. Only moderate benefit has been shown with the use of systemic or epidural glucocorticoids. Urgent surgical referrals are indicated in cases of rapidly progressive neurological impairment.

Table 8.7 Lumbar nerve root localization

Disc involved	L3–L4	L4–L5	L5–S1
Nerve root involved	L4	L5	S1
Pain	Posterolateral hip and thigh	Posterolateral thigh, leg, and dorsum of foot	Posterior thigh, lateral calf and foot, heel, and lateral toes
Motor weakness	Knee extension	Ankle dorsiflexion	Ankle plantar flexion
Sensory loss	Medial shin to knee	Dorsum of foot, web space of great toe, and lateral calf	Lateral border of foot and posterior calf
Reflex depression	Knee (patellar)	None	Ankle (Achilles)
Wasting in chronic disease	Thigh	Calf	Calf
Musculoskeletal testing	Squat and stand	Heel walking	Toe walking

Entrapment neuropathies of the lower extremities are reviewed in other chapters of this text. Neuromas of the foot are due to swelling and scar tissue formation on the small interdigit nerves. Treatment is with metatarsal supports, broad-toe shoes, exercise, NSAIDs, and rarely surgery.

8.6 Indications for Referral to Specialists, Role of Imaging, Red Flags

Patients presenting with neck or back pain with or without extremity pain may be managed conservatively without inpatient admission and imaging as long as red flags are absent. Most patients with acute low back pain have an excellent outcome with conservative treatment alone and do not require referral to a specialist. Motor weakness and sensory dysfunction as well as bowel/bladder dysfunction should always prompt further work-up. Other concerning "red flags" in the back pain patient include a fever, history of cancer, history of trauma, weight loss, immunosuppression, intravenous drug use, recent infection such as urinary tract infection, and saddle anesthesia. For patients with neck pain, the Neck Pain Task Force has recommended that the following be considered as red flags: pathologic fracture, neoplasm, systemic inflammatory diseases, infection, cervical myelopathy, and previous neck surgery.

Cauda equine syndrome (CES) is a rare but true lumbar spinal emergency and delays in diagnosis and treatment are a common source of litigation regardless of the clinical outcome. Studies have shown that CES has a disproportionately high rate of medicolegal consequences. CES is characterized by low back pain, sciatica, genital/saddle sensory disturbance, and bowel/bladder/sexual dysfunction. Patients with low back pain and bowel/bladder complaints, regardless of neurological examination, should undergo urgent lumbar MRI. If the facility does not have MRI or lacks urgent MRI capabilities, urgent transfer to another facility should be performed if this diagnosis is entertained. Patients who cannot have an MRI must be admitted for urgent CT myelography. Pain-associated urinary retention is not rare in patients with low back pain; however, this symptom should prompt urgent imaging to rule-out large lumbar disc herniations, which are the primary cause of CES. A meta-analysis of the literature suggests that motor–sensory as well as bowel–bladder function outcomes are improved when surgery is performed within 48 hours.

Consultation of a spine specialist (neurosurgeon or orthopedic spine surgeon) should be considered in all cases of spinal pain with "red flags" or when imaging shows acute traumatic findings, neoplasms, or severe degenerative disease. When the history includes recent trauma, CT is the imaging modality of choice and has been shown to be vastly superior to plain x-rays alone. All female patients of child-bearing age must have a negative pregnancy test prior to undergoing CT scanning and a pregnant patient with spine trauma should prompt a spine specialist consultation before any imaging; MRI is the imaging modality of choice for pregnant patients.

8.7 Spasticity and Intrathecal Baclofen

Spasticity refers to a velocity-dependent increase in tonic stretch reflexes (muscle tone) and exaggerated tendon jerks. There are myriad causes, including cerebral palsy, stroke, spinal cord injury, and traumatic brain injury. When spasticity is poorly controlled with medications and botulinum toxin injections or when side effects of medications limit their use, intrathecal baclofen (ITB) pump therapy may be offered to patients. Other surgical strategies exist for spasticity (e.g., selective dorsal rhizotomy); however, ITB has the benefits of being nonablative and titratable and has supplanted many of the older nerve-cutting surgeries for spasticity.

Baclofen is a GABA-B agonist and has both presynaptic and postsynaptic effects that reduce muscle spasms and spasticity. ITB via an implanted device is FDA-approved and has been effectively used to treat spasticity since the 1980s. ITB also has proven efficacy in cases of neuropathic pain such as complex regional pain syndrome. The implantable system consists of a pump that most commonly resides unilaterally in the lower abdomen and an intrathecal catheter. Side effects of ITB include sedation, flaccidity, confusion, hypotension, weight gain, constipation, nausea, urinary retention, and sexual dysfunction. The most feared complication of ITB is baclofen withdrawal, which can lead to respiratory depression, rhabdomyolysis, fever, muscle rigidity, disseminated intravascular coagulation, seizures, and death. One of the best early indicators of baclofen withdrawal is pruritus. Causes of baclofen withdrawal in ITB patients include pump malfunction, intrathecal catheter kink/occlusion, iatrogenic dose reduction, and exhausted pump battery. Since baclofen withdrawal is life-threatening, prompt recognition is key. Treatment consists of intensive care cardiorespiratory support along with oral baclofen, intravenous dantrolene, intravenous benzodiazepines, propofol infusion, and temporary ITB delivery.

8.8 Intrathecal Pump Therapy for Pain

Intrathecal drug delivery is also an option for patients with chronic intractable pain using the same pump/catheter systems used for ITB administration. Many different drugs may be administered intrathecally in such a fashion; however, the only FDA-approved intrathecal pump-delivered drugs for pain are morphine and ziconotide. Intrathecal delivery systems for pain have been successfully applied to patients with many different types of chronic pain, including patients with severe cancer-related pain. Usually systemic doses of opioids can be reduced by 50% or more in patients who undergo implantation of a pump/catheter system for pain. Since intrathecal administration of opioids can achieve effective pain relief at much lower doses than the same drug administered parenterally, intrathecal pump/catheter systems can be particularly useful in cancer patients who may develop significant side effects (e.g., sedation, constipation) from the large doses of opioids required to control malignant pain.

Respiratory depression is the most serious safety issue associated with the intrathecal administration of opioids such as morphine. Naloxone may be necessary to treat respiratory depression in patients receiving intrathecal opioids. The intrathecal pump may be "turned off" by reducing its drug delivery to the lowest basal rate or by performing an emergency shut off with the programmer.

One potential emergency complication of intrathecal pump therapy is a catheter-associated inflammatory mass or what is sometimes called a granuloma. These intradural masses develop at the tips of intrathecal catheters and have been most commonly associated with patients receiving high daily doses of intrathecal morphine. However, catheter-associated inflammatory masses have been reported in association with other intrathecal opioids and ITB as well. Pathologic analysis of these masses reveals granulation tissue and necrosis and cultures are negative for infection. In worst-case scenarios, catheter-associated inflammatory masses may cause spinal cord compression with paralysis and bowel/bladder dysfunction; such cases require emergency surgical resection via laminectomy and intradural exploration. Earlier clues are loss of analgesic effect despite escalating doses on the pump, new back pain, and lower extremity sensory loss. Catheter-associated inflammatory masses may be detected on MRI or CT myelography. In cases when such a mass is diagnosed before severe neurologic symptoms, discontinuation of the pump drug or replacement of the pump drug with saline may lead to shrinkage and disappearance of the mass without surgery. Although this complication of intrathecal drug delivery is not common, the possibility should be entertained in any patient with an implanted drug catheter system that presents with neurologic symptoms and signs or worsening pain despite recent attempts to increase the dosage of the pump drug or drugs.

8.9 Challenges and Future Direction

The emergency physician faces the challenge of appropriately managing pain during each shift worked. Emergency physicians are experts at treating acute nociceptive pain from trauma and injury. They have also been aware of the increasing addiction and deaths from opioid prescribing over the past decade. These challenges have led the emergency medicine specialty in several directions. First, alternative therapies for pain management have been explored to reduce use of addicting opioid analgesics. Fifty percent nitrous oxide, migraine cocktails, ketamine, propofol, hypnosis, and expanded use of nerve blocks and regional anesthesia have become new and exciting areas of research that can potentially reduce societal dependence and addiction while improving pain management. Many of these efforts are in the study phases, but should be learned by the reader as they become the standard of care for certain pain syndromes. Second, national and state organized emergency medicine societies have produced guidelines for pain management, especially chronic pain syndromes. These guidelines uniformly include emergency prescription of only short-acting opioids at the lowest dose, use of controlled substances databases, and more referrals to detoxification and chronic pain centers. These guidelines are being adopted across the United States and these efforts will likely change standard pain management in the ED over the next decade.

Pearls and Pitfalls

- The fifth, ninth, and tenth cranial nerves all provide sensory innervation of the external ear – explaining referral of otalgia to the head or throat.
- Search for indicators of multiple sclerosis in any patient under age 40 with trigeminal neuralgia.
- Pain around the stylomastoid foramen is characteristic of Bell's palsy.
- In radiculopathies from cervical or lumbar disc disease, the root affected generally carries the same number as the vertebral body inferior to the disc; that is, the C6–C7 disc affects the C7 root. The L4–L5 disc affects the L5 root.
- Of cervical radiculopathies, 90% affect the C6 or C7 nerve root; of all lumbar radiculopathies, 95% affect the L5 or S1 nerve root.

- Neurogenic claudication differs from ischemic claudication in that the former produces pain when the patient is standing still.
- An ipsilateral straight-leg-raise sign is 95% sensitive, but contralateral or "crossed" straight-leg-raise sign is more specific for lumbar disc herniation.
- A catheter-associated inflammatory mass may develop in some patients with intrathecal pumps and may cause neurologic weakness requiring emergency surgery.
- Baclofen withdrawal is a potentially life-threatening emergency seen in patients with ITB pumps; pruritus is a common early sign.

Bibliography

Ahn UM, Ahn NU, Buchowski JM, et al. Cauda equine syndrome secondary to lumbar disc herniation: a meta-analysis of surgical outcomes. *Spine* 2000;**25** (12):1515–1522.

American Society of Anesthesiologists Task Force on Neuroaxial Opioids, Horlocker TT, Burton AW, et al. Practice guidelines for the prevention, detection, and management of respiratory depression associated with neuraxial opioid administration. *Anesthesiology* 2009;**110**:218–230.

Arnold PM, Harsh V, Oliphant SM. Spinal cord compression secondary to intrathecal catheter-induced granuloma: a report of four cases. *Evid Based Spine Care J* 2011;**2** (1):57–62.

Baker K. Chronic pain syndromes in the emergency department: identifying guidelines for management. *Emerg Care Australia* 2005;**17**:57–64.

Bauman BH, McManus JG. Pediatric pain management in the emergency department. *Emerg Med Clin North Am* 2005;**23**:393–414.

Dillard J, Knapp S. Complementary and alternative pain therapy in the emergency department. *Emerg Med Clin North Am* 2005;**23**:529–549.

Ducharme J. The future of pain management in emergency medicine. *Emerg Med Clin North Am* 2005;**23**:467–475.

Fosnocht DE, Swanson ER, Barton E. Changing attitudes about pain and pain control in emergency medicine. *Emerg Med Clin North Am* 2005;**23**:297–306.

Gilmer-Hill H, Boggan JE, Smith KA, et al. Intrathecal morphine delivered via subcutaneous pump for intrathecal cancer pain: a review of the literature. *Surg Neurol* 1999;**51**:12–15.

Hansen, G. Management of chronic pain in the acute care setting. *Emerg Med Clin North Am* 2005;**23**:307–338.

Hassenbusch S, Burchiel K, Coffey RJ, et al. Management of intrathecal catheter-tip inflammatory masses: a consensus statement. *Pain Med* 2002;**3**(4):313–323.

Lawrence L. Legal issues in pain management: striking the balance. *Emerg Med Clin North Am* 2005;**23**:573–584.

Motov SM, Khan, Problems and barriers of pain management in the emergency department: are we going to get better? *J Pain Res* 2009;**2**:5–11.

Motov SM, Marshall JP. Acute pain management curriculum for emergency medicine residency programs. *Acad Emerg Med* 2011;**18**:S87–S91.

Perrone J, Mycyk MB, A challenging crossroads for emergency medicine: the epidemics of pain and pain medication deaths. *Acad Emerg Med* 2014;**21**:334–336.

Prager J, Deer T, Levy R, et al. Best practices for intrathecal drug delivery for pain. *Neuromodulation* 2014;**17**:354–372.

Richards, C. Establishing an emergency department pain management system. *Emerg Med Clin North Am* 2005;**23**:519–527.

Ross JC, Cook AM, Steward GL, et al. Acute intrathecal baclofen withdrawal: a brief report of treatment options. *Neurocrit Care* 2011;**14**(1):103–108.

Santana L, Quintero M. Management baclofen withdrawal syndrome. *Rev Columb Anesthesiol* 2012;**40**(2):158–161.

Smith HS, Deer TR, Staats PS, et al. Intrathecal drug delivery. *Pain Phys* 2008;**11**:S89–S104.

Thomas, S. Management of pain in the emergency department. *ISRN Emerg Med* 2013;**23**:1–19.

Todd, K. Treating chronic pain patients in the emergency department. *ACEP News*, 2008.

Tomycz ND, Ortiz V, McFadden KM, et al. Management of symptomatic intrathecal catheter-associated masses. *Clin Neurol Neurosurg* 2012;**114**(2): 190–195.

Venkat A, Fromm C, Isaacs E, Ibarra J. An ethical framework for the management of pain in the emergency department. *Acad Emerg Med* 2013;**20**: 716–723.

Dizziness

Kevin M. Kelly, Arthur Alcantara Lima,
and Thomas P. Campbell

9.1 Introduction

The evaluation of patients with the complaint of "dizziness" is a frequent occurrence in the ED. It accounts for 3.5–11% of ED visits. The word *dizziness* is a nonspecific term used by patients and healthcare professionals to describe a disturbed sense of wellbeing, usually perceived as an altered orientation in space. Vertigo is defined as an illusion of movement of oneself or one's surroundings. It is usually experienced as a sensation of rotation or, less frequently, as undulation, linear displacement (pulsion), or tilt. Although vertigo usually suggests a vestibular disorder that can involve the inner ear or brain, this symptom itself cannot reliably localize the disorder. Dizziness or vertigo can result from numerous disorders of a complex human balance system. Despite the inherent complexities, the ED evaluation of dizziness or vertigo can be simplified by a systematic approach in history-taking, physical examination, and laboratory testing. A useful diagnostic method is to determine whether the patient's symptoms are due to a disorder of the vestibular system or nonvestibular systems.

9.2 Anatomy

Dizziness or vertigo is frequently caused by a disorder of the vestibular system. The vestibular system is organized into peripheral and central components.

9.2.1 Peripheral Vestibular System

The peripheral vestibular system is composed of bilateral sensory organs, their afferent fibers, and brainstem efferent fibers that innervate the sensory organs. Figure 9.1 shows the location of the vestibular sensory organs within the inner ear. They are located in the bony labyrinth, which is a series of hollow channels connecting into a round chamber, called the vestibule, within the petrous portion of the temporal bone. The sensory organs within the bony labyrinth are three semicircular canals, the utricle, and the saccule, together constituting the membranous labyrinth. The semicircular canals are ring-shaped tubes aligned at right angles to each other, one in the horizontal plane (horizontal) and the other two in the vertical plane orthogonal to each other (superior and posterior). Each of the semicircular canals is able to interpret angular acceleration of the head relative to the plane of that canal by changes within the crista ampullaris, a neuroepithelial receptor organ in the ampullated end of the canal that is adjacent to the vestibule. Hair cells within the cristae sense displacement of fluid within the canals during head acceleration and transduce the stimulus into a generator potential. The utricle and saccule, commonly referred to as "otolithic organs," are saclike structures that communicate with each other and with the fluids of

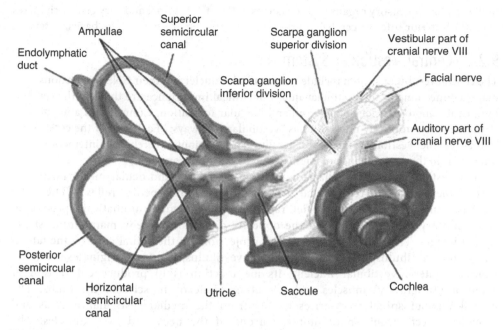

Figure 9.1 Illustration of the vestibular sensory organs in relation to the cochlea.

the cochlea. The utricle and saccule sense linear inertial forces (gravity) as well as linear head accelerations. They contain the maculae, receptor organs that consist of a gelatinous material containing calcium carbonate crystals (otoliths) overlying a membrane containing sensory hair cells. The hair cells sense displacement of the otolithic membrane during linear acceleration of the head and transduce the stimulus to a generator potential similar to that of the hair cells within the cristae.

The fluid within the membranous labyrinth that bathes the vestibular sensory organs is called endolymph. The membranous labyrinth is surrounded by a continuous space within the bony labyrinth, containing a chemically distinct second fluid-type called perilymph. The perilymph and the endolymph fluid compartments are continuous with those inside the cochlea, the auditory sensory organ. Perilymph chemically resembles extracellular fluid, having low potassium and high sodium concentrations. The endolymph is believed to be produced in specialized cells of the cochlea and vestibular labyrinth. The endolymph resembles intracellular fluid, having high potassium and low sodium.

The hair cells of the vestibular sensory organs are innervated by afferent bipolar cells of the vestibular ganglion (Scarpa's ganglion), located in the internal auditory canal of the petrous portion of the temporal bone. The central processes of these cells form the superior and inferior vestibular nerves, which occupy the posterior half of the internal auditory canal. Afferent fibers from the cochlea form the auditory nerve, which occupies the anteroinferior part of the internal auditory canal. The vestibular nerves and the auditory nerve emerge from the internal auditory canal and combine to constitute the eighth cranial nerve. Afferent vestibular axons enter the brainstem and synapse mostly in the vestibular nuclei, with a small component of fibers synapsing within the cerebellum directly. The blood supply of the vestibular sensory organs and the nerves within the internal auditory canal originates from the anterior inferior cerebellar artery (AICA), which arises from the basilar artery.

9.2.2 Central Vestibular System

The central vestibular system includes the vestibular nuclei and their CNS connections. The major connections of the vestibular nuclei of clinical importance are those to the cerebellum, ocular motor nuclei, spinal cord, and reticular formation. Connections among these structures are commonly referred to as "vestibular pathways." Each side of the cerebellum influences the vestibular nuclei bilaterally. The vestibular–cerebellar interactions are important in the maintenance of equilibrium and locomotion.

The vestibular nuclei, median longitudinal fasciculus, and ocular motor nuclei are part of the neuronal circuitry that underlies the vestibulo-ocular reflex (VOR). The VOR is primarily a response to brief, rapid head movements, automatically producing compensatory eye movements in the opposite direction, thereby maintaining stable retinal images. The vestibular nuclei send projections to the spinal cord by the lateral and medial vestibulospinal tracts. The lateral vestibulospinal tract originates primarily from the lateral vestibular nucleus; its main action is to produce contraction of extensor (antigravity) muscles and relaxation of flexor muscles of the limbs. The medial vestibulospinal tract arises mainly from the medial vestibular nucleus and provides direct inhibition of motor neurons of the neck and axial muscles. The vestibulospinal tracts are important in vestibular reflex reactions and in the maintenance of posture.

The blood supply of the central vestibular system originates primarily from the posterior circulation. The vestibular nuclei and the vestibulocerebellum are supplied by the vertebral arteries, which ascend along the ventrolateral aspects of the medulla and unite at the pontomedullary junction to form the basilar artery. The basilar artery runs along the ventral aspect of the pons and ends at the caudal midbrain. A posterior inferior cerebellar artery (PICA) arises from each vertebral artery approximately 1 cm inferior to the basilar artery and supplies the lateral surface of the medulla and part of the surface of the cerebellar hemisphere ipsilaterally.

9.3 History and Physical Examination

9.3.1 History

A carefully obtained history is critical in the evaluation of a patient's complaint of dizziness or vertigo. This is important diagnostically because vertigo usually results from vestibular system disorders, whereas nonvertiginous dizziness usually results from nonvestibular system disorders. Symptom description can also facilitate differentiating peripheral from central vestibular system disorders. Special attention is paid to the quality and time course of symptoms, associated symptoms, predisposing factors, precipitating factors, and exacerbating or mitigating factors. Importantly, given the vast differential diagnosis of dizziness and the challenging interview of the dizzy patient, diagnostic mistakes are common. Table 9.1 lists general properties of dizziness in vestibular and nonvestibular system dysfunction. Table 9.2 lists properties of vertigo and associated symptoms due to peripheral and central vestibular system dysfunction.

Table 9.1 Properties of dizziness due to vestibular and nonvestibular system dysfunction

Property	Vestibular	Nonvestibular
Description	Spinning, whirling, rotating, off-balance	Lightheaded, faint, dazed, floating
Time course	Episodic or constant	Episodic or constant
Associated symptoms	Nausea, vomiting, pallor, diaphoresis, hearing loss, tinnitus	Paresthesias, palpitations headache, syncope
Predisposing factors	Congenital inner ear anomaly, ototoxins, ear surgery	Syncope due to cardiovascular disease, psychiatric illness
Precipitating factors	Head or body position changes, ear infection or trauma hyperventilation	Body position changes, stress, fear, anxiety,

Table 9.2 Properties of vertigo and associated symptoms due to peripheral and central vestibular system dysfunction

Symptom	Peripheral	Central
Onset	Sudden	Insidious
Quality	Spinning, rotation	Disequilibrium
Intensity	Severe	Mild to moderate
Occurrence	Episodic	Constant
Duration	Seconds, minutes, hours, or days	Weeks or longer
Exacerbation by head movement	Moderate to severe	Mild
Nausea and vomiting	Severe	Mild
Imbalance	Mild	Moderate
Ear pressure or pain	Occasional	None
Hearing loss	Frequent	Rare
Tinnitus	Frequent	Rare
Neurologic symptoms	Rare	Frequent

Symptom Quality. The patient should be allowed to describe their symptoms in their own words, so that the examiner has an initial impression of the symptom quality. If the patient's description of symptoms is not clear, the patient can be asked if the symptoms resemble lightheadedness, faintness, imbalance, weakness, or a sensation of spinning or whirling. The patient should specify whether one symptom gave rise to another. Symptom intensity is graded as mild, moderate, or severe. However, patients are frequently too sick to describe their symptoms, have difficulty explaining their complaints, or provide vague information. Providers should be careful not to excessively direct the interview or over-rely on the symptom description, the latter especially when the rest of the clinical assessment is not congruent.

Symptom Time Course. Symptom onset is described as sudden or insidious. Symptoms are described as episodic or constant. The time course of symptom intensity includes the time to peak intensity, peak intensity duration, and the time of decreasing intensity.

Associated Symptoms. Numerous symptoms can be associated with dizziness or vertigo. Autonomic symptoms of nausea, vomiting, pallor, and diaphoresis often occur with vestibular disorders due to the numerous connections between brainstem vestibular and autonomic centers. The symptoms are generally more severe when the vestibular abnormality is peripheral than when it is central. These symptoms also can occur in other forms of dizziness where lightheadedness, shortness of breath, or palpitations may be prominent.

Symptoms associated with dizziness or vertigo can be due to the anatomical location of the abnormality and can occur in different combinations. Hearing loss, tinnitus, pressure, pain, hyperacusis (hypersensitivity to loud sounds), and diplacusis (distortion of pitch perception in one ear) are associated with inner ear lesions; hearing loss, tinnitus, and facial weakness with internal auditory canal lesions; hearing loss, tinnitus, facial weakness and/or numbness, and extremity incoordination with cerebellopontine angle lesions; diplopia, dysarthria, dysphagia, hiccups, perioral numbness, and extremity weakness and numbness with brainstem lesions; imbalance and incoordination with cerebellar lesions.

Other symptoms experienced with dizziness or vertigo can involve vestibular or nonvestibular systems depending on anatomical or physiological involvement. Headache can be associated with systemic illness or an intracranial process such as hemorrhage, mass lesion, or infection. Alteration or loss of consciousness can be associated with presyncope, syncope, hyperventilation, seizures, or vertebrobasilar insufficiency. Falling can be associated with labyrinthine disorders, vertebrobasilar insufficiency, syncope, seizures, or posterior fossa mass lesions.

Predisposing Factors. The patient's medical, surgical, and psychiatric history, family history, recent general health, medications, and substance abuse history are reviewed carefully. The medical and psychiatric history can reveal that symptoms are recurrent and attributable to a particular disease state that has been identified previously. Surgery may have been performed to treat a specific disorder associated with dizziness or vertigo. In other patients, symptoms can develop following surgery. The patient's family history is reviewed because several vestibular disorders have a genetic predisposition. These include migraine, Meniere's disease, and otosclerosis. The patient's recent general health is reviewed for any abnormality such as infection, mood disturbance, or trauma. Medication use is frequently associated with dizziness or vertigo and is reviewed carefully. Particular attention is paid to any new prescriptions, and to the use of antihypertensives, hypoglycemics, diuretics, or known ototoxins. Possible drug interactions or drug synergism is questioned. The patient is asked directly if any controlled substances or street drugs have been used and, if so, whether previous use was associated with similar symptoms.

Precipitating Factors. A detailed account of the circumstances at the onset of symptoms is elicited from the patient. General considerations include whether the patient was at rest, engaged in normal activity, exercising, straining, or sleeping at the time of onset. The patient is asked to identify any event that seemed to precipitate symptoms.

Exacerbating or Mitigating Factors. Worsening dizziness or vertigo with movement is a general characteristic of peripheral and central vestibular system disorders. Worsening symptoms with standing are often due to a nonvestibular disorder and can precede syncope. Vertigo worsened by loud noise (Tullio phenomenon), change in pressure in the ear canal, or Valsalva maneuvers suggests a disorder of inner ear fluid mechanics, such as Meniere's disease, otosyphilis, or perilymph fistula. Nonvertiginous dizziness worsened by Valsalva maneuvers can precede syncopal states, as described above. Exercise-induced worsening of symptoms can occur with perilymph fistula, other peripheral or central vestibular disorders, or nonvestibular disorders such as cardiopulmonary disease.

Vestibular Syndromes. In order to formulate a focused differential diagnosis, it has been proposed that patients with dizziness can be classified into groups, depending on the information obtained during the interview. Acute vestibular syndrome (AVS) includes those with sudden onset, continuous dizziness, frequently associated with severe nausea, vomiting, gait imbalance, and nystagmus. Causes of AVS include vestibular neuritis, acute labyrinthitis, and perhaps more importantly posterior circulation strokes. Spontaneous episodic vestibular syndrome (s-EVS) encompasses those with intermittent dizziness, without a specific trigger, usually lasting minutes to hours. Etiologies for s-EVS include vestibular migraine, Meniere's disease, or TIA. Lastly, triggered episodic vestibular syndrome (t-EVS) represents patients with intermittent dizziness brought about by a specific provoking factor such as sudden head motion, standing up, and Valsalva maneuvers. Benign paroxysmal positional vertigo (BPPV), central paroxysmal positional vertigo (CPPV), and orthostasis are in this category. Organizing symptoms into vestibular syndromes informs and facilitates a focused examination and diagnostic testing (Edlow et al., 2018).

9.3.2 General Physical Examination

General inspection of the patient can reveal apparent weakness or anxiety, tremulousness, relative immobility, instability, or vomiting. Vital signs can give evidence of infection, hypotension or hypertension, arrhythmias, or respiratory and/or metabolic disturbances. In particular, the patient is assessed for orthostatic hypotension and hyperventilation. The skin can reveal decreased turgor with dehydration, edema with fluid retention, pallor with anemia, a rash with infection, cyanosis with hypoxemia, or diaphoresis and pallor with autonomic nervous system changes. Abrasions, ecchymoses, or lacerations suggest trauma. The sinuses can be tender to percussion or the oropharynx erythematous, which are findings associated with local infection. The neck can reveal jugular venous distension or carotid bruits with cardiovascular disease, or a decreased range of motion with severe osteoarthritis.

Special attention is paid to the otoscopic examination of the external auditory canal and the tympanic membrane. The external auditory canal is inspected for cerumen, erythema, bloody or purulent otorrhea, CSF leak, or foreign body. The tympanic membrane can show amber or erythematous discoloration with middle ear disease, myringosclerosis from previous otitis media, evidence of prior trauma, retraction pockets, or cholesteatoma. Complete examination of the chest, abdomen and extremities may reveal medically related causes.

9.4 Neurological Examination

There are multiple available scoring predictors to determine the risk of central or vascular lesions being the cause of dizziness. The ABCD2 Score was originally developed as a tool to predict how likely TIAs are to evolve into strokes. Patients are scored depending on age, blood pressure, clinical presentation, history of diabetes, and duration of symptoms. Although its original purpose was not to stratify patients with dizziness, it has proven to be useful as a screening tool for dizziness in the ED setting. The Posterior Circulation Ischemia (PCI) score is another scoring system developed specifically to identify individuals with dizziness at risk for cerebral ischemia. In addition to high blood pressure and diabetes, symptoms such as tinnitus, ataxia, and difficulties with speech are taken into consideration. Unfortunately, the NIH Stroke Scale is not a good predictor of posterior circulation strokes in patients presenting with dizziness due to its overreliance on anterior circulation symptoms such as aphasia or hemiparesis. It must be emphasized that these screening tools do not substitute for a thorough history and physical examination.

A focused neurological examination is performed to assess mental status, the functioning of cranial nerves, motor and sensory systems, and muscle stretch reflexes. Particular attention is directed to the neuro-otologic examination of patients with a suspected vestibular disorder.

Mental Status. The mental status of the patient is determined as alert, confused, lethargic, stuporous, or comatose. Typically, patients presenting to the ED with the complaint of dizziness or vertigo are alert. Some may have an abnormal mental status at the time of presentation, which can deteriorate depending on the nature of the disorder (e.g., CNS infection or mass lesion, toxic or metabolic encephalopathies).

Cranial Nerves. The cranial nerve examination is focused and thorough, including ophthalmoscopy, visual acuity evaluation, visual field evaluation, pupil size, and pupil deviation. Ocular alignment and the range of ocular movements are assessed carefully. A skew deviation, or vertical misalignment of the eyes, and head tilt can be seen in patients with the complaint of vertical diplopia. This can be due to a fourth cranial nerve palsy or an otolith disorder involving peripheral or central vestibular pathways. Smooth pursuit movements are tested with the patient visually following a slowly moving finger. Abnormalities of pursuit can indicate central disorders (e.g., impaired downward tracking in cerebellar degeneration or craniocervical junction anomalies). Saccadic breakdown of pursuit movements becomes extremely common with advancing age. Saccades are rapid eye movements associated with changes in ocular fixation or eye position within the orbit. Dysmetria, or undershooting or overshooting of saccadic eye movements, is pathological if it persists with repeated testing (e.g., hypermetria with a midline cerebellar lesion).

Nystagmus. The evaluation of nystagmus is extremely important in the evaluation of a patient with a possible vestibular system disorder. Nystagmus is an involuntary rhythmic pattern of eye movements consisting of fast and slow components occurring in opposite directions. It is caused by physiological activation of the VOR, or by pathology in the peripheral or central vestibular system, and generally cannot be compensated by orbital eye movements. When the nystagmus is not particularly intense, it may be suppressed by gaze fixation. By convention, the direction of the fast component designates the direction of nystagmus. Physiological nystagmus occurs in healthy individuals and can be induced by head rotation, caloric irrigations, and rapidly moving (optokinetic) stimuli in the visual field. Two to three beats of "end-point nystagmus" is a normal finding when the eye position is moved eccentrically in the orbit to the extremes of ocular range of motion. Pathological nystagmus suggests an underlying abnormality and can be characterized as one of several types: spontaneous (eyes in primary position), gaze-evoked (induced by changes in gaze position), positional (not present in seated position but present in some other head positions), and rapid positioning (appears only with sudden changes in body position).

Head Impulse – Nystagmus – Test of Skew (HINTS) is a bedside oculomotor test that has been proposed to differentiate peripheral from central vertigo in patients with AVS. It is performed on patients with continuous (acutely symptomatic), not episodic, vertigo. If the study's results are benign and there are no other neurologic deficits, the test suggests a peripheral etiology. The majority of such patients will have vestibular neuritis, but the HINTS examination may help to identify the smaller number of patients who are experiencing central causes of vertigo, including possible stroke.

The first part of HINTS is the head impulse test, which involves a seated patient fixating on an object, usually the examiner's nose, followed by a quick movement of the head to the left or right then back to the neutral position. A corrective saccade indicates a positive test and is typically consistent with vestibular neuritis. Absence of the saccade is concerning for a central cause. The second part of HINTS (i.e., nystagmus) refers to a direction change of nystagmus on eccentric gaze. For example, when the patient looks to the left, the fast component beats to the left; when the patient looks to the right, the fast component beats to the right (www.youtube.com/watch?v=Dlwu6CpuHY4). This direction-changing nystagmus may indicate a stroke in a patient with AVS. The third part of HINTS, (i.e., test of skew) refers to vertical ocular misalignment during alternate cover testing and its presence is suggestive of brainstem strokes (www.youtube.com/watch?v=zgqCXef-qPs).

Using HINTS requires experience and practice, and it should only be used in patients with a first-time episode of constant vertigo from AVS as was required in the clinical studies involving the HINTS exam. For example, applying the head impulse test in a patient who is dizzy due to BPPV would result in a negative test predisposing to the incorrect conclusion that the dizziness is a manifestation of a central cause of vertigo. In general, performing both the HINTS and Hallpike (see below) test on the same patient is not appropriate. Instead, BPPV and AVS should be distinguished from each other by history and the presence of spontaneous nystagmus. The use of HINTS when done properly is superior to MRI in the first 24 hours when diagnosing posterior fossa infarcts.

In testing for pathological nystagmus, the eyes are examined in primary position and during horizontal and vertical gaze. Spontaneous nystagmus that is inhibited with visual fixation can be demonstrated by ophthalmoscopic visualization of the fundus of one eye while the patient covers the other eye. Gaze-evoked nystagmus can be assessed by having the patient change eye position by fixating on a target 30 degrees to the left, right, up, and down, and holding the eye position for 20 seconds. Positional nystagmus can be identified by placing the patient into right-ear-down and left-ear-down positions to see if nystagmus appears. Rapid positioning nystagmus can be induced by the Hallpike (Figure 9.2) or Nylen–Barany maneuver. These are relatively synonymous eponyms for a series of maneuvers that produce rapid changes in head position relative to gravity. These maneuvers

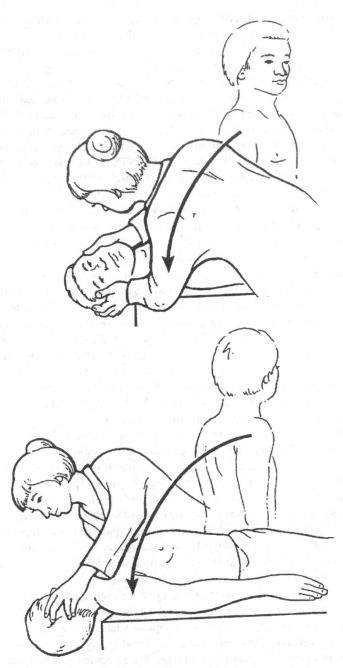

Figure 9.2 Illustrations of the technique for the Hallpike maneuver, for right side (top) and left side (bottom). Note the patient's eyes are open and fixated on the examiner. Reprinted with permission from: *Practical Management of the Balance Disorder Patient*, Shepard and Telian, 1996, Singular Publishing Group, San Diego.

Table 9.3 Properties of nystagmus due to peripheral and central vestibular system dysfunction

Nystagmus	Peripheral	Central
Spontaneous		
Quality	Horizontal or combined torsional	Vertical, horizontal, torsional
Fixation	Inhibits, unless severe	Little effect
Direction	Unidirectional	May change direction
Gaze-evoked type	None, although gaze in direction of fast phase intensifies nystagmus	Symmetrical, asymmetrical, dysconjugate, rebound (disappears or reverses)
Rapid positioning		
Quality	Torsional, never vertical	Horizontal or vertical
Latency	2–20 seconds	None
Duration	<30 seconds	>30 seconds
Direction	To downward ear	Up or variable, reversing
Fatigability	Usual	Unusual
Head position	One position	More than one position
Associated symptoms	Vertigo, nausea, vomiting	May have none

should be considered for patients with symptoms of BPPV or intermittent and fluctuating vertigo.

Classically, the patient is taken rapidly from sitting erect to a supine position, with the head extended and hanging over the edge of the table by 45 degrees in the center position. This position is maintained for 30 seconds, after which the patient is rapidly brought back to sitting erect. The maneuver is repeated with an additional 45 degree rotation of the head to the left and repeated again with head rotation to the right. The patient is observed for nystagmus in the head-hanging and sitting positions. In clinical use, it is best to ask the patient which of these positions is most likely to produce vertigo and perform that maneuver first. If nystagmus is observed, the movement is repeated to determine whether the response is fatigable – that is, less intense on the repeat trial. Table 9.3 lists properties of spontaneous, gaze-evoked, and rapid positioning nystagmus due to peripheral and central vestibular system dysfunction.

Bedside assessment of VORs can be done by the doll's eyes (oculocephalic) and cold caloric tests. These tests are most useful in the assessment of a comatose patient.

The corneal reflex tests the functional integrity of the trigeminal and facial nerves. A unilateral facial paralysis is due to an ipsilateral abnormality in the temporal bone, facial nerve, or brainstem.

Eighth cranial nerve function subserving hearing is evaluated by testing the auditory threshold by presenting a minimal stimulus to each ear, such as the rubbing of fingers, a whispered word, or a watch tick. If hearing loss is present, tests using a tuning fork can differentiate between conductive and sensorineural causes. In the Weber test, the vibrating tuning fork is applied to the middle of the forehead and the sound is normally heard in both ears. In conductive hearing loss, the sound is localized to the affected ear, and to the normal ear in sensorineural hearing loss. In the Rinne test, the vibrating fork is applied to the mastoid area until the sound extinguishes, and then held at the external auditory meatus. Air conduction is greater than bone conduction normally. In conductive hearing loss of the external or middle ear, bone conduction is greater than air conduction. In sensorineural hearing loss, the reverse is true, although air and bone conduction can be quantitatively reduced.

Palatal elevation and the gag reflex test the integrity of the glossopharyngeal and vagus nerves. The gag reflex is tested carefully to minimize the possibility of vomiting. Absent reflexes suggest impairment of the medulla. Tongue deviation with protrusion can be due to impairment of a cerebral hemisphere or a hypoglossal nerve lesion. Tongue deviation to the right suggests impaired function of the left cerebral hemisphere or the right hypoglossal nerve.

Motor System. Motor function is assessed initially by inspection of the patient. Tremor can be due to basal ganglial disease, cerebellar disease, or anxiety. Carpopedal spasm is seen with hyperventilation. Atrophy, fasciculations, and decreased strength occur with lower motor neuron impairments. Increased resistance to passive manipulation of the joints and weakness suggest contralateral upper motor neuron impairment. Decreased resistance to passive manipulation is seen in cerebellar disease. Abnormal cerebellar tests in an appendage generally suggest ipsilateral cerebellar hemisphere impairment, although unilateral dysmetria can be a sign of an acute ipsilateral disturbance of peripheral vestibular function. Abnormalities of station and gait not related to weakness can localize impairments to the midline cerebellum or to the vestibular system.

Sensory System. Sensory function impairments such as paresthesias or numbness can result in abnormal responses to testing by light touch or pinprick. Paresthesia or numbness that is generalized or occurs in the distal extremities bilaterally and around the mouth suggests hyperventilation. A "stocking glove" distribution pattern suggests a peripheral neuropathy. When unilateral, these abnormalities can suggest an ipsilateral mononeuropathy, radiculopathy or plexopathy, or contralateral cerebral hemisphere impairments. Impaired proprioception and vibration sense can suggest posterior column disease. Impaired proprioception can be tested with the Romberg test, which assesses the patient's ability to maintain balance with the feet together and the eyes closed. Significant swaying or inability to maintain the posture is a positive test sign. Repeated falling to one side can be seen with a severe acute unilateral labyrinthine disorder, although most patients with isolated unilateral vestibular disorders can perform the Romberg test without difficulty.

Muscle Stretch Reflexes. Muscle stretch reflex testing can reveal decreased reflexes (e.g., Achilles tendon reflex) in peripheral neuropathy. Increased reflexes can be seen in contralateral upper motor neuron impairment. Pendular reflexes can be seen in cerebellar disease.

9.4.1 Provocative Tests

Hyperventilation. Hyperventilation is frequently the cause of presyncopal dizziness. When hyperventilation is suspected from the patient's history, the patient is asked to hyperventilate for 1–3 minutes. Breathing should be rapid and deep, and encouragement is offered to promote a good effort by the patient. Following hyperventilation, the patient is asked to describe the way he or she feels, and to judge whether any unusual sensations resemble the previously experienced dizziness.

Valsalva Maneuver. The Valsalva maneuver is performed by having the patient forcibly exhale against a closed glottis, causing decreased cardiac output and cerebral hypoxia. The Valsalva maneuver can result in dizziness or syncope, vertigo can worsen with a perilymph fistula or a craniocervical junction anomaly (e.g., Arnold-Chiari malformation).

9.5 Differential Diagnosis

The differential diagnosis of dizziness or vertigo can be approached by determining whether the disorder is due to an abnormality of the vestibular system or of nonvestibular systems. Vestibular system disorders of particular importance to ED management are described.

9.5.1 Benign Positional Vertigo

Benign paroxysmal positional vertigo (BPPV) (also known as benign positional vertigo or positional vertigo) is a condition characterized by brief periods of vertigo induced by position changes of the head. Onset is usually in middle age and it is the most common cause of vertigo assessed in clinical practice. Vertigo is often precipitated by rolling over in bed, getting in or out of bed, bending over, or extending the neck. It typically lasts for only a few seconds but can persist for hours or days. The patient may recognize a critical head position that reproduces the vertigo. Following the first attack or a flurry of episodes, lightheadedness and nausea may persist for hours to days.

It is likely that dislodgement of calcium carbonate crystals from the otolithic membrane in the utricle results in gravity-sensitive particles settling onto the cupula (cupulolithiasis) or floating freely in the membranous portion (canalolithiasis) of the posterior semicircular canal. BPPV can be the sequela of head injury, degeneration due to aging, viral labyrinthitis, vestibular neuronitis, vascular disease of the inner ear, or any cause of peripheral vertigo.

Diagnosis is based on history and supported by a positive rapid positioning test (Hallpike maneuver). The patient with classic BPPV demonstrates torsional rotatory nystagmus, with a fast horizontal component that beats toward the ear that is placed downward. The nystagmus has the following additional features to support the diagnosis of BPPV: (1) it is latent, beginning 2–5 seconds after assuming the provocative position; (2) it is transient, disappearing within 20–30 seconds; (3) it has a crescendo and decrescendo in intensity; and (4) it fatigues with repeat trials, usually with complete resolution by the fourth repetition of the Hallpike maneuver. The dependent ear is generally the one that causes the symptoms, although bilateral disease can occur. Most patients with BPPV note resolution of symptoms without treatment. Although vestibular suppressants can provide temporary relief of associated nausea and lightheadedness, they usually do not prevent the motion-provoked spells of vertigo. Therefore, proper management includes discouraging the long-term use of such medications. Conventional vestibular rehabilitation training exercises are effective in treating this condition. A unique therapeutic procedure that can provide immediate relief of BPPV, the canalith repositioning (Epley) maneuver, has been developed (Figure 9.3). The procedure involves slowly bringing the patient's head through a series of movements designed to permit the removal of the offending otolith from the posterior semicircular canal. The rare patient who does not respond to conservative therapy is a candidate for surgical therapy.

9.5.2 Vestibular Neuronitis

Vestibular neuronitis is caused by damage to the sensory neurons of the vestibular ganglion, whereas vestibular neuritis is due to damage to the vestibular nerve. However, the pathologies are often considered in conjunction and are alternately known as acute vestibulopathy, acute vestibular neuritis, and vestibular neurolabyrinthitis. The condition is typically characterized by sudden, severe vertigo associated with nausea and vomiting in

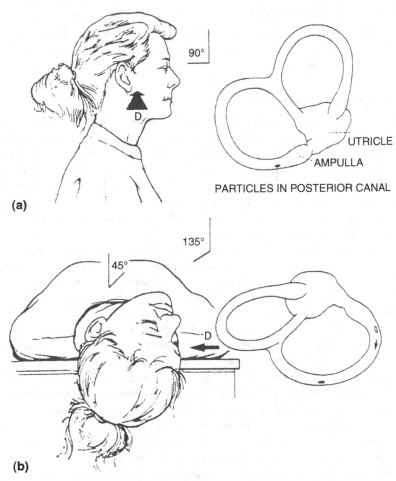

Figure 9.3 Particle repositioning maneuver for the right ear (a–d). The left side of each drawing shows the position of the patient. The arrow (d) represents the direction of view of the labyrinth depicted on the right side showing the relative position of the labyrinth and the movement of particles (dark oval, new position; open oval, previous position) in the posterior semicircular canal. (a) Patient sitting lengthwise on table. (b) Patient in Hallpike position placing the undermost (affected) ear in the earth-vertical axis. Nystagmus is exhibited in this position, possibly associated with vertigo. This position is maintained until the nystagmus is resolved. (c) Head is rotated to the left with the head turned 45 degrees downward. (d) Head and body are rotated until facing downward 135 degrees from the supine position and maintained for 1–2 minutes before the patient sits up. During b–d, particles gravitate in the posterior semicircular canal through the common crus and into the utricle. Reprinted with permission from Parnes LS, Price-Jones RG: Particle repositioning maneuver for benign paroxysmal vertigo. *Ann Otol Rhinol Laryngol* 1993;102:325–331.

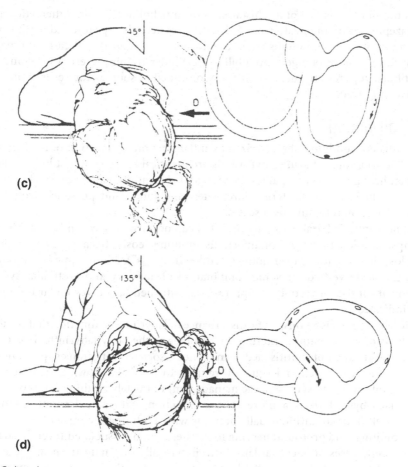

(c)

(d)

Figure 9.3 (cont.)

the absence of auditory symptoms. Symptoms usually peak within 24 hours, and patients can remain relatively immobile because symptoms often worsen with head movement. There can be truncal unsteadiness, imbalance, and difficulty focusing vision. Symptoms subside in several days and resolve within several weeks to 3 months. Recovery from any acute peripheral lesion depends on the process of vestibular compensation within the CNS. During the compensation process patients can have a sense of disequilibrium that is aggravated by rapid head movements. In general, vestibular neuronitis is a benign condition characterized by one episode of symptoms. However, 20–30% of patients have at least one recurrent attack of vertigo. There are several other more serious conditions that can mimic vestibular neuronitis.

Vestibular neuronitis is a diagnosis of exclusion, based on a compatible history, signs of an acute unilateral vestibular loss (vertigo and spontaneous nystagmus, usually with the fast phase away from the abnormal ear), and the absence of any central findings on the neurological examination, imaging studies, or on electronystagmography. Management includes the short-term use of antihistamines or anticholinergics, an antiemetic, and/or a benzodiazepine for tranquilization as needed. Corticosteroids appear to reduce the intensity and duration of acute symptoms when administered early in the disease. The patient is encouraged to avoid prolonged immobility. Vestibular training exercises are undertaken and vestibular suppressant medication is discontinued as soon as the severe initial symptoms have improved.

9.5.3 Labyrinthitis

Labyrinthitis is a condition characterized by inflammation or infection of the labyrinthine system. The symptoms of acute labyrinthitis are identical to those of vestibular neuronitis, except that hearing loss accompanies the vertigo. Labyrinthitis can be caused by numerous agents, including viruses, bacteria, spirochetes, and fungi, and possible involvement of systemic allergic or autoimmune diseases.

Viral labyrinthitis (viral neurolabyrinthitis) can occur with a systemic viral illness such as mumps, measles, influenza, or infectious mononucleosis. It can present with severe hearing loss that progresses over hours ("sudden deafness"), accompanied by tinnitus and ear fullness, acute vertigo, or some combination of auditory and vestibular symptoms. Management consists of vestibular suppressants, antiemetics, and vestibular training exercises as indicated.

Toxic labyrinthitis is a nonspecific disturbance of labyrinthine function that results from the products of inflammation entering the confines of the bony labyrinth. This occurs in response to acute or chronic otitis media, and is not associated with frank suppuration in the labyrinth. Inner ear function frequently returns to normal following treatment of the underlying infection and symptomatic management of the labyrinthine symptoms.

Bacterial labyrinthitis is a more serious infection, with actual suppuration of the labyrinth itself. This condition usually presents with a fulminant course of severe vertigo, nausea, vomiting, and profound hearing loss. There can be associated fever, headache, or pain. Unilateral cases of bacterial labyrinthitis typically originate from infection in the pneumatized spaces of the temporal bone (acute or chronic otitis media, mastoiditis); bilateral cases can result from bacterial meningitis. Diagnosis is commonly based on clinical information. Treatment consists of aggressive parenteral antibiotic therapy with agents that provide adequate penetration of the blood–brain barrier. Surgery can be required for treatment of middle ear or mastoid infection, and to drain the resulting abscess within the labyrinth in the critically ill patient with unilateral suppurative labyrinthitis.

Syphilitic labyrinthitis occurs as a late manifestation of either congenital or acquired syphilis. It begins with deteriorating inner ear function and, when untreated, progresses slowly to profound bilateral loss of auditory and vestibular function. This course is punctuated with episodic fluctuating and progressive sensorineural hearing loss and vertigo. The peak incidence of congenital syphilitic labyrinthitis is in the fourth or fifth decade of life. The acquired form peaks in the fifth or sixth decade. Pathological changes consist of an inflammatory infiltration of the labyrinth and osteitis of the otic capsule (osseous boundary of the labyrinth). This condition can occur despite prior treatment of syphilis, and may not be accompanied by neurosyphilis. Diagnosis is based on a history of unexplained vertigo, a course of fluctuating hearing loss, which is often bilateral, and a positive fluorescent treponemal antibody (FTA) test. Penicillin is the treatment of choice. Corticosteroid therapy may provide additional benefit, albeit often temporary, in some cases.

9.5.4 Meniere's Disease

Meniere's disease (endolymphatic hydrops) is characterized by fluctuating hearing loss, tinnitus, and episodic vertigo. Onset of the syndrome is usually in the third or fourth decade of life. The patient typically becomes symptomatic in one ear, with the development of a sensation of fullness or pressure, hearing loss, and tinnitus. Episodes of spontaneous, intense vertigo that peak within minutes and subside over several hours usually follow these symptoms, but can precede them. Nausea, vomiting, diaphoresis, and pallor usually occur. Following an acute attack of vertigo, the patient can feel unsteady for several days. The syndrome follows a remittent course, with relapses having variable severity and periodicity. Tinnitus can resolve or decrease between episodes. When persistent, the tinnitus typically increases in intensity immediately prior to or during a recurrent attack. Hearing loss is reversible in the early stages of the disease, but a gradually worsening residual hearing loss occurs with repeated attacks. Approximately one-third of patients experience symptoms in both ears. The paroxysmal episodes cease spontaneously late in the course of the disease.

The characteristic histopathological finding in Meniere's disease is a distension of the entire endolymphatic system. The increased volume of endolymph likely results from retention of sodium in the endolymphatic compartment and possibly impaired resorption of endolymph due to dysfunction of the endolymphatic duct and sac. The mechanism responsible for the fluctuating course of severe symptoms is not known completely, but may be due to episodic ruptures of the delicate membranes separating endolymph and perilymph, such as Reissner's membrane, located between the scala media and the scala vestibuli in the cochlea. This would result in an admixture of the two fluid compartments and a potassium intoxication of the neural processes that lead to the afferent fibers of the eighth nerve until the fluid balance is restored. Several diseases can result in Meniere's disease, including temporal bone trauma, otological surgery such as stapedectomy, and viral, toxic, bacterial, or syphilitic labyrinthitis. However, the cause is idiopathic in most cases.

Diagnosis is based on a characteristic history and documentation of fluctuating hearing by audiometry. Electronystagmography can show a peripheral spontaneous nystagmus acutely and vestibular paresis on caloric testing in chronic cases. Acute management is largely empirical and involves the use of vestibular suppressants and antiemetics. A low-salt diet and diuretic use is recommended for maintenance therapy. Surgical options in refractory cases include endolymphatic shunts and ablative procedures, with the latter providing more reliable results.

9.5.5 Perilymph Fistulas

Perilymph fistulas are defects of the otic capsule or its oval or round windows. These defects allow leakage of perilymph from the inner ear into the middle ear space. Perilymph fistulas can occur secondary to congenital defects of the inner ear; following stapedectomy surgery for otosclerosis; following pressure changes in the middle ear associated with nose blowing, sneezing, or barotrauma as in SCUBA diving; or with sudden increases in CSF pressure associated with lifting, coughing, or straining.

Perilymph fistulas are commonly experienced as an audible "pop" in the ear followed by hearing loss and vertigo. Diagnosis is made from the history and supported by a positive fistula test or Valsalva maneuver. Management is conservative except in cases of penetrating otologic trauma because most perilymph fistulas heal spontaneously. Bed rest, sedation, head elevation, and the avoidance of straining are recommended. Surgical exploration and repair can be indicated with persistent auditory and vestibular symptoms.

9.5.6 Cerebellopontine Angle Tumors

Tumors of the cerebellopontine angle (CPA) typically begin in the internal auditory canal and slowly grow into the CPA, compressing the seventh and eighth cranial nerves. The most common CPA tumor is the vestibular schwannoma (acoustic neuroma), which usually arises from Schwann cells of the vestibular nerve but can also arise from the facial, acoustic, or trigeminal nerves. Vestibular schwannomas account for over 90% of tumors of the CPA. Unilateral hearing loss and tinnitus are the most frequently experienced symptoms. A progressive unilateral hearing loss in a patient with dizziness is considered diagnostic of a vestibular schwannoma until proven otherwise by MRI, which is extremely sensitive in identification of these tumors. With few exceptions, such as small tumors in the elderly, treatment is surgical removal.

9.5.7 Vascular Disease

The vertebrobasilar circulation supplies blood to the labyrinth, eighth cranial nerve, and brainstem. Hypoperfusion of the vertebrobasilar system, or vertebrobasilar insufficiency (VBI), can lead to widespread or focal ischemia and/or stroke of the vestibular system. VBI is a common cause of vertigo that has an abrupt onset, lasts for minutes, and can occur with nausea and vomiting. Other associated symptoms include diplopia, visual field defects, and headache. The common cause of VBI is atherosclerosis of the subclavian, vertebral, and basilar arteries. Occasionally, VBI can be precipitated by postural hypotension or by decreased cardiac output. VBI due to compression of the vertebral arteries by bony cervical spine spurs is a rare occurrence.

There are several clinical syndromes of abnormalities of the vertebral and basilar arteries and their branches. Certain syndromes are of particular importance in the ED evaluation of vertigo. Occlusion of the AICA can result in labyrinthine ischemia or infarction. There is usually a sudden profound loss of auditory and vestibular function. Ipsilateral facial numbness and weakness, ipsilateral Horner's syndrome, ipsilateral cerebellar signs, paresis of lateral gaze, and nystagmus can occur. Occlusion of the PICA, known as the lateral medullary or Wallenberg's syndrome, results in infarction of the lateral medulla. There is usually a sudden onset of vertigo, nystagmus, diplopia, dysphagia, nausea, and vomiting. Ipsilateral abnormalities include Horner's syndrome, palatal paralysis, loss of pain and temperature sensation of the face, facial and lateral rectus weakness, and cerebellar signs. There is contralateral loss of pain and temperature sensation of the body.

Acute management of vertigo due to vascular disease is usually directed at correcting the underlying disorder, whenever possible. General medical stabilization includes oxygenation, control of blood pressure, and fluid balance regulation.

9.6 Laboratory Studies

Ordering of laboratory studies in the ED for a patient with dizziness or vertigo is guided by information obtained from the history and physical examination. Routine hematological and chemical tests for consideration include a complete blood count with white blood cell differential counts, serum electrolytes, glucose, blood urea nitrogen, and creatinine. Other studies include FTA, cardiac enzymes, carboxyhemoglobin, and ethanol levels. Urine can be obtained for routine and microscopic tests and for a toxicology screen. Arterial blood gases, pulse oximetry, chest radiograph, or electrocardiogram may be required.

9.7 Imaging Studies

Imaging studies of the skull and brain may be indicated in the evaluation of a patient with dizziness or vertigo. The three most important imaging techniques used for this purpose are CT of the head, CT angiography of the head and neck, and MRI of the brain. In the emergency setting, CT is useful to rule-out a suspected infarct or hemorrhage. Definitive diagnostic imaging is usually performed later with gadolinium-enhanced MRI as the ideal study for neoplasm, thin-cut CT without contrast for temporal bone lesions, and MRA for vascular pathology. Algorithms for consideration of diagnostic studies for patients presenting with initial acute persistent vertigo, spontaneous recurrent vertigo, and provoked recurrent vertigo are shown in Figure 9.4.

One important challenge in the ED is the patient with AVS, in which an ischemic stroke is suspected. Although MRI is a valuable diagnostic tool, providers should not over-rely on negative imaging if the clinical assessment is consistent with cerebral ischemia. Different cohorts have shown the false negative rate for MRI in assessing posterior circulation strokes can be up to 19%. If used appropriately, the HINTS exam can have better sensitivity than MRI. Therefore normal imaging should not preclude lifestyle counseling and pharmacologic treatment/prophylaxis of ischemic strokes in patients with risk factors and suggestive clinical assessments.

9.8 Management

9.8.1 Initial Stabilization

A patient who presents to the ED acutely ill with vertigo accompanied by severe nausea and vomiting requires immediate stabilization. These symptoms can cause the patient to be extremely frightened and can compromise the emergency physician's ability to obtain an adequate history and physical examination. The patient is given calm verbal reassurance and is allowed to assume a body position that minimizes symptoms. All unnecessary external stimuli (e.g., excessive light, noise) are removed from the examination room. When tolerated by a vomiting patient, a semiprone position can provide some airway protection against aspiration of gastric contents. Oxygen can be administered by nasal cannulae, and a peripheral intravenous line is established. Oropharyngeal suctioning can be performed when necessary. Any trauma associated with the patient's presentation is treated as a high priority.

9.8.2 Pharmacological Treatment

Vestibular Suppressants. The main categories of vestibular suppressants (Table 9.4) are antihistamines, anticholinergics, benzodiazepines, and monoaminergics. These medications

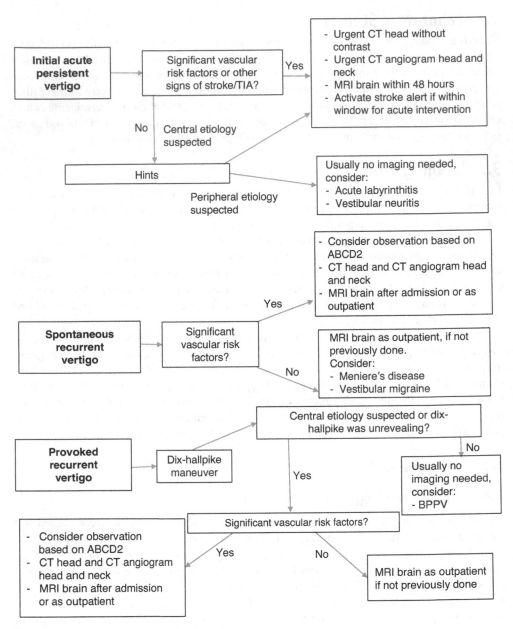

Figure 9.4 Approach to diagnostic imaging in vertigo.

are commonly used to suppress vertigo associated with peripheral vestibular disorders. In experimental studies, these medications alter and usually suppress the level of tonic activity in vestibular neurons. Antihistamines suppress vestibular end organs and inhibit central cholinergic pathways. The macular end organs (utricle and saccule) are typically more suppressed than the semicircular canals. Therefore, antihistamines are often more effective in treating

Table 9.4 Symptomatic treatment of vestibular disorders: medications, dosing, and routes of administration

Vestibular suppressants

Antihistamines

    Meclizine (Antivert) 12.5–25 mg PO q4–6 h

    Dimenhydrinate (Dramamine) 50 mg PO, IM q4–6 h

    Promethazine (Phenergan) 25–50 mg PO, PR, IM q4–6 h

    Cyclizine (Marezine) 50 mg PO, IM q4–6 h

    Diphenhydramine (Benadryl) 25–50 mg PO, IM, IV q4–6 h

    Astemizole (Hismanal) 10 mg PO qd

Anticholinergics

    Scopolamine (Transderm Scop) 1 disc delivers 0.5 mg q3d

Benzodiazepines

    Diazepam (Valium) 5–10 mg PO, IM, IV q4–6 h

Monoaminergics

    Ephedrine 25 mg PO, IM q4–6 h

    Antiemetics

    Ondansetron (Zofran) 4–8 mg ODT PO then 4 mg q8 h

Phenothiazines

    Prochlorperazine (Compazine) 5–10 mg PO, IM q6 h or 25 mg PR q12 h

    Thiethylperazine (Torecan) 10 mg PO, PR, IM q8–24 h

    Promethazine (Phenergan) 12.5–25 mg PO, PR, IM, IV q4–6 h

Butyrophenones

    Droperidol (Inapsine) 2.5–5 mg IM, IV

Benzamides

    Trimethobenzamide (Tigan) 250 mg PO q6–8 h or 200 mg PR, IM q6–8 h

Psychotherapeutic agents

Benzodiazepines

    Alprazolam (Xanax) 0.25–0.50 mg PO q8 h

    Chlordiazepoxide (Librium) 25–50 mg PO q6–8 h

    Diazepam (Valium) 2–10 mg PO q6–12 h

    Lorazepam (Ativan) 2–3 mg PO q8–12 h

Tricyclic antidepressants

    Amitriptyline (Elavil) 50–100 mg PO qd

    Imipramine (Tofranil) 50–150 mg PO qd

    Nortriptyline (Pamelor) 25 mg PO q6–8 h

Notes: Recommended pharmacological regimen for the vertiginous patient to provide acute and short-term vestibular suppression, control of nausea and vomiting, and sedation:
Diazepam 2–10 mg PO, IM, IV q4–6 h
Promethazine 12.5–25 mg PO, PR, IM, IV q4–6 h
Dosing and route of administration are determined by body weight, severity of symptoms, and response to therapy. Therapy is intended to provide prompt control, continued relief, and convenience at the lowest effective dose to allow for vestibular compensation.

motion sickness than acute, severe vertigo. The side effects of antihistamines include dry mouth, drowsiness, blurred vision, and urine retention, but are generally well tolerated by patients. Anticholinergics inhibit activation of central cholinergic pathways and are similar to the antihistamines with regard to effectiveness in treating motion sickness and side effects. Benzodiazepines suppress central and peripheral vestibular pathways, provide tranquilization, and are often beneficial when antihistamines and anticholinergics are ineffective. Benzodiazepines can cause confusion, drowsiness, and ataxia and are used judiciously because of abuse potential. Monoaminergics suppress activity within vestibular neurons and can cause hypertension, nervousness, palpitations, and insomnia.

The use of vestibular suppressants is guarded because of their ability to retard CNS compensatory mechanisms needed to restore vestibular balance. Abnormal vestibular inputs must be recognized by the CNS in order for it to initiate adaptive changes. Recognition of a vestibular deficit by the CNS results from the integration of visual, proprioceptive, and vestibular sensory feedback information produced when the patient attempts to use his or her vestibular reflexes. Research in animals and humans suggests that compensation can be affected directly by the experience of the animal or patient immediately after loss of function. Therefore, suppression of vestibular symptoms by medications or immobilization can limit the potential of the CNS to establish, modify, and maintain the compensatory mechanisms necessary for full recovery.

Antiemetics. The main categories of antiemetic medications are the phenothiazines, butyrophenones, and benzamides. These medications are effective in treating nausea and vomiting by antagonism of dopamine receptors in the chemoreceptor trigger zone of the vomiting center in the lateral reticular formation of the medulla. Phenothiazines can also suppress vestibular nuclei and central vestibular pathways, likely due to their antihistaminic or anticholinergic activity. Side effects include sedation, hypotension, and extrapyramidal symptoms.

Psychotherapeutic Agents. Psychotherapeutic medications include benzodiazepines and tricyclic antidepressants. Benzodiazepines can be used acutely in the ED to treat moderately severe anxiety syndromes that cause dizziness. However, continued outpatient use of these medications is under the supervision of the patient's physician because of abuse potential. Tricyclic antidepressant medication can be instituted in the ED in consultation with the patient's family physician or psychiatrist to treat major depression that causes dizziness. The side effects of these medications are orthostatic hypotension and anticholinergic symptoms.

Pathophysiological treatment of vertigo is performed under the direction of an otolaryngologist, otologist, or neurologist. Such treatment can involve the use of diuretics, vasodilators, corticosteroids, or antibiotics, depending on the final diagnosis.

Surgical treatment is indicated for some patients with vertigo who do not respond adequately to conservative management. The best surgical candidates are those who have unstable labyrinthine disease that leads to fluctuating or progressively deteriorating inner ear function.

9.8.3 Emergency Treatment of the SCUBA Diver with Vertigo

Transient vertigo during self-contained underwater breathing apparatus (SCUBA) diving that resolves with equalization of pressure in the middle ear cleft is known as alternobaric vertigo and requires no treatment except to avoid diving when eustachian tube function may be impaired. Distinguishing between inner ear barotrauma, perilymphatic fistula, and inner ear decompression sickness can be complex, and is best done by an otolaryngologist in consultation with a diving medicine expert.

9.8.4 Vestibular Rehabilitation

Vestibular rehabilitation is an exercise-based physical therapy program designed to facilitate CNS compensatory mechanisms in patients with vestibular pathology. Rehabilitative therapy can be beneficial for patients with acute or chronic symptoms of vestibular dysfunction. Patient assessment and the development of a training program are usually done by a properly trained physical or occupational therapist, who designs a customized program tailored to the needs of the individual patient.

Pearls and Pitfalls

- Carefully obtain clinical information. Timing of symptoms, associated complaints, and provoking maneuvers can facilitate determining whether dizziness is caused by a disorder of the peripheral or central vestibular system or nonvestibular systems. Overreliance on symptom quality can be misleading.
- Vertigo usually suggests a vestibular system disorder but cannot reliably localize it.
- The neuro-otologic examination is important in assessing a patient with dizziness or vertigo.
- The Hallpike maneuver can diagnose benign paroxysmal positional vertigo; the particle repositioning maneuver can treat it.
- The HINTS exam can reliably differentiate between peripheral and central pathology in patients with acute vestibular syndromes.
- MRI of the brain has a significant rate of false negatives for posterior circulation strokes and should not preclude appropriate risk factor management and treatment.
- Symptomatic treatment of severe vertigo in the ED usually includes vestibular suppressant and antiemetic medications.

Bibliography

Chen R, Su R, Deng M, et al. A posterior circulation ischemia risk score system to assist the diagnosis of dizziness. *J Stroke Cerebrovasc Dis* 2018;**27** (2):506–512.

Cheung CS, Mak PS, Manley KV, et al. Predictors of important neurological causes of dizziness among patients presenting to the emergency department. *Emerg Med J* 2010;**27** (7):517–521.

Choi JH, Oh EH, Park MG, et al. Early MRI-negative posterior circulation stroke presenting as acute dizziness. *J Neurol* 2018;**265**(12):2993–3000.

Crespi V. Dizziness and vertigo: an epidemiological survey and patient management in the emergency room. *Neurol Sci* 2004;**25**(1):S24–S25.

Edlow JA, Gurley KL, Newman-Toker DE. A new diagnostic approach to the adult patient with acute dizziness. *J Emerg Med* 2018;**54** (4):469–483.

Epley JM. The canalith repositioning procedure: for treatment of benign paroxysmal positional vertigo. *Otolaryngol Head Neck Surg* 1992;**107**(3):399–404.

Kattah JC, Talkad AV, Wang DZ, Hsieh YH, Newman-Toker DE. HINTS to diagnose stroke in the acute vestibular syndrome: three-step bedside oculomotor examination more sensitive than early MRI diffusion-weighted imaging. *Stroke* 2009;**40**(11):3504–3510.

Kerber KA. Vertigo and dizziness in the emergency department. *Emerg Med Clin North Am* 2009;27(1):39–50.

Kerber KA, Newman-Toker DE. Misdiagnosing dizzy patients: common pitfalls in clinical practice. *Neurol Clin* 2015;33(3):565–575.

Lammers W, Folmer W, Van Lieshout EM, et al. Demographic analysis of emergency department patients at the Ruijin Hospital, Shanghai. *Emerg Med Int* 2011;**2011**:748274.

Martin-Schild S, Albright KC, Tanksley J, et al. Zero on the NIHSS does not equal the absence of stroke. *Ann Emerg Med* 2011;**57** (1):42–45.

Navi BB, Kamel H, Shah MP, et al. Application of the ABCD2 score to identify cerebrovascular causes of dizziness in the emergency department. *Stroke* 2012;**43** (6):1484–1489.

Navi BB, Kamel H, Shah MP, et al. Rate and predictors of serious neurologic causes of dizziness in the emergency department. *Mayo Clin Proc* 2012;**87** (11):1080–1088.

Newman-Toker DE, Cannon LM, Stofferahn ME, et al. Imprecision in patient reports of dizziness symptom quality: a cross-sectional study conducted in an acute care setting. *Mayo Clin Proc* 2007;**82**(11):1329–1340.

Oppenheim C, Stanescu R, Dormont D, et al. False-negative diffusion-weighted MR findings in acute ischemic stroke. *AJNR Am J Neuroradiol* 2000;**21**(8):1434–1440.

Parnes LS, Price-Jones RG. Particle repositioning maneuver for benign paroxysmal positional vertigo. *Ann Otol Rhinol Laryngol* 1993;**102**(5):325–331.

Schneck MJ. Current stroke scales may be partly responsible for worse outcomes in posterior circulation stroke. *Stroke* 2018;**49**(11):2565–2566.

Smith DB. Dizziness: a clinical perspective. In Kaufman AI, Smith DB (eds.) *Neurologic Clinics: Diagnostic Neurotology*. W. B. Saunders, 1990.

Tintinalli J, Ma OJ, Yealy D, et al. *Tintinalli's Emergency Medicine: A Comprehensive Study Guide*, 9th ed. McGraw-Hill, 2019.

Chapter 10

Gait Disturbances

Jon S. Brillman and Troy Desai

10.1 Introduction

Abnormalities of gait are commonly seen in the emergency department (ED) and often reflect some disorder of the nervous system. Station and gait are unique to each individual and reflects gender, age, body habitus, mood, and even culture. The goal of evaluation is to determine what part(s) of the nervous system are involved by the type of gait observed. The evaluation is individualized depending on the patient's ability to ambulate safely. Patients may be observed standing with eyes open, eyes closed, and ambulating. They may be asked to walk on their toes, heels, or tandem walk, or hop on one foot at a time. The use of assistive devices may be indicated. Different types of gait disturbance are described with regard to neuroanatomical localization and specific neurological disorders (Figure 10.1).

10.2 ED Evaluation and Management

10.2.1 Senescent Gait (Early Gait Apraxia)

This gait is observed commonly in patients of advanced age and is characterized by small, uncertain steps. Generally the foot is planted flat without springing from the heel to the ball of the foot and there is reduced associated arm movement. This is seen in cerebral atrophy but also reflects loss of joint mobility, tightness of the hamstrings, and loss of proprioception.

10.2.2 Advanced Senescent Gait (Late Gait Apraxia)

Patients with advanced senescent gait are usually demented. They may have Alzheimer's disease or cerebral atrophy from other causes or subcortical involvement from multiple strokes. Communicating hydrocephalus (normal pressure hydrocephalus) may produce this type of gait, but under those circumstances the degree of cognitive dysfunction is variable. Steps are extremely small and hesitant and the feet tend to be "magnetized" to the floor. Patients may be tipped over easily forward or backward.

10.2.3 Parkinson's Disease and Parkinsonian Conditions

The gait of patients with Parkinson's disease and related disorders is stereotyped but may be confused with senescent gait. Patients take slow, small, shuffling steps and have diminished swing of one upper extremity initially, which may also have a tremor. Over time they may develop a flexion of all limbs and trunk and a tendency to lean forward and accelerate with walking, a disturbance referred to as "festination." As with patients with gait apraxia they are easily tipped in one direction or another. Characteristically, patients may get stuck in

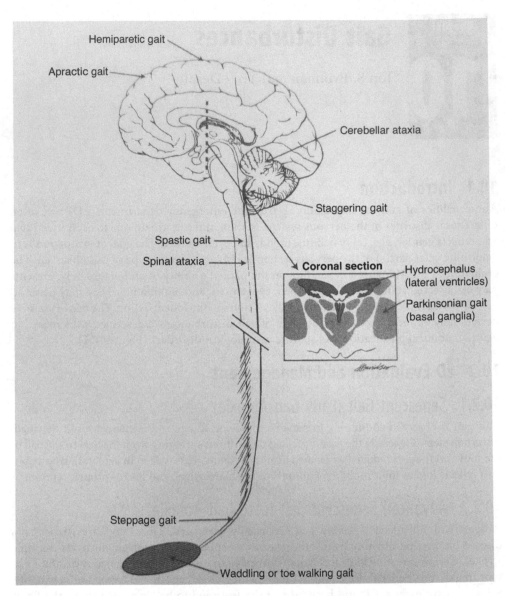

Figure 10.1 Gait disturbance.

doorways or with other obstacles. Turning is accomplished with very small steps and is segmented. Tremor, rigidity, and other parkinsonian features may also be seen.

10.2.4 Hemiparetic Gait

The most frequent cause of hemiparetic gait is cerebral infarction, and may represent a chronic problem. The arm may be adducted and fingers and wrist flexed with hyperextension and plantar inversion of the foot. The advancing foot may catch on the floor because of weakness of dorsiflexion, or extensor hypertonia. To avoid tripping, and to conserve energy, the patient swings the affected leg out in a circumducting fashion.

10.2.5 Spastic Gait

Patients with spastic gait have problems involving bilateral cerebral hemispheres or the spinal cord. Children diagnosed with cerebral palsy may have a spastic gait. Under these circumstances, the characteristic gait is "wooden-legged" or stiff. Patients may drag their legs along the floor. Because of increased tone of the hip adductors, they have a narrow gait and the legs may even cross the midline to the other side. This is referred to as "scissoring" of gait with the thighs rubbing together during walking.

10.2.6 Ataxic Gait

Ataxia is a disordered balance not associated with specific neuroanatomical localization. Frequently it is seen in cerebellar disease but may also be seen with spinal cord disease and frequently coexists with spasticity. Ataxic gait refers to a wide base of gait that the patient requires to maintain balance. Severe peripheral neuropathies with large fiber involvement and loss of proprioception may be associated with ataxic gait because the feet have difficulty with spatial organization. Ataxic gait is seen with dorsal column disease and pancerebellar disease. Midline (vermian) cerebellar disorders are seen in patients with drug intoxication or alcoholism and may be associated with difficulty with tandem walking. The Romberg sign refers to the patient's ability to maintain their balance with upright stance until their eyes are closed, after which they begin to sway back and forth. Closure of the eyes removes visual cues, thus causing the patient to rely more on proprioceptive clues, which may be impaired by abnormalities of large peripheral nerve fibers or dorsal columns, as seen in vitamin B12 deficiency.

10.2.7 Staggering Gait

Staggering gait is observed commonly in EDs and is characteristic of alcoholic intoxication and seen in patients who have taken sedative drugs. It can be distinguished from a cerebellar ataxic gait because it is wide-based and associated with pitching and reeling to one side, loss of balance, and a need to grasp and hold onto objects. Associated features of intoxication are frequently present.

10.2.8 Steppage Gait

Steppage gait is observed in patients who have foot drop due to peripheral neurologic disorders. It is usually unilateral and caused by an injury to the common peroneal nerve at the level of the fibular head in the lateral portion of the knee. Injury to this nerve can be due to direct trauma and is commonly seen in cachectic bedridden patients. The steps are normal but the advancing foot cannot be dorsiflexed and must be elevated by excessive flexion of the hip and knee so the foot can clear the floor, curbsides, or steps. The affected foot will slap the ground and often make an audible noise. Occasionally, foot drop results from an L5 radiculopathy due to a herniated disc at the L4–L5 level. Bilateral foot drops suggest a more severe disease process such as Charcot–Marie–Tooth, amyotrophic lateral sclerosis, or polio.

10.2.9 Waddling Gait

Waddling gait is characteristic of patients who have hip girdle weakness. It is seen in hip dislocations usually in adults and is characteristic of polymyositis and muscular dystrophy. Patients with waddling gait shift their weight from side to side in an exaggerated fashion. When the leg is planted on the floor the ipsilateral hip drops (Trendelenburg sign), and the opposite hip rises. The trunk tends to tilt to the side of the patient's step. The alteration in trunk movement results in the waddling feature.

10.2.10 Hysterical Gait

Hysterical gait is a gait abnormality that cannot be explained satisfactorily by a specific neuroanatomical localization or disease process. As is the case with other hysterical disorders, associated features of emotional disturbance can be elicited in a nonthreatening manner by the examiner. Gait may be bizarre, pitching and starting to one side or the other, wavering suddenly from left to right, or with twirling motions with the arms outstretched and flopping about (astasia-abasia). Frequently, patients suddenly topple or fall into a position where they may take a step and push the other leg. In hysterical hemiparesis there is absence of circumducting gait, hyperactive deep tendon reflexes, and an extensor plantar response (e.g., Babinski sign). A diagnosis of hysterical gait is not made when there is objective evidence of nervous system dysfunction.

10.2.11 Antalgic Gait

Antalgic gait results from a shortened stance phase of a painful limb. Because of pain, the patient will consciously or subconsciously limit time spent bearing weight on the affected limb. Osteoarthritis is a common cause. Sometimes called coxalgic gait, it commonly refers to hip disease and the compensatory gait of decreased stride length and stance phase that minimizes discomfort in the affected hip joint.

10.3 Management of Gait Abnormality

In the ED, the initial concern is to determine whether a gait abnormality is a chronic condition or an acute change that requires further evaluation, treatment, and/or hospital admission. Emergent conditions such as stroke, cerebral hemorrhage, myelitis, and other potential causes need to be considered. If there is sudden worsening of a chronic gait abnormality, infection and other systemic causes must be investigated; there also may be progression of the chronic underlying neurologic condition. A safety assessment must be undertaken. Care providers in the ED may prescribe assistive devices or physical therapy. The patient and caregivers should be educated regarding fall prevention. Depending on the underlying etiology, medications such as amantadine, dalfampridine, and antispasmodics may be prescribed. Although typically beyond the purview of the emergency physician, ankle–foot orthoses (AFOs) and other braces as well as external peroneal nerve stimulators may be indicated. Referral to neurology or physiatry is often advisable.

Pearls and Pitfalls

- Advanced senescent gait may be similar to that seen in normal pressure hydrocephalus where cognitive dysfunction is variable.
- Universal flexion is typically associated with the gait of Parkinson's disease.
- Circumduction is a characteristic sign of hemiparetic gait.
- Chronic spasticity of both lower extremities can result in "scissoring" of gait.
- Sensory ataxias are caused by dorsal column and peripheral nerve disease.
- Steppage gait is caused by foot drop.
- Hysterical gait cannot be diagnosed in the presence of nervous system dysfunction.
- Patients should be educated on preventing falls.
- Physical therapy and assistive devices should be prescribed as needed.
- Referral to neurology or physiatry should be considered.

Bibliography

Ropper AH, Samuels MA, Klein J, Prasad S (eds.). *Adams and Victor's Principles of Neurology*, 11th ed. McGraw-Hill, 2019.

Chapter

Ischemic Stroke and Transient Ischemic Attack

Crystal Wong, Melani S. Cheers, Molly A. McGraw, Lauren King Palmer, and Russell Cerejo

11.1 Introduction

In the United States, one stroke occurs every 40 seconds on average. Ischemic stroke is a leading cause of serious long-term disability and the fifth leading cause of death. Every year, 795,000 people experience a new or recurrent stroke. In 2018, stroke accounted for 1 of every 19 deaths. Stroke typically occurs suddenly, with symptoms of motor weakness, impaired speech, vision loss, or numbness, and can lead to significant disability. The financial burden of stroke, including direct medical costs and potential wages lost, is greater than $30 billion per year. Time-based acute stroke treatments improve functional outcome and reduce mortality, which makes rapid recognition of stroke of utmost importance.

11.2 Pathophysiology

Of all strokes encountered in the emergency department (ED), 87% are ischemic and the rest are hemorrhagic, including intracerebral hemorrhage (ICH) and subarachnoid hemorrhage (SAH). Brain ischemia events manifest as transient ischemic attack (TIA) or ischemic stroke.

TIA is traditionally defined as focal neurologic symptoms or signs lasting less than 24 hours. However, with advances in technology and more widespread availability of CT and MRI, up to one-third of individuals who meet the traditional definition for TIA have evidence of infarct on imaging. As a result, the American Stroke Association (ASA) endorses the following revised, tissue-based definition of TIA: "a transient episode of neurological dysfunction caused by focal brain, spinal cord, or retinal ischemia, without acute infarction."

Ischemic stroke is defined by central nervous system infarct accompanied by focal neurologic symptoms, whether or not they are transient or persist beyond 24 hours. "Silent strokes" are often incidental findings on imaging, representing infarcts that are not associated with any known symptoms.

Brain ischemia occurs when the arterial blood supply is interrupted by vessel occlusion, most frequently by a thrombus, resulting in focal neurologic deficits. Ischemic strokes and TIAs are primarily caused by large artery atherosclerosis, cardiac embolism, and small-vessel disease. However, other less common etiologies include arterial dissection, prothrombotic states, vasculopathies, genetic and metabolic disorders, hypoperfusion states, and idiopathic causes.

Atherosclerotic plaque rupture of a major intra- or extracranial artery and subsequent thrombus formation can lead to vessel occlusion or embolization to distal branches. Cardiac sources of embolism include atrial fibrillation, atrial flutter, and intracardiac thrombus in the setting of reduced ejection fraction. Less common but important sources of embolization include air, fat, bacterial vegetations, tumor cells, atherosclerotic plaque debris, and particulate matter from intravenous drug use.

Lacunar stroke, due to small-vessel disease, is another common cause of stroke, accounting for 20–30% of all ischemic strokes. Chronic hypertension leads to the development of lipohyalinosis, microatheroma, fibrinoid necrosis, or Charcot–Bouchard aneurysms in the small penetrating arteries. These changes may eventually result in occlusion of the vessel. Although small-vessel disease is most strongly associated with hypertension, other risk factors include dyslipidemia, tobacco abuse, and diabetes.

11.3 Stroke Syndromes

Ischemic stroke types are often categorized as anterior circulation strokes or posterior circulation strokes. The anterior circulation refers to the internal carotid arteries and their branches, and the posterior circulation refers to the vertebral and basilar arteries and their branches. The most common anterior circulation strokes involve ischemia in the distribution of the middle cerebral artery (MCA). Left MCA syndromes manifest one or more symptoms of right hemibody weakness, right hemisensory loss, aphasia, or left gaze preference or deviation. Right MCA syndromes produce similar symptoms as left MCA syndromes, only on the contralateral side; additionally, aphasia is usually absent and left hemineglect can be seen instead. If the area of MCA ischemia is large, a contralateral homonymous hemianopia may be present, as well as drowsiness or depressed mental status. Amaurosis fugax, or sudden transient monocular blindness, may result from occlusion of the ophthalmic branch of the internal carotid artery, and can indicate the presence of underlying carotid disease. When monocular blindness persists, permanent infarction of the retina has occurred. Common anterior and posterior circulation stroke syndromes are listed in Table 11.1.

Table 11.1 Common anterior and posterior circulation stroke syndromes

Syndrome	Arterial occlusion site	Symptoms
Left MCA syndrome (anterior circulation)	Left middle cerebral artery	Right hemibody weakness Right hemisensory loss Right homonymous hemianopia Aphasia Left gaze preference or deviation
Right MCA syndrome (anterior circulation)	Right middle cerebral artery	Left hemibody weakness Left hemisensory loss Left homonymous hemianopia Left extinction or hemineglect Right gaze preference or deviation
Amaurosis fugax (anterior circulation)	Central retinal artery, ophthalmic artery, internal carotid artery	Sudden, transient monocular blindness (ipsilateral)

Table 11.1 (cont.)

Syndrome	Arterial occlusion site	Symptoms
Cerebellar ischemia (posterior circulation)	Posterior inferior cerebellar artery, anterior inferior cerebellar artery, superior cerebellar artery	Gait ataxia Ipsilateral limb ataxia Vertigo Nausea and/or vomiting Nystagmus
Occipital lobe ischemia (posterior circulation)	Posterior cerebral artery	Contralateral hemianopia

Symptoms of posterior circulation ischemia are various and differ in important ways from those of the anterior circulation. It is highly important to identify the presence of posterior circulation ischemia, which is sometimes the result of vertebral or basilar artery thrombus. If occlusions at these sites go undetected and untreated, they may result in rapid progression of neurologic symptoms, leading to significant disability or death. Gait ataxia, vertigo, vomiting, and nystagmus may result from cerebellar or brainstem ischemia. Occipital lobe involvement often results in contralateral hemianopia alone. Arm or leg ataxia is usually specific to the ipsilateral cerebellar hemisphere. Other signs of brainstem dysfunction include dysconjugate extraocular movements, gaze paresis, dysarthria, dysphagia, crossed symptoms (ipsilateral facial motor or sensory deficit with contralateral arm or leg involvement), and quadriplegia. Brainstem ischemia may also produce nonspecific signs such as depressed mental status, coma, respiratory insufficiency, cardiac arrhythmias, and labile blood pressure. Common posterior circulation stroke syndromes are listed in Table 11.1. Selected uncommon brainstem stroke syndromes are listed in Table 11.2.

Small-vessel stroke often presents as one of several well-described lacunar syndromes (Table 11.3). Pure motor stroke, or hemiparesis alone, is usually seen with infarction of the corona radiata, internal capsule, pons, or medulla. Pure sensory strokes are attributable to the thalamus or pons. Mixed motor and sensory ("sensorimotor") strokes involve the thalamus and adjacent internal capsule. Infarction of the corona radiata, internal capsule, or pons can result in ataxic hemiparesis (motor weakness with limb ataxia) or dysarthria clumsy hand syndrome (dysarthria with ataxic arm). Lacunar stroke syndromes are summarized in Table 11.3.

11.4 Diagnosis

As the range and effectiveness of time-critical treatments for acute ischemic stroke continues to increase, it is becoming more important to prioritize recognition and rapid triage of acute stroke patients. Any suspicion that the patient is having a stroke should trigger prompt evaluation and diagnosis. The ASA recommends specific time goals for management of stroke patients in the ED to help hospitals formulate effective processes to streamline and optimize care (Table 11.4).

The most important piece of information to obtain in the patient's clinical history is the time of symptom onset, which can immediately determine if time-based interventions

Table 11.2 Selected uncommon clinical stroke syndromes

Syndrome	Arterial occlusion site	Clinical manifestations
Lateral medullary syndrome (Wallenberg syndrome)	Posterior inferior cerebellar artery (often lesion in vertebral artery)	(a) Ipsilateral limb ataxia, (b) ipsilateral loss of facial cutaneous sensation, (c) hiccup, (d) ipsilateral Horner syndrome, (e) nausea/vomiting/nystagmus, (f) contralateral loss of pain and temperature sensation, (g) dysphagia, (h) hoarseness with ipsilateral vocal cord paralysis, (i) loss of ipsilateral pharyngeal reflex
Lateral inferior pontine syndrome	Anterior inferior cerebellar artery	(a–f) above, plus: (g) ipsilateral facial paralysis, (h) deafness and tinnitus, (i) ipsilateral gaze paralysis
Lateral midpontine syndrome	Short circumferential artery	(a–f) above, plus: (g) trigeminal nerve impairment: chewing difficulty (bilateral lesions) or ipsilateral jaw deviation with mouth opened (unilateral lesions)
Lateral superior pontine syndrome	Superior cerebellar artery	(a–f) above, plus: (g) no specific cranial nerve signs
Medial medullary syndrome	Paramedian branches of basilar artery	(a) Contralateral hemiparesis, (b) contralateral loss of proprioception and vibratory sensory function, (c) ipsilateral limb ataxia, (d) ipsilateral tongue weakness
Medial inferior pontine syndrome	Paramedian branches of basilar artery	(a–c) above, plus: (d) ipsilateral gaze paralysis, (e) ipsilateral lateral rectus paralysis, (f) gaze-evoked nystagmus
Medial superior pontine syndrome	Paramedian branches of basilar artery	(a–c) above, plus: (d) internuclear ophthalmoplegia, (e) palatal myoclonus
Ventral midbrain syndrome (Weber syndrome)	Paramedian branches of basilar artery	(a) Contralateral paresis, (b) contralateral supranuclear facial paresis, (c) ipsilateral oculomotor nerve palsy
Central midbrain syndrome (tegmental syndrome)	Paramedian branches of basilar artery	(a) Ipsilateral oculomotor nerve palsy, (b) hemichorea of contralateral limbs, (c) contralateral loss of cutaneous sensation and proprioception
Dorsal midbrain syndrome (Parinaud syndrome)	Usually caused by compression by	Paralysis of upward gaze

Table 11.2 (cont.)

Syndrome	Arterial occlusion site	Clinical manifestations
	extra-axial lesion (pinealoma)	
Locked-in syndrome	Basilar artery occlusion causing bilateral ventral pontine lesions	Complete quadriplegia, inability to speak, and loss of all facial movements despite normal level of consciousness: patients may communicate with eye or eyelid movements

Reprinted from *Emergency Medicine Clinics of North America*, Vol 20, Thurman RJ, Jauch EC, Acute ischemic stroke: emergent evaluation and management, 609–630, 2002, with permission from Elsevier.

Table 11.3 Lacunar stroke syndromes

Syndrome	Site of brain ischemia	Symptoms
Pure motor stroke	Internal capsule, pons, corona radiata, medulla	Contralateral hemibody weakness
Pure sensory stroke	Thalamus, pons	Contralateral hemisensory loss
Mixed motor and sensory (sensorimotor) stroke	Thalamus and adjacent internal capsule	Contralateral hemibody weakness Contralateral hemisensory loss
Ataxic hemiparesis	Pons, corona radiata, internal capsule	Contralateral hemibody weakness Contralateral limb ataxia
Dysarthria clumsy hand	Pons, corona radiata, internal capsule	Dysarthria Contralateral arm ataxia

should be considered. If the exact time of onset cannot be established, an acceptable surrogate is the time the patient was last known to be normal (LKN), or at their baseline neurologic status. When ascertaining the time of onset or LKN, it is critical to determine that time as accurately as possible, which may involve detailed questioning or the use of environmental cues. For example, patients exhibiting a right MCA syndrome often have decreased or absent insight to their condition and cannot give an accurate history. Thus, it may be necessary to ask more specific questions, such as, "Did you have problems dropping things from your hand at that time?" or "Did the person with whom you were talking notice anything wrong with your speech?" Other patients may have been seated and did not notice their symptoms until they tried to stand, making it crucial to determine the last time they were able to walk or use their legs normally. Patients who "woke up" with symptoms may

Table 11.4 Recommended time goals by the ASA for ED-based acute ischemic stroke care

Event	Time goal (from time of arrival)
Evaluate patient (by emergency physician)	≤10 minutes
Notify stroke team	≤15 minutes
Initiate CT scan	≤25 minutes
Interpret CT scan (by radiology)	≤45 minutes
Initiate treatment with IV tPA	≤60 minutes
Initiate mechanical thrombectomy (groin puncture)	≤90 minutes

IV tPA = intravenous recombinant tissue plasminogen activator.

have been able to walk or groom themselves shortly before the onset of symptoms. Finally, some patients may have symptoms that resolve before recurring. In such cases, the resolution of symptoms effectively "resets" the clock and the time of symptom recurrence should be used for considering acute stroke therapy.

Other aspects of clinical history may provide clues that the patient's neurologic symptoms are due to a stroke mimic or require further investigation. Seizures can produce a postictal "Todd's" paralysis. A sudden, thunderclap headache may suggest SAH and require additional diagnostic testing. Stroke symptoms in the context of tearing chest pain may indicate aortic dissection. Patients with migraine headaches may have a pattern of focal neurologic symptoms associated with prior migraines. A diabetic who uses insulin may be hypoglycemic, which can cause stroke-like symptoms that resolve after achieving normoglycemia.

The examination of the patient should be focused and brief, and should be performed only after the patient is stabilized from the standpoint of airway, breathing, and circulation. The general physical exam should include cardiac auscultation, palpation of peripheral pulses, and evaluation for signs of trauma. A cardiac murmur may indicate the presence of endocarditis. An irregularly irregular heart rhythm is often associated with atrial fibrillation. Unequal extremity pulses may alert the examiner to the possibility of aortic dissection. External signs of trauma may overlie bone fractures or soft tissue injuries that may preclude the use of thrombolytics.

The National Institutes of Health Stroke Scale (NIHSS) is the most commonly used method of rapidly evaluating stroke patients and can be performed within minutes. It was originally formulated as a standardized scale for use in clinical research. It is a 15-item scale that encompasses key components of the neurologic examination, with scores ranging from 0 to 42. Because it can be administered rapidly and has high inter-rater reliability among neurologists and non-neurologists alike, it is now widely used to assess the location and severity of stroke in the acute setting. The components of the NIHSS are presented in Table 11.5. Links to the National Institute of Neurological Disorders and Stroke (NINDS) version of the NIHSS can be found at https://stroke.nih.gov/resources/scale.htm. The American Heart Association provides video demonstrations of the NIHSS and online training (https://learn.heart.org/nihss.aspx) free of charge for CME credit.

Table 11.5 The NIH Stroke Scale (adapted). The patient should be scored on actual performance, not what the clinician believes the patient is capable of doing. NINDS material for testing language and dysarthria (items 9, 10) can be found at www.stroke.nih.gov/documents/NIH_Stroke_Scale_508C.pdf

Item	Title and description	Response and score
1a	**Level of consciousness (LOC):** **Assess the patient's level of alertness and degree of consciousness.**	0 = **Alert** 1 = **Drowsy.** Arousable by minor stimulation to participate in the examination. 2 = **Not alert.** Requires repeated stimulation to attend, or requires strong or painful stimulation to make nonstereotyped movements. 3 = **Unresponsive.** Does not respond to examiner. Reflex motor or autonomic responses may be present.
1b	**LOC orientation questions:** **Ask the patient the month and his/her age.** Do not give the patient "clues" to the right answer. Aphasic and obtunded patients who are unable to answer the questions should score 2. Patients who cannot answer the questions for reasons other than aphasia (such as endotracheal intubation or language barrier) should score 1.	0 = **Answers both questions correctly.** 1 = **Answers one question correctly.** 2 = **Answers neither question correctly.**
1c	**LOC response to commands:** **Ask the patient to open and close the eyes, and form a fist with and release the nonparetic hand.** Substitute another one-step command if the hands cannot be used, such as in patients with trauma or amputation. For patients who do not seem to understand the commands, pantomiming the movements for them to mimic is permitted. Only the first attempt should be scored.	0 = **Performs both tasks correctly.** 1 = **Performs one task correctly.** 2 = **Performs neither task correctly.**

Table 11.5 (cont.)

Item	Title and description	Response and score
2	**Best gaze:** **Test the horizontal eye movements by asking the patient to track your finger or an object.** Reflexive eye movements may be scored as well. Isolated peripheral nerve paresis (III, IV, or VI) or a gaze deviation that the patient can overcome should score 1.	0 = **Normal.** 1 = **Partial gaze palsy.** Abnormal gaze is present in one or both eyes, but forced deviation or total gaze paresis is absent. 2 = **Forced deviation or total gaze palsy.**
3	**Visual:** **Test all four quadrants of the visual fields using finger counting or visual threat.** If the patient looks at the finger in the quadrant appropriately, this may be scored as normal.	0 = **No visual loss.** 1 = **Partial hemianopia.** 2 = **Complete hemianopia.** 3 = **Bilateral hemianopia** (blind).
4	**Facial palsy:** **Ask the patient to smile or show their teeth, raise the eyebrows, and close the eyes.** Pantomime may be used for patients in whom comprehension is impaired. Noxious stimuli may be used in poorly responsive patients to induce facial grimace.	0 = **Normal.** 1 = **Minor paralysis** (mild asymmetry). 2 = **Partial paralysis** (severe or total paralysis of lower face). 3 = **Complete paralysis** of upper and lower face on one or both sides.
5	**Motor arm:** **5a. Left arm** **5b. Right arm** **If the patient is sitting, the arm is held extended, palm down, at 90 degrees. If supine, the arm is held extended at 45 degrees.** Pantomime and encouragement may be used, but not noxious stimuli. Each arm should be tested individually. Untestable in the presence of amputation or joint fusion.	0 = **No drift.** Arm holds without drift for 10 seconds. 1 = **Drift.** Arm holds initial position, but drifts down before 10 seconds without hitting the bed. 2 = **Some effort against gravity,** but arm falls to the bed before 10 seconds. 3 = **No effort against gravity,** but some movement is present. 4 = **No movement.**

6	Motor leg:	0 = No drift. Leg holds without drift for 5 seconds.
	6a. Left leg	1 = Drift. Leg holds initial position, but drifts down before
	6b. Right leg	5 seconds without hitting the bed.
	The patient should be supine with leg held at 30 degrees.	2 = Some effort against gravity, but leg falls to the bed before
	Pantomime and encouragement may be used, but not	5 seconds.
	noxious stimuli. Each leg should be tested individually.	3 = No effort against gravity, but some movement is present.
	Untestable in the presence of amputation or joint fusion.	4 = No movement.
7	Limb ataxia:	0 = Absent.
	Perform finger–nose–finger and heel–shin on both sides	1 = Present in one limb.
	to test for cerebellar ataxia. Ataxia should be scored only if	2 = Present in two limbs.
	out of proportion to the degree of limb weakness. If the	
	patient cannot perform this item because of aphasia or	
	paralysis, ataxia is considered to be absent.	
	Untestable in the presence of amputation or joint fusion.	
8	Sensory:	0 = Normal.
	Sensation may be tested with pinprick in the awake	1 = Mild-to-moderate sensory loss, but the patient is aware of
	patient, or with noxious stimulus in the aphasic or poorly	the stimulus.
	responsive patient. Patients who have bilateral sensory loss	2 = Severe to total sensory loss. The patient is not aware of the
	or are unresponsive should score 2.	stimulus, or has bilateral sensory loss.
9	Best language:	0 = No aphasia.
	Language expression and comprehension often become	1 = Mild-to-moderate aphasia. Some impairment of language
	evident during the course of history-taking and examination	expression or comprehension. Can still express ideas but has
	of the patient. Ask the patient to name objects or read a series	some difficulty with conversation.
	of sentences using materials from the NINDS website.	2 = Severe aphasia. The amount of information exchanged is
	Unresponsive patients will score 3.	limited and fragmentary. The burden of communication lies
		with the examiner.
		3 = Mute, global aphasia. No information exchanged with
		speech or comprehension.

Table 11.5 (cont.)

Item	Title and description	Response and score
10	**Dysarthria:** The quality of the patient's speech becomes evident during the course of history-taking and examination. To further assess dysarthria, have the patient read a series of short phrases using materials from the NINDS website.	0 = **Normal.** 1 = **Mild-to-moderate dysarthria.** Some words are slurred but speech is still intelligible. 2 = **Severe dysarthria.** The patient is mute or the speech is slurred to the point of being unintelligible. 3 = **Intubated or other physical barrier.**
11	**Extinction and inattention:** **Double simultaneous stimulation may be used in tactile (sensory) and visual field testing for this item.** The score should be normal if the aphasic patient cannot participate in giving responses to double simultaneous stimulation, but appears to attend to both sides.	0 = **Absent.** 1 = **Mild hemi-inattention or extinction** to bilateral simultaneous stimulation in one modality (visual, tactile, auditory, spatial). 2 = **Severe hemi-inattention or extinction to more than one modality.** Patient completely neglects one side of space or has extinction to two or more modalities.

Level of consciousness is determined by evaluating the patient's degree of alertness and whether or not he can answer orientation questions and follow commands accurately. An aphasic patient, however, will score poorly in this section due to inability to understand the questions and commands. Testing horizontal gaze by asking the patient to track the examiner's finger may reveal a gaze deviation or dysconjugate eye movements. The presence of decreased visual fields on one side, assessed by counting fingers or testing blink to visual threat, may indicate occipital lobe ischemia. Facial palsy can be assessed when the patient smiles or grimaces to a noxious stimulus. Arm or leg weakness may be gauged by the patient's ability to elevate and maintain the limb's position against gravity and whether it drifts downward or falls to the bed. Limb ataxia produces abnormal finger-to-nose or heel-to-knee-to-shin testing. Sensation may be evaluated using light touch or pinprick, or with noxious stimuli in the aphasic or poorly responsive patient. Problems with language expression or comprehension become evident when the aphasic patient attempts to interact with the NINDS materials for the NIHSS (e.g., describing what she sees in the picture, naming objects in the diagram, and reading sentences aloud). Aphasia may also be assessed by the patient's ability to provide a history and to understand and obey commands during the examination. The presence of dysarthria may be noted in the course of the interview and by having the patient read from a series of phrases. Finally, visual or tactile extinction or inattention may be detected by presenting double simultaneous stimuli to both modalities, such as by having the patient count fingers in bilateral visual fields or the examiner touch both arms simultaneously.

11.5 Neuroimaging

If clinical history and physical exam are suggestive of acute stroke, the patient should immediately undergo neuroimaging. The most rapid, commonly used, and widely available modality is noncontrast CT of the head. While it is poorly sensitive for acute ischemic stroke, it is the gold standard for detecting acute ICH, which can present with symptoms similar to those of ischemic stroke. In addition, the noncontrast head CT provides sufficient neuroimaging information as part of the evaluation for treatment with thrombolytics. Even in cases of acute ischemia, early ischemic changes may be present in up to 75% of patients within 3 hours of symptom onset. Such changes include loss of differentiation of the gray–white matter junction, sulcal effacement, and a hyperdense artery indicating vessel occlusion (Figure 11.1a). A hypodense area may be seen in the territory of the infarct within 12–24 hours, and a well-demarcated hypodensity is visible after 24 hours (Figure 11.1b).

Brain MRI is not commonly used for diagnostic evaluation when considering acute stroke therapies. Compared to CT, MRI is more costly and thus not always staffed 24 hours a day at some institutions; there are more barriers to use due to contraindications such as metallic implants and devices and claustrophobia; it is prone to patient motion artifacts; and it requires a much longer time for image acquisition. For these reasons, noncontrast head CT is often preferred for assessing patients for acute stroke treatment. However, MRI is far more sensitive at detecting ischemic stroke of all sizes and is just as sensitive as CT for the presence of hemorrhage. Some centers utilize MRI as their first-line acute stroke imaging modality and have abbreviated MRI protocols to avoid prolonged scan times.

Noninvasive CT angiography (CTA) or MR angiography (MRA) can identify the presence of a large artery occlusion that may be amenable to endovascular clot retrieval. CTA is most commonly used in the emergency setting since it shares many of the same time

(a)   (b)

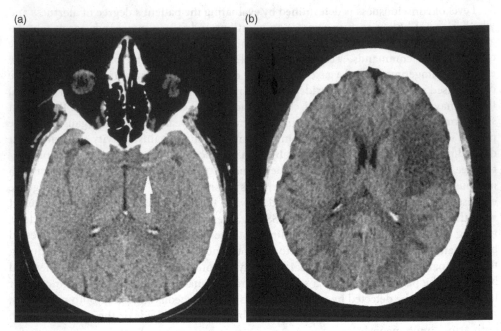

Figure 11.1 (a) Hyperdense left MCA sign (arrow) on noncontrast head CT. (b) Hypodense infarct in the left frontal lobe on noncontrast head CT.

and ease-of-use advantages as noncontrast CT. However, the presence of an allergy to iodine or renal impairment may pose significant risk to the patient and may preclude use of this imaging modality. Alternatively, MRA may be considered in the patient who cannot undergo CTA safely, although it is subject to the same limitations as MRI.

Advanced imaging modalities, such as CT or MR perfusion and multiphase CTA, are used to assess cerebral perfusion and the size of the core infarct or the robustness of the collateral circulation, respectively. These studies often require specialized software to post-process the source images and neuroradiology expertise and experience in interpretation. They are most commonly used as an adjunct to stratify an individual patient's potential risks vs benefit of undergoing endovascular clot retrieval.

11.6 Ancillary Testing

Additional nonradiologic testing is helpful and often necessary. A complete metabolic panel can reveal hypo- or hyperglycemia or impaired renal function. Anemia can be seen on a complete blood count, and systemic anticoagulation may be detected by a prolonged prothrombin time (PT) or activated partial thromboplastin time (aPTT). There is a limited role for coagulation tests such as thrombin time, ecarin clotting time, and the anti-factor Xa activity assay to assess the activity of direct thrombin inhibitors or direct factor Xa inhibitors, since such tests are not widely available on an emergency basis. Cardiac biomarkers are often elevated in acute stroke due to a neurogenic catecholamine surge, but can also indicate concurrent myocardial infarction that should be confirmed on EKG. Young patients without obvious stroke risk factors should undergo a urine drug screen. Women of child-bearing age

Table 11.6 Recommended diagnostic studies for evaluation of patients with suspected acute ischemic stroke derived from ASA 2013 Early Management of Patients with Acute Ischemic Stroke Guidelines

Must have results prior to administering IV tPA	Noncontrast head CT or brain MRI
	Blood glucose
May administer IV tPA while results are pending*:	Serum electrolytes
	Renal function tests
	Complete blood count (including platelet count)
	Markers of cardiac ischemia
	PT/INR
	aPTT
	EKG

* Treatment with IV tPA should not be delayed while awaiting results of these tests unless there is suspicion for a bleeding diathesis, thrombocytopenia, or if the patient has received anticoagulation agents such as heparin, vitamin K antagonist, direct thrombin inhibitor, or direct factor Xa inhibitor.
aPTT, activated partial thromboplastin time; EKG, electrocardiogram; INR, international normalized ratio; IV tPA, intravenous recombinant tissue plasminogen activator; PT, prothrombin time.

should have a pregnancy test before undergoing neuroimaging or acute stroke therapies. Chest x-ray can provide information about lung opacities or reveal a widened mediastinum in cases concerning for aortic dissection, which should be confirmed with a CTA.

Lumbar puncture should be performed if the clinical presentation is concerning for SAH. Sentinel SAH is not well-detected on noncontrast head CT, and often precedes a later, larger aneurysmal SAH. The sensitivity of head CT for detecting SAH also declines after the first 24 hours if the patient presents for evaluation after that time period. If the patient had recently suffered a sentinel SAH, the cerebrospinal fluid (CSF) should contain red blood cells that do not clear between tubes one and four, and an elevated protein level. Xanthochromia may be present, which is detected as a yellowish tint when the CSF sample is held against a white surface, although spectrophotometry is much more sensitive than visual inspection alone.

Table 11.6 provides a summary of the recommended diagnostic studies for evaluation of acute ischemic stroke.

11.7 Management

Initial management should begin with correcting hemodynamic and cardiac abnormalities and treating respiratory insufficiency. Cardiac monitoring can reveal the presence of dangerous arrhythmias or atrial fibrillation. Supplemental oxygen should be used, if necessary, to keep oxygen saturation above 94%. Endotracheal intubation may be used for respiratory failure or airway protection, but only if absolutely necessary.

Hypotension, if present, should be treated promptly in order to minimize hypoperfusion to the region of brain ischemia. Blood pressure is commonly elevated in acute ischemic stroke, possibly as a physiologic response to increase or maintain cerebral perfusion. However, severe hypertension may cause hypertensive encephalopathy and cardiac or renal complications. It is unclear whether lowering very high blood pressure or allowing permissive hypertension affects outcome. Currently, the ASA recommends not treating hypertension unless the blood pressure is greater than 220/120 mm Hg. However, if the patient appears to be a candidate for intravenous thrombolytic acute stroke treatment, the blood pressure should be maintained below 185/110 mm Hg.

Hyperthermia is associated with poor neurologic outcome, but it is unclear whether treating hyperthermia improves outcome. Inducing hypothermia confers neuroprotective benefits in the setting of cardiac arrest, but its utility in stroke neuroprotection has not been established. Hypoglycemia can cause stroke-like symptoms and seizures, and should be corrected as soon as possible since prolonged hypoglycemia can lead to irreversible brain injury. Hyperglycemia, if present in the first 24 hours, is associated with worse clinical outcome, although it is unclear if aggressive early lowering of blood sugar improves outcome. The ASA recommends maintaining blood sugars in the range of 140–180 mg/dL in acute ischemic stroke.

Aspirin use within 24–48 hours of onset of acute ischemic stroke has been shown to reduce death and disability. The benefit of giving clopidogrel or aspirin with dipyridamole within this time period has not been established. There is no role at this time for administering intravenous antiplatelet agents such as glycoprotein IIb/IIIa receptor blockers. Studies do not demonstrate any benefit in using intravenous unfractionated heparin (UFH), which was standard practice for treating acute ischemic stroke in the past. UFH has been associated with an increased risk of bleeding, and heparin exposure increases the risk of developing heparin-induced thrombocytopenia. At this time, UFH is not recommended for treatment of acute ischemic stroke.

11.8 Acute Stroke Intervention

Time-based interventions have been shown to improve functional outcome after acute ischemic stroke. The two primary forms of stroke intervention, intravenous fibrinolysis and endovascular mechanical thrombectomy, will be discussed in the following sections.

Rapid evaluation and treatment are crucial to maximize the chances of attaining the best outcome possible. For every 30-minute delay in reperfusion, the relative likelihood of achieving a good outcome is reduced by 10%. All patients who present with ischemic stroke symptoms should be evaluated for both thrombolysis and endovascular treatment, which can be administered alone or in combination. Treatment with thrombolysis should not be delayed in eligible patients when they are being evaluated for endovascular clot retrieval. Figure 11.2 summarizes the potential pathways for acute stroke interventions and reflects the ASA 2019 Early Management of Patients with Acute Ischemic Stroke as well as the practice at our institution.

11.8.1 Intravenous Thrombolysis

Intravenous alteplase, or recombinant tissue plasminogen activator (IV tPA), was first approved by the FDA in 1996 for treatment of acute ischemic stroke, and it remains the standard of care today. Alteplase chemically lyses clots by converting plasminogen to plasmin, which binds to thrombus and dissolves its fibrin network. In the 1996 landmark NINDS trial, using alteplase to treat acute ischemic stroke resulted in better functional outcomes.

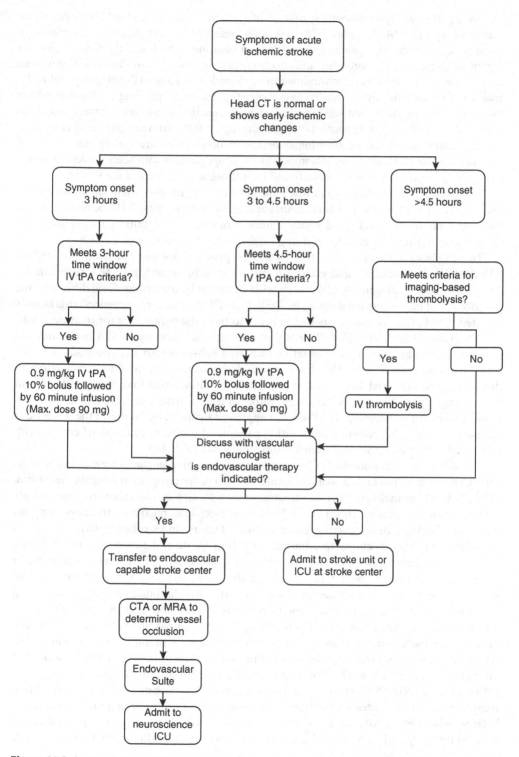

Figure 11.2 Acute ischemic stroke management decision tree based on the ASA 2019 Guideline Statement for Early Management of Patients with Acute Ischemic Stroke, and the practice at our institution.

Every patient who presents with symptoms of acute ischemic stroke should be evaluated for treatment with IV tPA. The phrase "time is brain" refers to the fact that for every minute of brain ischemia the average patient loses 1.9 million neurons. In addition, the time window for administering the medication safely and effectively is only 3 hours from the time of symptom onset or LKN (in select cases, the window can be extended to 4.5 hours). Subgroup and meta-analyses of multiple thrombolysis trials have shown that the earlier the drug is administered, the higher the chances the patient will experience a good functional outcome. Current guidelines recommend that the "door to needle time" (i.e., the time it takes from arriving at the hospital to starting treatment) should be 60 minutes or less in order to ensure speedy evaluation and treatment (Table 11.4). Therefore it is imperative to triage patients with acute stroke symptoms as rapidly as possible in order to identify and treat those who are eligible for IV tPA.

The most pertinent information when considering thrombolysis includes the following: LKN time, relevant medical history, neurologic examination using NIHSS, blood glucose level, and noncontrast CT head result. These components are critical to guiding early clinical decision-making and determining eligibility for treatment with IV tPA.

The eligibility criteria and IV tPA treatment protocol are derived from the original NINDS trial. The inclusion and exclusion criteria for administering IV tPA based on the ASA 2019 Early Management of Patients with Acute Ischemic Stroke Guidelines and the practice at our institution are detailed in Table 11.7. Of the standard exclusion criteria, only elevated blood pressure may be treated in order to meet the parameters for treatment with IV tPA (Table 11.8). The ECASS III trial showed that administering IV tPA between 3 and 4.5 hours after time of symptom onset or LKN in a subset of patients also leads to better functional outcomes. The ECASS III study included patients with similar characteristics to those in the NINDS trial, but excluded additional conditions that may increase the risk of hemorrhage: age > 80 years, NIHSS > 25, warfarin use regardless of INR, and a history of stroke and diabetes. Although IV tPA is not approved by the FDA for use in the 3–4.5 hour time window, the ASA recommends treating patients who meet the ECASS III criteria with IV tPA who present within the extended time window (Table 11.9).

The WAKE UP trial published in 2018 demonstrated positive outcomes for patients presenting >4.5 hours from last known well, but within 4.5 hours after recognition of stroke symptoms.

The ASA 2019 guidelines states that treatment with IV tPA can be considered in patients after additional eligibility criteria have been met. Decisions regarding treatment rely on results of additional neuroimaging, patient clinical factors, and stroke severity.

Relative contraindications to administering IV tPA do not necessarily preclude the patient from receiving the medication (Tables 11.7 and 11.9). If considering treatment in the presence of one or more relative contraindications, the risks of treatment must be weighed against the potential benefit in each case. Mild (nondisabling) or rapidly improving symptoms (with minor residual deficit) remains a common reason for withholding thrombolytic treatment since the risk of giving IV tPA is generally believed to outweigh the benefit in these patients. However, up to 30% of patients with mild or rapidly improving symptoms who are not treated have been found to have poor outcomes. Thus, treatment of this subset of patients is a subject of current study in randomized, controlled trials. Some patients with an NIHSS score <4 should be considered for treatment in the case of disabling symptoms, such as severe motor limb weakness or isolated homonymous hemianopia. Patients who present with seizure may be considered for treatment if it appears that the residual neurologic symptoms are likely due to brain ischemia rather than a postictal state.

Table 11.7 Intravenous tPA inclusion and exclusion criteria for the 3 hour time window of stroke symptom onset. These criteria are derived from the ASA 2019 Guideline Statement for Early Management of Patients with Acute Ischemic Stroke and from our institution's practice, and may vary from practice to practice based on case mix and experience

Inclusion criteria	Disabling ischemic stroke symptoms (NIHSS score ≥4, but some disabling symptoms may score <4)
	Symptom onset <3 hours from initiating treatment
	Age ≥18 years
Exclusion criteria	Prior intracranial hemorrhage
	Prior myocardial infarction in past 3 months
	Prior gastrointestinal or urinary tract hemorrhage in past 21 days
	Prior severe head trauma, intracranial surgery, or intraspinal surgery in past 3 months
	Presence of intracranial neoplasm, arteriovenous malformation, or aneurysm
	Major surgery or serious trauma in past 14 days
	Arterial puncture at noncompressible site in past 7 days
	Lumbar puncture in past 7 days
	Evidence of active bleeding or trauma on examination
	Active internal bleeding
	Uncontrolled hypertension at time of treatment (SBP >185 mm Hg or DBP >110 mm Hg)
	Receiving warfarin and INR >1.7
	Receiving heparin in past 48 hours and elevated aPTT
	Receiving direct thrombin inhibitor or direct factor Xa inhibitor within past 48 hours
	Receiving direct thrombin inhibitor or direct factor Xa inhibitor > past 48 hours with elevated INR, aPTT, TT, ECT, or factor Xa activity assay
	Platelet count <100,000/mm^3
	Noncontrast head CT shows intracranial hemorrhage or infarction with hypodensity >1/3 cerebral hemisphere
	Symptoms suggest subarachnoid hemorrhage
Relative exclusion criteria	Seizure at onset with postictal residual neurological impairment
	Prior ischemic stroke in past 3 months
	Minor neurological deficit (NIHSS score <4, excluding disabling symptoms such as hemianopia or severe limb weakness)
	Neurological deficits rapidly improving (clearing spontaneously)
	Blood glucose <50 or >400 mg/dL
	Pregnancy

NaPTT, activated partial thromboplastin time; ECT, ecarin clotting time; IHSS, National Institutes of Health Stroke Scale; INR, international normalized ratio; TT, thrombin time.

Table 11.8 Recommended treatment of blood pressure before and after thrombolytic therapy, based on ASA 2019 Guidelines for Early Management of Patients with Acute Ischemic Stroke and our institution's practice

Blood pressure parameters	Potential treatment approaches
If eligible for IV tPA	
SBP >185 mm Hg or DBP >110 mm Hg	Labetalol 10–20 mg IV over 1–2 minutes, can give 1–2 doses
	Nicardipine 5 mg/h IV continuous infusion, increase by 2.5 mg/h every 5–15 minutes until desired BP is achieved, maximum rate 15 mg/h
	May also use other agents when appropriate, such as clevidipine, enalapril, hydralazine, nitro paste
SBP >185 mm Hg or DBP >110 mm Hg despite BP treatment	Do not administer IV tPA
If after administering IV tPA:*	
SBP >180 mm Hg or DBP >105 mm Hg	Labetalol 10–20 mg IV over 1–2 minutes; may repeat dose every 10–20 minutes to a maximum dose of 300 mg
	Labetalol IV continuous infusion 2–8 mg/min
	Nicardipine 5 mg/h IV continuous infusion, increase by 2.5 mg/h every 5–15 minutes until desired BP is achieved, maximum rate 15 mg/h
BP still not controlled despite BP treatment or DBP >140 mm Hg	Consider using IV sodium nitroprusside

* After initiating treatment with IV tPA, monitor BP every 15 minutes for 2 hours, then every 30 minutes for 6 hours, then every hour for 16 hours. Elevated BP after treatment with IV tPA should be treated aggressively since higher BP is associated with increased risk of symptomatic intracranial hemorrhage.
IV tPA, intravenous recombinant tissue plasminogen activator.

Table 11.9 Additional inclusion and exclusion criteria for treatment with thrombolysis within the 3–4.5 hour time window of stroke symptom onset based on ASA 2019 Guideline Statement for Early Management of Patients with Acute Ischemic Stroke and from our institution's practice

Inclusion criteria	Disabling ischemic stroke symptoms (NIHSS score ≥4, but in some cases <4)
	Symptom onset within 3–4.5 hours from initiating treatment
Relative exclusion criteria	Age >80 years
	NIHSS >25
	Any oral anticoagulation use regardless of INR or other coagulation studies
	History of both diabetes and prior ischemic stroke

INR, international normalized ratio; NIHSS, National Institutes of Health Stroke Scale.

Novel oral anticoagulants (NOACs) present a special challenge in the evaluation of a stroke patient for thrombolysis. Direct thrombin inhibitors and direct factor Xa inhibitors do not result in reliable alterations of traditional coagulation tests, such as PT, INR, and aPTT. Thrombin time, ecarin clotting time, and anti-factor Xa activity assays provide more accurate information about the activity and circulating concentration of NOACs, but it can take hours for results to become available, limiting their usefulness in the emergency setting. The ASA recommends that thrombolysis should be considered in a patient taking a NOAC only if the last dose was ingested more than 48 hours ago, the traditional coagulation tests (PT/INR, aPTT) are normal, and renal and hepatic function are normal.

Table 11.6 lists diagnostic studies that should be performed when evaluating a patient for treatment with IV tPA. Note that thrombolytic therapy may be initiated before results are received for serum electrolytes, renal function, complete blood count with platelets, cardiac ischemia markers, PT/INR, aPTT, and electrocardiogram unless the patient is suspected to have a bleeding disorder, thrombocytopenia, or is taking an anticoagulant agent that may lead to abnormal findings. Retrospective reviews have found that the likelihood of unsuspected coagulopathy or thrombocytopenia in patients who have received thrombolysis is very low. If the patient receives IV tPA and subsequent test results reveal a coagulopathy or low platelet count, the infusion should be stopped immediately and the patient should be monitored closely for signs of bleeding. If the patient's coagulopathy places him at high risk of bleeding, consider administering cryoprecipitate to restore fibrinogen levels, and platelets if appropriate.

Treating acute ischemic stroke with IV tPA can be associated with some important complications. Since tPA lowers fibrinogen levels, symptomatic ICH, defined as ICH leading to neurologic deterioration, can occur in up to 6% of patients who receive the medication. Studies have shown that deviating from the NINDS treatment protocol is associated with higher rates of symptomatic ICH. Extracranial hemorrhage is also a real risk, particularly in patients with a recent history of trauma or recent arterial puncture. Additionally, procedures such as placement of a Foley catheter or intravenous lines should be performed prior to administering the drug and avoided afterwards, if possible, to minimize bleeding risk. Up to 5% of patients who receive IV tPA develop orolingual angioedema (i.e., swelling of the tongue, lips, or oropharynx), which can lead to airway obstruction. The risk is higher in patients taking an angiotensin-converting enzyme inhibitor (ACE-I) prior to treatment.

Patients who receive IV tPA should be admitted to an ICU at a stroke center that is experienced in caring for tPA-treated patients. ICU care should include close monitoring of vital signs and for any change in neurologic status or signs of bleeding. In the first 24 hours, when the risk of hemorrhagic complications is highest, specific measures need to be taken to reduce this risk. Blood pressure should be monitored frequently and maintained below 180/105 mm Hg (Table 11.8). Antiplatelet or anticoagulant agents should not be administered during this time. Nonemergent procedures, such as endoscopy, should be deferred until the 24 hours have passed. Patients who complain of headache or have worsening of neurologic symptoms should immediately undergo noncontrast head CT. If the imaging shows ICH, the tPA infusion – if still running – should be stopped, and cryoprecipitate may be given to restore depleted fibrinogen levels. Angioedema should also be treated with discontinuation of drug infusion and by administering ranitidine, diphenhydramine, and methylprednisolone. In severe cases of angioedema with impending airway compromise, epinephrine should be used and emergent endotracheal intubation should be considered. Icatibant, a selective bradykinin B2 receptor antagonist has been successfully used in hereditary angioedema and ACE-I-related angioedema.

11.8.2 Endovascular Thrombectomy

While thrombolysis for acute ischemic stroke has been shown to be effective in improving outcomes, this approach alone leads to recanalization of the occluded artery only 30% of the time on average. Smaller arteries, such as distal MCA branches, enjoy a rate of recanalization of up to 40%, but proximal large intracranial artery occlusions (i.e., the internal carotid artery terminus) experience recanalization as low as 8% of the time. The larger the size of the affected artery and the greater the thrombus length, the less likely it is that IV tPA alone will restore blood flow. Recanalization of the occluded artery is strongly associated with better functional outcomes and reduced mortality.

Endovascular methods of clot retrieval have not been shown to be effective until relatively recently. Prior trials investigating catheter-based thrombectomy in acute stroke suffered from slow recruitment due to the availability of open-label treatment outside of research studies and use of older-generation devices with relatively low recanalization rates. Furthermore, enrollment into these trials did not require imaging evidence of a large vessel occlusion, which likely further diluted the treatment effect.

In 2015, five trials were published showing that endovascular stroke therapy, when used in addition to IV tPA, was as safe as and more effective than treatment with IV tPA alone. The number of patients who need to be treated (NNT) with endovascular therapy for one patient to achieve functional independence in these studies ranges from 3 to 7, compared with IV tPA alone with an NNT of 8–14. The newer endovascular trials heavily or exclusively utilized the newest generation of clot removal devices – termed retrievable stents, or stent retrievers – that are associated with reported recanalization rates upward of 80%. The retrievable stent, tethered to a wire, is deployed within the thrombus. Its self-expanding radial force displaces the thrombus against the artery wall and traps the clot into the stent struts. The device, along with thrombus, is then withdrawn into the catheter (Figure 11.3). In addition to higher recanalization rates, retrievable stents have the advantage of transiently restoring blood flow prior to the actual removal of clot, which is not feasible with older-generation devices.

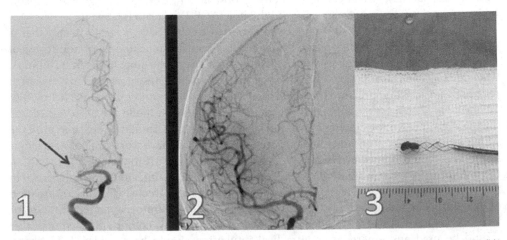

Figure 11.3 (1) AP projection digital subtraction angiography of the right internal carotid artery showing MCA (M1 segment) occlusion (arrow). (2) Recanalization of the right M1 segment occlusion after mechanical thrombectomy. (3) Stent retriever with clot attached to the stent retriever

These studies have demonstrated that treatment with endovascular clot retrieval results in better functional outcomes when compared to using IV tPA alone, despite risks that are unique to catheter-based treatments. Procedure-related complications, such as arterial dissection, vessel perforation, and formation of groin hematoma, do occur but are rare. Endovascular thrombectomy is associated with a statistically significant higher risk of ischemic stroke in a different arterial territory due to distal embolization of thrombus or plaque. However, the rates of mortality, overall serious adverse events, and symptomatic intracranial hemorrhage are similar to those of IV tPA alone.

Since 2015, the ASA recommends that patients with acute ischemic stroke should undergo endovascular clot retrieval if the patient meets the following criteria (Table 11.10): excellent prestroke functional status, eligible to receive IV tPA within the 4.5 hour time window, presence of an internal carotid artery or proximal MCA occlusion, NIHSS score ≥6, age ≥18 years, Alberta Stroke Program Early CT Score (ASPECTS) ≥6 (few early ischemic changes on head CT), and the potential to initiate the procedure within 6 hours of stroke onset. While this population represents only 10% of all patients with ischemic stroke, these patients tend to experience the most severe and disabling strokes, which likely contribute in a significant manner to overall stroke morbidity and mortality. There are insufficient data regarding the benefit of treatment in patients who do not meet all of the endovascular inclusion criteria, but treatment may still be considered in these patients, such as those who cannot receive IV tPA safely, with arterial occlusions at other sites, or who have poor ASPECTS scores. In early 2018, the ASA/AHA guidelines for acute endovascular stroke therapy were revised after the publication of two trials (DAWN and Defuse 3), which showed benefit of endovascular therapy in an extended time window up to 24 hours using perfusion imaging. CT or MRI perfusion can help identify the core or infarcted tissue as well as the penumbra or area at risk. The Defuse 3 trial enrolled patient up to 16 hours from LKN and used core – penumbra mismatch imaging criteria for selecting patients. The DAWN trial enrolled patients up to 24 hours from LKN and used clinical-imaging mismatch to select patients. The 2018 guidelines recommend endovascular therapy for patients with acute ischemic stroke from an ICA terminus or M1 segment occlusion meeting DAWN or DEFUSE 3 criteria (Table 11.11) within the 6–24 hour time period.

Table 11.10 ASA 2018 inclusion criteria for endovascular treatment of acute ischemic stroke 0–6 hours. Patients who do not meet all inclusion criteria may still benefit from endovascular thrombectomy and their individual cases should be discussed with a vascular neurologist

- Prestroke mRS score of 0–1 (no disability at baseline)
- Symptomatic occlusion of the internal carotid artery or proximal MCA (M1 segment)
- Age ≥18 years
- NIHSS score ≥6
- ASPECTS ≥6 (few early ischemic changes on head CT)
- Treatment can be initiated (defined by groin arterial puncture) within 6 hours of symptom onset

ASPECTS, Alberta Stroke Program Early CT Score, a grading system of early ischemic changes on noncontrast head CT; mRS, modified Rankin Score, a scale used to measure the degree of disability or dependence in activities of daily living; NIHSS, National Institutes of Health Stroke Scale.

Table 11.11 ASA 2018 inclusion criteria for endovascular treatment of acute ischemic stroke 6–24 hours based on DAWN and DEFUSE criteria

6–16 hours DEFUSE criteria	6–24 hours DAWN criteria
Age 18–90 years	Age ≥18
NIHSS ≥6	
Prestroke mRS ≤2	Prestroke mRS 0–1
ICA or M1 occlusion	Symptomatic occlusion of the internal carotid artery or proximal MCA (M1 segment)
Mismatch profile on CT perfusion or MRI: Ischemic core volume is <70 mL mismatch ratio is >1.8 and mismatch volume is >15 ml	Mismatch profile (CT perfusion or MRI): A. Age ≥80 y/o, NIHSS ≥10 + core <21 mL B. Age <80 y/o, NIHSS ≥10 + core <31 mL C. Age <80 y/o, NIHSS ≥20 + core <51 mL

mRS, modified Rankin Scale; NIHSS, National Institute of Health Stroke Scale.

Endovascular thrombectomy should always be considered in basilar artery occlusion, as long as an extensive infarct has not already developed. Untreated basilar artery occlusion is associated with a mortality rate of >80% and a high risk of significant disability.

Every patient who presents with acute ischemic stroke who is a candidate for IV tPA treatment should receive the drug as quickly as possible, even if endovascular intervention is being considered. Such patients should also undergo CTA or MRA to identify the presence of a large artery occlusion. However, advanced imaging studies should not be performed if doing so will prolong the transfer of the patient to a center that offers endovascular stroke treatment. Transport to the tertiary care center or comprehensive stroke center should be arranged without delay since a shorter time to treatment is associated with better functional outcome. Pre-hospital notification should be used to alert the receiving hospital so that the treatment team can mobilize in anticipation of the patient's arrival. Processes at the tertiary care center should be streamlined in order to obtain any necessary advanced imaging and to transfer the patient to the endovascular suite as quickly as possible.

The decision tree in management of acute ischemic stroke is detailed in Figure 11.2.

11.9 TIA Management

While TIA does not result in permanent brain infarction, 10–15% of people who experience TIA will have a stroke in the first 90 days, of which 50% occur within the first 48 hours. Up to 50% of people who present with stroke have had a TIA in the last 30 days. Forty-one percent of TIAs last less than one hour. The estimated incidence of TIA is 200,000–500,000 per year.

The $ACBD_2$ score is a validated prediction tool that assesses the patient's risk of stroke within the next 48 hours (Tables 11.12).

Whether the patient with TIA is hospitalized varies between hospitals and practitioners. While the $ACBD_2$ score predicts short-term stroke risk after TIA, its usefulness in assisting with triage decisions has not been demonstrated. Additionally, the benefit of hospitalization after TIA has not been studied. In our practice, we admit all patients who present with TIA. Advantages of hospitalization include clinical monitoring and the ability to administer thrombolytics or initiate endovascular thrombectomy in the event

Table 11.12a ACBD$_2$ score used in transient ischemic attack (TIA) risk stratification

Risk factor	Points
Age	
<60 years	0
≥60 years	1
Blood pressure (initial)	
<140/90 mm Hg	0
≥140/90 mm Hg	1
Category	
Speech impairment without focal weakness	1
Focal weakness	2
Duration	
<10 minutes	0
10–59 minutes	1
≥60 minutes	2
Diabetes	
No	0
Yes	1

Table 11.12b Risk of stroke within the next 48 hours based on ACBD$_2$ score

Score	48-hour risk of stroke
0–1	0%
2–3	1.3%
4–5	4.1%
6–7	8.1%

of an acute stroke. One analysis showed that hospitalizing TIA patients whose 24-hour risk of stroke was greater than 4% was cost-effective because of the ability to administer acute stroke treatment in-house. Continuous cardiac monitoring may result in detection of atrial fibrillation or flutter. Rapid diagnostic evaluation is another benefit of hospitalization and can include brain MRI, CTA or MRA, echocardiogram, and assessment of risk factors such as dyslipidemia and diabetes. In patients with a high ABCD$_2$ score (≥4), short-term use of aspirin and clopidogrel may be beneficial. Although UFH has not been shown to be beneficial in treating acute stroke, there may be a role for UFH or systemic anticoagulation in TIA in the presence of a causative large artery thrombus to prevent clot propagation or embolization.

11.10 Stroke Systems of Care

Implementing pre-hospital strategies for stroke management has increased the number of patients who can receive time-based acute stroke treatments. Education of 911 dispatchers, emergency medical services (EMS) staff, and the general public has led to a more widespread awareness of stroke, resulting in early recognition of stroke symptoms and rapid activation of pre-hospital EMS stroke protocols. Field management of stroke patients includes maintaining airway, breathing, and circulation; managing hypotension and hypoglycemia; starting an intravenous line; and in some systems obtaining blood samples prior to hospital arrival. A brief, relevant history should be obtained from the patient or witnesses, especially the time of onset or LKN. Ideally, EMS should obtain the contact information, such as cell phone numbers, from key observers who may be able to provide the treating physician with more detailed information. Various pre-hospital stroke screens are available for assessing the patient for stroke symptoms. The patient should be transported as rapidly as possible to the nearest primary stroke center (PSC) or thrombectomy-capable stroke center (TSC) or comprehensive stroke center (CSC), or if none is nearby, the closest stroke-ready hospital. In addition, there are pre-hospital stroke severity scales that help EMS providers determine the possibility of suspected large vessel occlusion and may improve triage to the appropriate stroke center. Air transport is recommended, if available, to transport the patient to the nearest stroke-capable hospital if it is greater than 1 hour away by ground. Pre-hospital notification should be sent to the receiving hospital in order to facilitate rapid assessment upon patient arrival.

Hospitals that experience high stroke volume, have dedicated stroke units, and are certified stroke centers have better clinical outcomes than comparable centers without such characteristics. An acute stroke-ready hospital (ASRH) has the ability to stabilize the patient and provide acute stroke treatment (i.e., thrombolytics) prior to transfer to the nearest PSC, TSC, or CSC. ASRHs are usually smaller rural or suburban facilities that enjoy telemedicine or telephone consultation support and expertise from a PSC or CSC.

PSCs are typically designated and certified through the Joint Commission and are equipped to care for the majority of stroke patients. Some centers provide ICU level of care. Having PSC designation is associated with higher rates of IV tPA administration as well as lower mortality and improved outcome.

CSCs also undergo a certification process through the Joint Commission and have the experience and expertise to manage the most complex stroke patients, such as those who may be a candidate for endovascular thrombectomy or those with intracranial hemorrhage. CSCs have capabilities commonly seen in tertiary care hospitals. These centers provide endovascular and neurosurgical interventions on a 24-hour basis and have neuroscience ICUs staffed by intensivists. Vascular neurologists are available around the clock for emergency consultations, treatment decisions, and patient management issues. Other advantages include the ability to perform specialized procedures such as hemicraniectomy, ventricular drain placement, conventional cerebral angiography, endovascular thrombectomy, carotid endarterectomy, and carotid stent placement.

TSCs are hospitals with capabilities between those of a PSC and a CSC. These centers, in addition to intravenous thrombolysis, are also capable of endovascular therapy for acute ischemic stroke.

11.11 Telemedicine and Telestroke

The American Telemedicine Association defines telemedicine as "the use of medical information exchanged from one site to another via electronic communications to improve a patient's clinical health status." The growth of telemedicine over time has led to the widespread use of this technology in the evaluation and management of acute stroke patients, otherwise known as telestroke.

Prior to the advent of telestroke, neurologists provided telephone consultations to emergency physicians to assist in decision-making with regard to use of thrombolytics in acute stroke patients. In 1999, Levine and Gorman demonstrated that IV tPA can be administered safely to patients when remotely evaluated by a stroke expert using state-of-the-art video telecommunication systems. The lack of access to stroke expertise and experience in using IV tPA is a known barrier to treating ischemic stroke patients with thrombolytics, resulting in low treatment rates. Evaluating patients using a telestroke system has the potential to increase the use of IV tPA in eligible patients by providing 24-hour expert stroke coverage in hospitals that would otherwise lack such resources. The NIHSS easily lends itself as a rapidly administered and standardized tool in assessing stroke patients via telecommunication systems. Continued advances in technology result in higher speeds of data transfer, higher resolution video, and increasing portability and mobility, thus improving the quality and versatility of telestroke communications over time.

Today, a telestroke system involves two-way high-resolution audiovisual communication with a mobile platform on the patient end and a computer or tablet on the physician end. The hub-and-spoke model is the most common setup, with a CSC or tertiary care center acting as the hub for multiple outlying, smaller spoke hospitals, allowing the spokes to access the hub's resources and specialty expertise. Telestroke is often used in conjunction with teleradiology, in which neuroimaging is interpreted remotely on an emergency basis by a radiologist in order to assist in acute stroke management decisions.

11.12 Cerebral Venous Thrombosis

Cerebral infarcts do not always have an arterial etiology and may occur from thrombosis of the dural sinuses and cerebral veins (Figure 11.4a). Occlusion of these vessels compromises the drainage of blood from the brain, leading to increased pressure and local brain edema. Buildup of venous pressure may cause hemorrhage by breakage of capillaries and arterioles. Brain infarction occurs if the arterial perfusion pressure cannot overcome the increased venous pressure in the affected territory (Figure 11.4b).

Infarcts due to cerebral venous thrombosis (CVT) are not common, accounting for up to 1% of all strokes. Women are three times more likely than men to develop CVT, and in one cohort study 78% of CVT occurred in patients younger than 50 years of age. Common risk factors for developing CVT include dehydration, traumatic head injury, pregnancy, oral contraceptive use, meningitis, otitis or mastoid infections, prothrombotic state induced by malignancy, and primary hypercoagulable conditions.

Because venous occlusions develop and propagate more slowly than arterial occlusions, symptoms may have a slower onset and progress over days to months before the problem is recognized, which can lead to delays in diagnosis. Headache is the most common symptom of CVT, with an incidence of nearly 90%, and may be the only symptom in some patients. Manifestations of headache range from thunderclap headache to migraine. Increased intracranial pressure causes blurry vision from papilledema and diplopia from a sixth

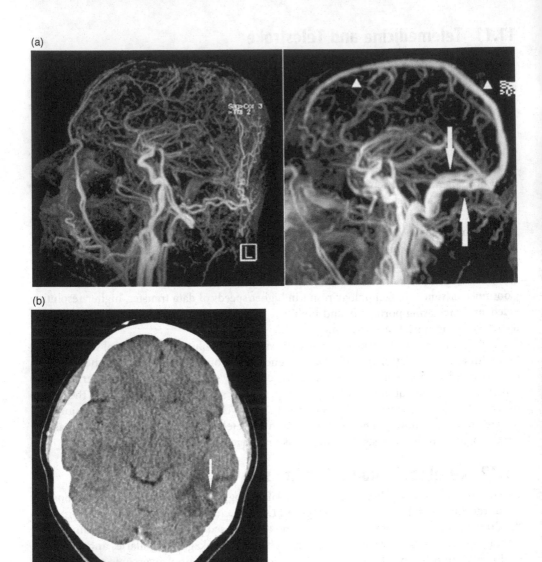

Figure 11.4 (a) Magnetic resonance (MR) venogram 3D reconstruction, lateral view, of thrombosis of the superior sagittal sinus and bilateral transverse and sigmoid sinuses (left) and recanalized dural sinuses after 12 months of treatment with warfarin (right). Large arrows indicate transverse sinuses and small arrowheads indicate superior sagittal sinus (right), which were not visualized on the initial MR venogram (left). (b) Cerebral venous sinus thrombosis with stroke and small hemorrhage (arrow) in the left temporal lobe on noncontrast head CT.

nerve palsy. Focal neurologic symptoms may develop in the territory affected by venous congestion or infarct. New-onset seizures are common, occurring in 40% of patients. When the deep cerebral veins are occluded, bilateral thalamic involvement may result in a depressed level of consciousness, often to the point of stupor or coma.

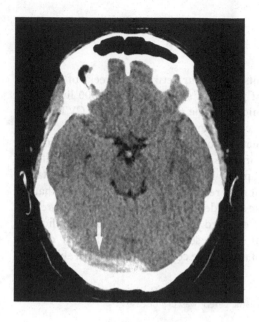

Figure 11.5 Hyperdense signal from thrombus in the right transverse dural venous sinus (arrow) on noncontrast head CT.

Head CT or brain MRI may detect venous congestion, infarct, or hemorrhage, but cannot definitively rule out CVT. A dural sinus thrombus may have a bright, or hyperdense, appearance on noncontrast head CT (Figure 11.5) or cause the appearance of absence of a flow void on MRI. A CT or MR venogram should be done to directly visualize the presence of venous thrombus. There is little utility in performing a lumbar puncture in CVT unless there is a clinical suspicion for meningitis.

Systemic anticoagulation appears to be safe and effective in the treatment of CVT, even in the presence of hemorrhage, based on data from several randomized clinical trials and observational studies. However, up to 13% of patients have poor outcome despite treatment with anticoagulation, thought to be due to a very extensive thrombus burden that responds poorly to medical therapy. In such severe cases, endovascular administration of local tPA or endovascular mechanical clot retrieval can be considered. Surgical decompression or evacuation of clot in intracranial hemorrhage may be necessary as a life-saving measure in the case of impending herniation syndromes from cerebral edema or hematoma-induced mass effect.

There does not appear to be any role for aspirin use in CVT. Although steroids can decrease vasogenic edema, they may increase hypercoagulability and their use is associated with an increased risk of mortality and disability. If seizure is present, the patient should be treated with antiepileptic medication. If infection is the etiology of CVT, the appropriate antibiotics should be used. Obstruction of CSF outflow may result in intracranial hypertension, which can be reduced with acetazolamide, which decreases CSF production. Severe cases that are refractory to acetazolamide should be treated with serial lumbar punctures or a lumboperitoneal shunt. If papilledema and vision loss continue to progress despite the above therapies, optic nerve sheath fenestration may be necessary.

11.13 Pediatric Stroke

11.13.1 Stroke in Neonates

Perinatal stroke refers to cerebrovascular events that occur between 28 weeks of gestation and the first 28 days of life. The incidence of perinatal stroke is 1 per 3,500 live births. Eighty percent of perinatal strokes are ischemic, with the remainder due to CVT or ICH (excluding SAH or intraventricular hemorrhage of prematurity).

Seizure is a common presentation for perinatal stroke, with ischemic stroke accounting for 10% of neonatal seizures. However, many infants are asymptomatic at birth, although developmental delay or early handedness can appear later on. The nature of fetal gestation and the process of birth present conditions that may result in risk factors for stroke that are unique to neonates. Major risk factors for stroke include intrauterine asphyxia, birth-related complications (e.g., placental abruption, umbilical cord prolapse), respiratory insufficiency from meconium aspiration, and left-to-right shunts seen in congenital heart disease. Perinatal stroke may also occur as the result of any of the conditions listed in Table 11.13.

Table 11.13 Risk factors for pediatric cerebrovascular disease

Congenital and acquired heart disease

Tetralogy of Fallot

Transposition of great vessels

Tricuspid atresia

Atrial and ventricular septal defects

Cardiomyopathies

Endocarditis

Pulmonary arteriovenous fistula

Cardiac myxoma

Coarctation of the aorta

Systemic vascular disease

Hypertension

Diabetes

Dehydration

Systemic disorders

Sjögren's syndrome

Scleroderma

Crohn's disease

Ulcerative colitis

Cryoglobulinemia

Migraine (vasospastic)

Table 11.13 (cont.)

Infectious

Facial, otitic, or sinus infections

Venous dural sinus occlusion and infection

Mycotic aneurysm

Vasculitis

Behçet's syndrome

Takayasu arteritis

Polyarteritis nodosa

Drug abuse (cocaine, heroin)

Acquired immunodeficiency syndrome (AIDS)

Bacterial meningitis

Varicella

Rheumatoid arthritis

Tuberculous meningitis

Vasculopathies

Systemic lupus erythematosus

Neurofibromatosis

Marfan syndrome

Ehlers–Danlos syndrome

Pseudoxanthoma elasticum

Moyamoya syndrome

Fibromuscular dysplasia

Polycystic kidney disease

Genetic and metabolic

Hyperhomocysteinemia

Homocystinuria

Menkes' kinky hair syndrome

Hypoalphalipoproteinemia

Familial hyperlipidemias

Methylmalonic aciduria

MELAS syndrome (mitochondrial encephalopathy, lactic acidosis, and stroke-like episodes)

Cytochrome oxidase deficiency

Fabry disease

Paroxysmal nocturnal hemoglobinuria

Table 11.13 (cont.)

Hematologic disorders and coagulopathies

Sickle cell anemia

Leukemia

L-arginase and aminocaproic acid treatment

Radiation vasculopathy

Antithrombin III deficiency

Protein C deficiency

Protein S deficiency

Factor V Leiden mutation

Prothrombin gene mutation

Antiphospholipid antibody syndrome

Malignancy/cancer

Thrombocytosis

Polycythemia vera

Thrombotic thrombocytopenic purpura

Disseminated intravascular coagulation

Venous sinus thrombosis

Hormonal contraceptive use

Congenital cerebrovascular anomalies

Arteriovenous malformation

Cavernous malformation

Cerebral aneurysm

Trauma

Child abuse

Intraoral trauma

Traumatic arterial dissection

When stroke is suspected in a neonate, cranial ultrasound, which is widely available, may be used to detect intracranial hemorrhage or ischemia. However, it may not be able to detect all ischemic lesions. CT is fast and also widely available, but it may miss early ischemic lesions in acute and hyperacute stroke. Additionally, CT exposes the neonate to ionizing radiation, which is associated with an increased risk of lifetime cancer in children who are exposed to even low radiation doses. MRI is an alternative to ultrasound and CT, and has the advantages of being very sensitive for detecting ischemia and avoiding exposure to harmful radiation. MR angiogram and MR venogram may be used to evaluate for the presence of an arterial or venous occlusive lesion.

Management of perinatal stroke typically involves supportive medical care. The use of thrombolytics and endovascular mechanical thrombectomy is not recommended outside of clinical trials as the safety and efficacy of these treatments in this population have not been established. Systemic anticoagulation is not commonly used unless there is concern for potential thrombus propagation or high risk of embolism. In CVT, systemic anticoagulation is shown to be safe and effective in small studies. Serial imaging for clot propagation is recommended if systemic anticoagulation is not used. In cases of ICH or intraventricular hemorrhage, placement of a ventricular drain or clot evacuation may be considered in the presence of elevated intracranial pressure, although it is not clear that these procedures improve outcome. Correction of low platelet counts, clotting factor deficiencies, and vitamin K deficiency is also recommended for perinatal ICH.

Long-term sequelae of neonatal stroke can take several forms. Sensory impairment may manifest as difficulty with visuospatial tasks. Cognitive impairment and speech abnormalities may develop. Cerebral palsy is a common sequela of stroke, often characterized by hemi- or quadriparesis. Even in the event of initial severe motor weakness, most neonates learn to walk independently before two years of age. Although most do not go on to develop seizure disorders, the presence of poststroke epilepsy may indicate a higher risk for neurodevelopmental abnormalities.

11.13.2 Stroke in Children and Adolescents

Ischemic stroke affects 1–2/100,000 children in the western developed countries per year while hemorrhagic stroke has an incidence of 1–1.7/100,000 per year. Of all childhood stroke, 55% are ischemic and 45% are hemorrhagic, compared with 85% ischemic in the adult population. Even when infarct is present on neuroimaging, focal neurologic symptoms are often transient in nature. The risk of clinical or radiologic recurrence of ischemic stroke is 6–14% even on antithrombotic medications. The strongest predictor of recurrence is presence of arteriopathy. While the most common causes of stroke in children are sickle cell disease and congenital or acquired heart disease, up to one-third of ischemic strokes have no identifiable cause.

Risk factors and etiologies of ischemic stroke in children are numerous and are summarized in Table 11.13. The most common causes are cardiac embolism, arterial dissection, CVT, coagulopathy, and arteriopathy.

Sickle cell disease causing ischemic stroke in children has reported incidences from 285 to as high as 600 per 100,000 per year. Some develop a progressive vasculopathy that leads to stenosis or occlusion of the distal internal carotid arteries, known as moyamoya syndrome. The proximal MCAs and posterior circulation are less commonly affected. CVT may also develop and cause venous infarcts. Treatment of acute ischemic stroke in a patient with sickle cell disease involves hydration; correction of hypoxia, hypotension, hypovolemia; and maintenance of normoglycemia. Although regular periodic blood transfusions have been shown to reduce the risk of stroke in these patients, studies have not proven the utility of blood transfusions in the setting of acute stroke. However, using exchange transfusion to reduce sickle hemoglobin to less than 30% of total hemoglobin may be considered.

Moyamoya can occur outside of the context of sickle cell disease. It is the most common cause of pediatric stroke in Japan (incidence 3 per 100,000 per year) and accounts for 6% of childhood stroke in the west (0.086 per 100,000 per year). The term "moyamoya" in Japanese roughly translates to "puff of smoke," which refers to the angiographic appearance of fine, delicate collateral circulation that forms over time. Vasculitis of intracranial arteries may cause ischemic stroke or ICH and is most commonly caused by autoimmune (lupus, Takayasu arteritis) or infectious (varicella zoster, tuberculosis) etiologies.

Cervical and intracranial arterial dissection may occur as the result of trauma, collagen disorders such as Ehlers–Danlos type IV and Marfan syndrome, aortic coarctation, polycystic kidney disease, or fibromuscular dysplasia. The dissection flap and false lumen may be seen on CT or MR angiogram, and fat-saturated T1 MRI sequences may detect the presence of blood in the dissected vessel wall. Optimal treatment is unclear and based on the adult literature, and secondary stroke reduction with either antiplatelet therapy or anticoagulation may be considered.

Congenital cardiac disease may result in right-to-left shunts and chronic cyanosis, as well as emboli in the heart or pulmonary artery, which can lead to ischemic stroke. Other cardiac sources of embolus include valvular disease, infectious endocarditis, cardiomyopathy with low ejection fraction, cardiac myxoma, and paradoxical embolism with right-to-left shunts.

Hypercoagulable disorders may be inherited or acquired and include antithrombin III deficiency, protein C or S deficiencies, factor V Leiden mutation, hyperhomocysteinemia, and polycythemia vera. Pregnancy should be considered as a possible cause of a prothrombotic state in teenage girls. CVT presents similarly to that of adults, and is treated with 3–6 months of systemic anticoagulation.

Intracranial hemorrhage in children is most commonly caused by arteriovenous malformations (AVMs) or cavernous malformations. AVMs are usually present at birth, and while they tend to present in adulthood, up to 20% are symptomatic in childhood. This condition is treated with microsurgical obliteration, stereotactic radiotherapy, endovascular embolization, or a combination of the aforementioned therapies. Cavernous malformations may be sporadic or familial, and can increase in size over time due to recurrent hemorrhage and subsequent tissue fibrosis and calcification. These are also treated with microsurgery or radiotherapy. Cerebral aneurysms are the most common cause of SAH in children and may be due to an underlying collagen disorder, coarctation of the aorta, polycystic kidney disease, or mycotic aneurysm.

If stroke is suspected in the pediatric patient, obtaining an accurate recent history and past medical history is fundamental to eliciting the potential etiology. The presence of headache may suggest ICH, SAH, or CVT. A history of congenital heart disease may point to a cardiac embolic source. Recent fevers or sickness exposures may reveal an infectious etiology. Arterial dissection or ICH may occur in the setting of trauma, and illegal drug use may cause stroke by vasoconstriction or particulate emboli. The use of oral contraceptives or pregnancy may induce a prothrombotic state.

In the general physical exam, elevated blood pressure may indicate SAH or increased intracranial pressure. Papilledema on fundoscopy or a bulging fontanelle in infants is also highly suggestive of increased intracranial pressure. Cardiac murmurs and arrhythmias may be auscultated in congenital or acquired heart disease. Diminished peripheral pulses may be present in coarctation of the aorta. The skin should be examined for signs of varicella infection or neurocutaneous disorders.

Findings on the neurologic exam may differ from the adult in that it should be tailored to the patient's present level of consciousness and developmental stage. Children and infants with stroke may have seizures as their primary symptom. Acute hemiplegia is the most common sign of acute ischemic stroke in children, and it often resolves with little or no residual symptoms within a matter of weeks. Sensory and cognitive symptoms are unusual unless the infarct involves bilateral structures. Extrapyramidal signs, such as dystonia, chorea, and athetosis, are more often seen in children than adults.

As with neonates, the use of diagnostic CT in children entails exposure to ionizing radiation, which is associated with an increase in the lifetime risk of cancer. However, CT is easily and quickly obtained, and is very sensitive for ICH. Brain MRI may be obtained if head CT is nondiagnostic or as an alternative in order to avoid exposure to radiation. MRA or CTA may be performed to identify the site of arterial occlusion or underlying vascular malformation. In addition to a complete metabolic panel and complete blood count, laboratory testing may include a toxicology screen, sickle cell screen, pregnancy test, homocysteine level, coagulation studies, and lumbar puncture when appropriate.

Management of pediatric stroke involves treating the underlying etiology. The use of thrombolytics has not been studied in a controlled trial in this population and is not recommended. Endovascular mechanical thrombectomy has not been studied in children but may be considered in select cases. Aspirin may be used in children who are at risk of recurrent stroke. Systemic anticoagulation is rarely used unless there is a specific indication. Infectious etiologies should be treated with antibiotics, and seizures should be controlled with antiepileptic agents. Increased intracranial pressure should be addressed urgently in order to prevent life-threatening herniation syndromes.

Pearls and Pitfalls

- "Time is brain." Patients with symptoms of acute stroke should be evaluated immediately to determine if they are candidates for IV thrombolysis or endovascular mechanical thrombectomy.
- Use questions about environmental cues to establish the time of onset of acute stroke symptoms as precisely as possible since some stroke syndromes reduce patient insight, which can result in unreliable answers to direct questions about timing. The time window for IV tPA is 4.5 hours from last known normal.
- If a patient has acute stroke symptoms that resolve, the time of symptom recurrence may be used as the new time of symptom onset.
- Rapidly improving symptoms may be considered a contraindication to IV tPA only if the residual symptoms are mild.
- Patients with relative contraindications to receiving IV tPA may be considered for treatment on a case-by-case basis if the potential benefit of treatment is believed to outweigh the risk.
- Basilar artery occlusions can present with atypical symptoms such as confusion, depressed level of consciousness, bilateral weakness, gait ataxia, gaze paresis, and vomiting. There should be a low threshold to evaluate a patient for suspected basilar artery occlusion, regardless of time of symptom onset, since untreated occlusions have a mortality rate of 80% or higher.
- Patients who do not meet all of the inclusion criteria for endovascular clot retrieval may still benefit from the procedure, and their cases should be discussed with a vascular neurologist.
- The time window for mechanical thrombectomy for large vessel occlusion strokes is 24 hours; however, the sooner therapy can be initiated the better.
- Transfer to another center for endovascular clot retrieval should occur without delay.
- Stroke can occur at any stage in life, from infants to children to adults of any age.

Bibliography

Barrett KM, Levine JM, Johnston KC. Diagnosis of stroke and stroke mimics in the emergency setting. *Continuum Lifelong Learning Neurol* 2008;14(6):13–27.

Benjamin E, Muntner P, Alonso A, et al. Heart disease and stroke statistics – 2019 update. *Circulation* 2019;139:10.

Berkhemer OA, Fransen PS, Beumer D, et al. A randomized trial of intraarterial treatment for acute ischemic stroke. *N Engl J Med* 2015;372(1):11–20.

Broderick JP, Palesch YY, Demchuk AM, et al. Endovascular therapy after intravenous t-PA versus t-PA alone for stroke. *N Engl J Med* 2013;368(10):893–903.

Campbell BC, Donnan GA, Lees KR, et al. Endovascular stent thrombectomy: the new standard of care for large vessel ischaemic stroke. *Lancet Neurol* 2015;14(8):846–854.

Campbell BC, Mitchell PJ, Kleinig TJ, et al. Endovascular therapy for ischemic stroke with perfusion-imaging selection. *N Engl J Med* 2015;372(11):1009–1018.

Caplan, LR. *Caplan's Stroke: A Clinical Approach*, 4th ed. Saunders Elsevier, 2009.

Ciccone A, Valvassori L, Nichelatti M, et al. Endovascular treatment for acute ischemic stroke. *N Engl J Med* 2013;368(10):904–913.

del Zoppo GJ, Poeck K, Pessin MS, et al. Recombinant tissue plasminogen activator in acute thrombotic and embolic stroke. *Ann Neurol* 1992;32(1):78–86.

Demaerschalk BM, Berg J, Chong BW, et al. American telemedicine association: telestroke guidelines. *Telemed e-Health* 2017;23(5):376–389.

DeMyer, WE. *Technique of the Neurologic Examination: A Programmed Text*, 5th ed. McGraw-Hill, 2004.

Easton JD, Saver JL, Albers GW, et al. Definition and evaluation of transient ischemic attack: a scientific statement for healthcare professionals from the American Heart Association/American Stroke Association Stroke Council; Council on Cardiovascular Surgery and Anesthesia; Council on Cardiovascular Radiology and Intervention; Council on Cardiovascular Nursing; and the Interdisciplinary Council on Peripheral Vascular Disease. American Academy of Neurology affirms the value of this statement as an educational tool for neurologists. *Stroke* 2009;40(6):2276–2293.

Emberson J, Lees KR, Lyden P, et al. Effect of treatment delay, age, and stroke severity on the effects of intravenous thrombolysis with alteplase for acute ischaemic stroke: a meta-analysis of individual patient data from randomised trials. *Lancet* 2014;384 (9958):1929–1935.

Ferriero D, Fullerton H, Bernard T, et al. Management of stroke in neonates and children. *Stroke* 2019;50:3.

Fonarow GC, Zhao X, Smith EE, et al. Door-to-needle times for tissue plasminogen activator administration and clinical outcomes in acute ischemic stroke before and after a quality improvement initiative. *JAMA* 2014;311(16):1632–1640.

Goyal M, Demchuk AM, Menon BK, et al. Randomized assessment of rapid endovascular treatment of ischemic stroke. *N Engl J Med* 2015;372(11):1019–1030.

Hacke W, Donnan G, Fieschi C, et al. Association of outcome with early stroke treatment: pooled analysis of ATLANTIS, ECASS, and NINDS rt-PA stroke trials. *Lancet* 2004;363(9411):768–774.

Hacke W, Kaste M, Bluhmki E, et al. Thrombolysis with alteplase 3 to 4.5 hours after acute ischemic stroke. *N Engl J Med* 2008;359(13):1317–1329.

Higashida R, Alberts MJ, Alexander DN, et al. Interactions within stroke systems of care: a policy statement from the American Heart Association/American Stroke Association. *Stroke* 2013;44(10):2961–2984.

Jauch EC, Saver JL, Adams HP, et al. Guidelines for the early management of patients with acute ischemic stroke: a guideline for healthcare professionals from the American Heart Association/American Stroke Association. *Stroke* 2013;44(3):870–947.

Jovin TG, Demchuk AM, Gupta R. Pathophysiology of acute ischemic stroke.

Continuum Lifelong Learning Neurol 2008;14 (6):28–45.

Jovin TG, Chamorro A, Cobo E, et al. Thrombectomy within 8 hours after symptom onset in ischemic stroke. *N Engl J Med* 2015;372(24):2296–2306.

Kernan WN, Ovbiagele B, Black HR, et al. Guidelines for the prevention of stroke in patients with stroke and transient ischemic attack: a guideline for healthcare professionals from the American Heart Association/American Stroke Association. *Stroke* 2014;45(7):2160–2236.

Khatri P. Evaluation and management of acute ischemic stroke. *Continuum (Minneap Minn)* 2014;20(2):283–295.

Khatri P, Levine J, Jovin T. Intravenous thrombolytic therapy for acute ischemic stroke. *Continuum Lifelong Learning Neurol* 2008;14(6):46–60.

Kidwell C, Jahan R, Gornbein J, et al. A trial of imaging selection and endovascular treatment for ischemic stroke. *N Engl J Med* 2013;368(10):914–923.

Levine SR, Gorman M. "Telestroke": the application of telemedicine for stroke. *Stroke* 1999;30(2):464–469.

Mohr JP, Wolf PA, Grotta JC, et al. *Stroke: Pathophysiology, Diagnosis, and Management*, 3rd ed. Elsevier Saunders, 2011.

Mozaffarian D, Benjamin EJ, Go AS, et al. Heart disease and stroke statistics – 2015 update: a report from the American Heart Association. *Circulation* 2015;131(4):e29–e322.

Mutgi SA, Zha AM, Behrouz R. Emerging subspecialties in neurology: telestroke and teleneurology. *Neurology* 2015;84(22):e191–e193.

National Institute of Neurological Disorders and Stroke rt-PA Stroke Study Group. Tissue plasminogen activator for acute ischemic stroke. *N Engl J Med* 1995;333 (24):1581–1587.

National Institute of Neurological Disorders and Stroke (NINDS). NIH stroke scale. Available at: www.ninds.nih.gov/doctors/NIH_Stroke_Scale.pdf.

Nogueira RG, Lutsep HL, Gupta R, et al. Trevo versus Merci retrievers for thrombectomy revascularization of large vessel occlusions in acute ischaemic stroke (TREVO 2): a randomized trial. *Lancet* 2012;380 (9849):1231–1240.

Powers WJ, Derdeyn CP, Biller J, et al. 2015 AHA/ASA Focused update of the 2013 guidelines for the early management of patients with acute ischemic stroke regarding endovascular treatment: a guideline for healthcare professionals from the American Heart Association/American Stroke Association. *Stroke*. 2015;46:3020–3035.

Powers WJ, Rabinstein AA, Ackerson T, et al. 2018 guidelines for the early management of patients with acute ischemic stroke: a guideline for healthcare professionals from the American Heart Association/American Stroke Association. *Stroke* 2018;49(3): e46–e99.

Rha J, Saver JL. The impact of recanalization on ischemic stroke outcome: a meta-analysis. *Stroke* 2007;38(3):967–973.

Roach ES, Golomb MR, Adams R, et al. Management of stroke in infants and children: a scientific statement from a Special Writing Group of the American Heart Association Stroke Council and the Council on Cardiovascular Disease in the Young. *Stroke* 2008;39(9):2644–2691.

Rohan V, Baxa J, Tupy R, et al. Length of occlusion predicts recanalization and outcome after intravenous thrombolysis in middle cerebral artery stroke. *Stroke* 2014;45 (7):2010–2017.

Rudkin S, Cerejo R, Tayal A, Goldberg MF. Imaging of acute ischemic stroke. *Emerg Radiol* 2018;1:1–4.

Saposnik G, Barinagarrementeria F, Brown RD Jr, et al. Diagnosis and management of cerebral venous thrombosis: a statement for healthcare professionals from the American Heart Association/American Stroke Association. *Stroke* 2011;42(4):1158–1192.

Saver JL. Time is brain – quantified. *Stroke* 2006;37(1):263–266.

Saver JL, Fonarow GC, Smith EE, et al. Time to treatment with intravenous tissue plasminogen activator and outcome from acute ischemic stroke. *JAMA* 2013;**309**(23):2480–2488.

Saver JL, Goyal M, Bonafe A, et al. Stent-retriever thrombectomy after intravenous t-PA vs. t-PA alone in stroke. *N Engl J Med* 2015;**372**(24):2285–2295.

Saver JL, Jahan R, Levy EI, et al. Solitaire flow restoration device versus the Merci Retriever in patients with acute ischaemic stroke (SWIFT): a randomized, parallel-group, non-inferiority trial. *Lancet* 2012;**380**(9849):1241–1249.

Thurman RJ, Jauch EC. Acute ischemic stroke: emergent evaluation and management. *Emerg Med Clin N Am* 2002;**20**(3):609–630.

Wardlaw JM, Murray V, Berge E, et al. Recombinant tissue plasminogen activator for acute ischaemic stroke: an updated systematic review and meta-analysis. *Lancet* 2012;**379**(9834):2364–2372.

Warner JJ, Harrington RA, Sacco RL, Elkind MS. Guidelines for the early management of patients with acute ischemic stroke: 2019 update to the 2018 guidelines for the early management of acute ischemic stroke. Stroke. 2019 Dec;50(12):3331–2.

Wijdicks EF, Scott JP. Outcome in patients with acute basilar artery occlusion requiring mechanical ventilation. *Stroke* 1996;**27**(8):1301–1303.

Chapter 12

Intracranial Hemorrhage

Crystal Wong, Khaled Aziz, and Bertram Richter

12.1 Introduction

Nontraumatic intracerebral hemorrhage (ICH) affects more than one million people per year worldwide and accounts for 10% of strokes in the United States. Aneurysm rupture is the most common cause of nontraumatic subarachnoid hemorrhage (SAH) and is often associated with significant morbidity and mortality. Subdural and epidural hemorrhages may be induced by head trauma and can be life-threatening if not closely monitored and treated. The widespread use of systemic anticoagulant agents for cardiac and prothrombotic conditions raises the risk of all types of intracranial hemorrhage and presents unique challenges in acute management. Treatment of intracranial hemorrhage is geared toward minimizing hematoma expansion, reducing increased intracranial pressure (ICP), and surgically treating aneurysms, vascular malformations, and herniation syndromes.

12.2 Intracerebral Hemorrhage

The most common risk factor for ICH is long-standing hypertension. Very high blood pressure can lead to increased arterial pressure and rupture (Figure 12.1). Chronic high blood pressure can lead to vasculopathy of the small, penetrating arteries of the brain in the form of lipohyalinosis and Charcot–Bouchard aneurysms, which also increase the risk of bleeding. Characteristic sites for hypertension-related ICH are the cerebellum, pons, basal ganglia, and thalamus.

Cerebral amyloid angiopathy (CAA) is a frequent cause of ICH located in the lobes of the brain in patients 65 years of age or older (Figure 12.2). Autopsy or biopsy reveals beta-amyloid deposition in the leptomeningeal and cortical arteries. Trauma can result in frontal or temporal lobe contusions and hemorrhage. Systemic anticoagulation may lead to spontaneous ICH in some patients, even if coagulation targets are at goal and no dosing errors have occurred. Bleeding diatheses such as hemophilia, thrombocytopenia, and disseminated intravascular coagulation are also risk factors for ICH but are often accompanied by extracranial bleeding events as well. Illegal substance use should be considered in younger patients with ICH. Sympathomimetic drugs such as amphetamines and cocaine can cause vasoconstriction and fusiform dilatation, which gives a beading appearance on conventional angiogram.

Vascular malformations often present with ICH; arteriovenous malformations (AVMs) are the most common type. Cavernous malformations, neoplasms, vasculitis, and vasculopathies can also cause ICH. The most important prognostic factors in ICH

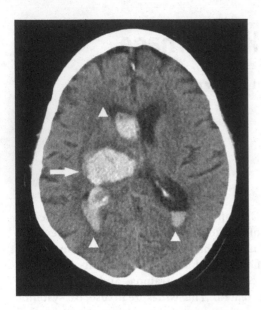

Figure 12.1 Right thalamic hemorrhage (large arrow), a common site for hypertension-related ICH. Arrowheads indicate intraventricular blood.

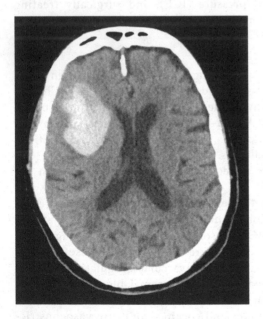

Figure 12.2 Right frontal lobar hemorrhage, likely related to CAA.

include hematoma size, location, and level of consciousness. The ICH score is a simple, validated prediction model for 30-day mortality risk after initial presentation with ICH (Table 12.1).

Table 12.1 ICH score with 30-day mortality risk. ICH volume is calculated using the ABC/2 method: A (greatest diameter on the slice in which the ICH appears largest) × B (diameter perpendicular to A) × C (number of axial slices multiplied by slice thickness) ÷ 2. The group that developed the ICH score did not have any patients in their cohort with a score of 6, but because patients with an ICH score of 5 had a 100% mortality risk at 30 days, they postulated that the outcome for patients with a score of 6 would be similarly poor

ICH score component	Points
Glasgow Coma Scale score	
3–4	2
5–12	1
13–15	0
ICH volume in cm³	
≥30	1
<30	0
IVH present	
Yes	1
No	0
Infratentorial origin of ICH	
Yes	1
No	0
Age in years	
≥80	1
<80	0

ICH score	30-day mortality risk (%)
0	0
1	13
2	26
3	72
4	97
5	100
6	100 (estimated)

12.3 Diagnosis

It is critical to diagnose ICH as quickly as possible since the risk for rapid clinical deterioration in the acute phase is high. More than 20% of patients with ICH will decline by 2 or more points on the Glasgow Coma Scale before reaching the hospital, and hematoma expansion occurs in more than 30% of patients within the first 3 hours. The severity of neurologic symptoms and degree of deterioration are highly predictive of the severity of long-term outcome.

In many cases, it is impossible to distinguish between ischemic stroke and ICH by history and examination alone. However, several features are more characteristic of ICH and can indicate increased ICP: systolic blood pressure (SBP) >220, severe headache, depressed mental status, and nausea and vomiting.

Noncontrast head CT is the gold standard for detecting ICH and can be quickly obtained. Brain MRI is just as sensitive for ICH as head CT, but has a longer image acquisition time and may be contraindicated in some patients. CT or MR angiography can be helpful in identifying the etiology of ICH, such as vascular malformations, moyamoya, and cerebral venous sinus thrombosis. Catheter angiography may be performed if there is a high suspicion for a vascular malformation that was not visualized with noninvasive imaging.

12.4 Management

Once a patient is found to have an ICH, he should be transferred immediately to a tertiary care center that has access to multiple specialty resources such as vascular neurology, neurological surgery, and neuroradiology. The patient should be medically stabilized prior to transfer. Increased ICP may result in cardiac arrhythmias. Nausea and vomiting are common, and combined with depressed mental status may lead to aspiration and respiratory insufficiency requiring mechanical ventilation. Treatment of extreme hypertension, blood glucose abnormalities, seizure, and hemostatic abnormalities should also be initiated prior to transfer.

Monitoring of ICH patients in a neuroscience ICU is associated with lower mortality rates. The neuroscience ICU offers the ability to monitor ICP, manage cerebral perfusion pressure, and practice established protocols for managing ICH-related complications such as severe hypertension and hyperglycemia.

Treatment of ICH is aimed at minimizing the risk of hematoma enlargement or recurrent hemorrhage and relieving increased ICP. Severe hypertension is associated with hematoma expansion, clinical worsening, and increased risk of death or disability. Elevated SBP is thought to be caused by a combination of sympathetic nervous system activation and increased ICP. Rapid lowering of blood pressure in ICH was once felt to be dangerous due to inducing hypoperfusion of a theoretical ischemic penumbra surrounding the hematoma. However, observational neuroimaging studies have not demonstrated the presence of such a penumbra. In 2013, INTERACT2 showed that there was no difference in mortality or adverse outcomes with rapid lowering of SBP to <140 mm Hg within 1 hour of presentation in patients with an initial SBP of 150–220 mm Hg. In addition, there appeared to be a modest benefit in improved functional outcome in the secondary end-point analyses. Thus, rapid lowering of SBP to <140 mm Hg is considered to be safe in this population.

Hyperglycemia is associated with increased mortality and poor outcome. However, it is unclear if aggressively treating hyperglycemia (such as with insulin infusion) is beneficial, possibly because inadvertently inducing hypoglycemia may raise the risk of mortality. The goal should be to achieve normoglycemia. Fever is also associated with worse clinical outcome in animal models of brain injury. However, there are no data that show that therapeutic cooling or treating fever with antipyretics improves clinical outcome.

Seizures can occur in up to 16% of ICH patients within the first week of onset. Data on use of prophylactic antiepileptic medications in ICH are mixed. Some studies show that using prophylactic antiseizure medications decreased the incidence of clinical seizures after ICH. However, seizures are not associated with worse outcome or increased mortality. Other studies have shown increased mortality and disability and no reduction in seizure incidence with use of prophylactic antiepileptic medications. The American Stroke Association recommends using antiseizure medications only to treat clinical or electrographic seizures.

Hemostatic abnormalities should be corrected and any antiplatelet or anticoagulation agents should be discontinued, if possible. It is unclear if platelet dysfunction from antiplatelet medications or other causes is associated with hematoma expansion or worsened neurological outcomes. Platelet transfusion has not been demonstrated to provide benefit in these cases and is not routinely recommended, but may be considered in those who are at high risk of hematoma expansion, such as cases with severe thrombocytopenia. In patients who are receiving intravenous unfractionated heparin (UFH), the infusion should be stopped and protamine may be given to reverse the anticoagulation. Refer to Sections 12.4.1 and 12.4.2 on management of ICH in the setting of warfarin and novel oral anticoagulant (NOAC) use for discussion on reversal methods for these agents.

Mass effect from ICH may cause herniation syndromes or obstruction of cerebral spinal fluid (CSF) outflow and subsequent hydrocephalus. These conditions require surgical management, which is discussed in more detail later in this chapter, and includes insertion of an external ventricular drain (EVD) for hydrocephalus, clot evacuation, and decompressive craniectomy. In some cases of intraventricular hemorrhage (Figure 12.3), administering

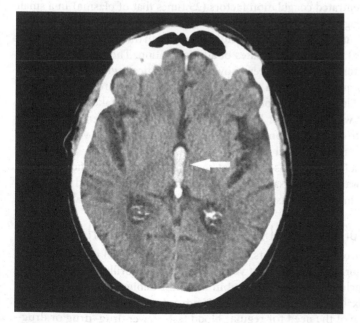

Figure 12.3 Intraventricular hemorrhage occluding the third ventricle (arrow).

recombinant tissue plasminogen activator (rtPA) via the EVD may be considered as an off-label treatment to help dissolve a clot that is obstructing CSF drainage; however, the safety and efficacy of this method have not been demonstrated in clinical trials.

12.4.1 Management of Warfarin-Related ICH

Warfarin is a vitamin K antagonist that is used to induce systemic anticoagulation in a number of conditions, including venous thromboembolism, atrial fibrillation, mechanical heart valves, and prothrombotic states. The fact that a patient on warfarin is at high risk of thrombosis is problematic when facing hemorrhagic complications. In warfarin-related ICH, the drug should be discontinued and its effects reversed as quickly as possible to reduce the risk of hematoma expansion.

Intravenous vitamin K may be used to rapidly induce formation of vitamin K- dependent clotting factors. However, it can take hours to see any effect, and there is a small risk of anaphylaxis when vitamin K is administered intravenously. Fresh frozen plasma (FFP) has been the mainstay for many years to reverse the international normalized ratio (INR) in the acute setting, but this treatment can also take hours. One study showed that up to 17% of patients taking warfarin who received FFP still had a 24-hour INR greater than 1.4. In addition, FFP carries the risk of transfusion reaction or allergic reaction, and there is a risk of volume overload in patients with congestive heart failure.

Over the last several years, prothrombin complex concentrate (PCC) has had increasingly more use in the treatment of warfarin-related hemorrhage. PCC was originally formulated to treat patients with hemophilia B, or factor IX deficiency. Three-factor PCC contains factors II, IX, and X, which also happen to be vitamin K- dependent clotting factors. Four-factor PCC also contains factor VII, and activated four-factor PCC contains activated factor VII. Four-factor PCC was approved by the FDA for warfarin reversal in the United States in 2013. Because PCC contains concentrated coagulation factors (25 times that of plasma) in a small volume, it has several advantages over FFP. PCC does not require thawing or cross-matching, can be rapidly administered, and reduces the risk of fluid overload. In the majority of patients, the INR can be reduced to <1.4 within 30 minutes of administration. The risk of thrombo-embolic events with four-factor PCC has not been shown to be statistically greater than that of FFP, but they occurred in patients with a higher baseline risk for thromboembolism. Therefore the patient's individual risk for thromboembolic events must be taken into account when considering treatment with four-factor PCC. Whereas PCC has not been shown to be superior to FFP with regard to clinical outcome, using PCC avoids the time and volume issues with FFP and results in more rapid reversal of INR.

Recombinant factor VIIa (rFVIIa) is used to treat congenital factor VII deficiency, and has been studied for use in warfarin reversal. However, a phase III study showed no clinical benefit. rFVIIa is not recommended for use in warfarin anticoagulation reversal.

12.4.2 Management of Novel Oral Anticoagulant-Related ICH

New, nonwarfarin oral anticoagulation agents, otherwise known as novel oral anticoagu-lants (NOACs), have been formulated in recent years to treat atrial fibrillation and venous thromboembolism. They include the direct thrombin inhibitor dabigatran, and factor Xa inhibitors rivaroxaban, apixaban, and edoxaban. Their advantages over warfarin include standard dosing, elimination of the need for regular blood tests, fewer drug–drug or drug–food interactions, enhanced rapid time of onset of anticoagulation, and shorter half-life when discontinuing the medication. They have been shown to be as effective as warfarin in preventing ischemic stroke, and some agents are associated with lower rates of certain bleeding complications, such as gastrointestinal and intracranial hemorrhage. However, NOACs are contraindicated in patients with severe liver or kidney disease and may raise the risk of thrombotic events when abruptly discontinued.

To date, there are two FDA-approved reversal agents for use in NOAC-related hemorrhage: idarucizumab for dabigatran and andexanet alfa for apixaban and rivaroxaban. The use of PCCs and rFVIIa in reversing the anticoagulation effects of NOACs, in conjunction with the approved FDA reversal agents, has been studied in animal models and healthy human subject trials with mixed results. Case reports using these agents also report conflicting findings, although some suggest there may be a clinical benefit. Thus, the use of these agents may be considered in selected patients, such as those with potentially life-threatening hemorrhage, although the safety and efficacy of this mode of treatment must be balanced with an increased risk of thrombosis. The number of NOACs and reversal agents is a rapidly evolving field and should be reviewed frequently for the most up-to-date evidence and practice.

12.5 Aneurysmal SAH, SDH, and EDH

Subarachnoid hemorrhage (SAH) is defined as the presence of blood in the space between the arachnoid and pia mater. Although trauma is the most common cause, SAH may occur spontaneously. In nontraumatic SAH, ruptured cerebral aneurysms are identified in approximately 85% of cases. Approximately 5% of the general population harbors an intracranial aneurysm. The overall incidence of aneurysmal SAH ranges between 2 and 16 cases per 100,000, with a 1:1.24 female predilection. In the United States the incidence of aneurysmal SAH is reported to be 9.7 per 100,000. Aneurysmal SAH remains a complex clinical challenge. Ongoing research and a multidisciplinary approach to treatment are necessary to continue to improve survival and quality of life for those afflicted.

12.5.1 Cerebral Aneurysms

Cerebral aneurysms are dilations of intracranial blood vessels resulting from weakness in the vessel wall. The exact pathophysiology of cerebral aneurysms remains poorly understood. Presumptive causative features are genetic predisposition in the form of focal lack or deficiency of the muscular tunica media of the vessel wall (termed "medial gap"), hypertensive atherosclerotic changes, infection, trauma, and smoking. A number of conditions are associated with development of cerebral aneurysms: autosomal dominant polycystic kidney disease, fibromuscular dysplasia, arteriovenous malformations, and connective tissue diseases, such as Ehlers–Danlos, Marfan syndrome, and pseudoxanthoma elasticum.

Several categories of cerebral aneurysm may be distinguished. Saccular aneurysms, or berry aneurysms, are attributed to a focal lack or deficient tunica media resulting in a dilated outpouching of the vessel filled with blood. Its wall is composed of hyalinized intima and adventitia. They most commonly occur at vessel branch points, the location of most hemodynamic stress. Their location in order of frequency is as follows: 85–95% occur in the carotid system, with 30% found in the anterior communicating artery (ACom), 25% in the posterior communicating artery (PCom), and 20% in the middle cerebral artery (MCA); 5–15% are found in the posterior circulation, with 10% on the basilar artery and 5% on the vertebral artery. Multiple aneurysms are present in 20–30% of patients. Fusiform dolichoectatic aneurysms are the widening of an entire segment of a blood vessel. Microaneurysms, or Charcot–Bouchard aneurysms, are believed to result from chronic hypertension and typically affect the small blood vessels supplying the basal ganglia and thalamus. Rupture of these aneurysms commonly results in intraparenchymal hemorrhage of the surrounding brain tissues. A vascular infundibulum refers to a funnel-shaped initial segment of an artery that is <3 mm at its widest portion and triangular in shape. While an infundibulum may bleed, they present significantly less risk of rupture compared to saccular aneurysms.

12.5.2 Differential Diagnosis

By far the most common cause of SAH is trauma, detectable with CT scan in up to 60% of patients with traumatic brain injury. However, as spontaneous SAH may precede a traumatic event, an index of suspicion must remain high in the setting of imaging findings suspicious for underlying vascular abnormalities. Table 12.2 lists diagnoses that should be considered when evaluating a spontaneous SAH.

12.5.3 Clinical Features

The most common presenting symptom of aneurysmal SAH is sudden-onset headache, often described as the "worst headache of my life" or "thunderclap headache," which occurs in up to 97% of cases. Often this headache is associated with nausea, vomiting, and photophobia. This headache may spontaneously resolve in sentinel hemorrhages, which are present in 30–60% of SAH, and are representative of spontaneous aneurysmal leak,

Table 12.2 Spontaneous SAH: differential diagnosis

Ruptured intracranial aneurysm – up to 85%
Cerebral arteriovenous malformation (AVM) – 4–5%
AVM may have associated aneurysms
Dural arteriovenous fistula (DAVF)
Vasculitis
Intracranial neoplasm
Cerebral artery dissection
Superficial artery/vein rupture
Rupture of infundibulum
Coagulation disorders: blood dyscrasias, thrombocytopenia
Dural sinus thrombosis
Spinal AVM – commonly cervical spine
Sickle cell anemia
Pituitary apoplexy
No identifiable cause – 14–22%

enlargement, or hemorrhage within the aneurysm wall. Neck or back pain may be experienced due to tracking of blood into the spinal subarachnoid space. Pooling of blood in the lumbar cistern may result in lower extremity pain. Diplopia may result from a focal cranial nerve deficit, especially from compression of the oculomotor nerve. Sudden onset of a cranial nerve III palsy may represent a suddenly enlarging posterior communicating artery aneurysm. Transient loss of consciousness results from a sudden rise in ICP.

Clinical signs following SAH include meningiomas, focal neurologic deficit, hypertension, obtundation or coma, and ocular hemorrhage. Nuchal rigidity typically occurs within the first 24 hours after SAH and may manifest with a positive Kernig or Brudzinski sign. Hypertension results from cerebral autoregulation to maintain adequate cerebral perfusion in response to increased ICP. Coma and obtundation are also attributable to increased ICP, damage to brain tissue from intracerebral hemorrhage and parenchymal destruction, hydrocephalus, ischemia, seizure, or low blood flow as a result of reduced cardiac output due to stunned myocardium (see Section 12.5.6.5). Intraocular hemorrhage may occur as a result of increased ICP following SAH. Three types of intraocular hemorrhage are described: subhyaloid (preretinal hemorrhage near the optic disc), intraretinal hemorrhage, and intravitreal hemorrhage, termed Terson syndrome. Terson syndrome occurs in 13% of patients with SAH and is associated with more severe SAH and significantly increased risk of death.

12.5.4 Work-up of SAH

12.5.4.1 Imaging and Diagnostic Studies

Presence of SAH is usually established with a noncontrast CT scan. The sensitivity of a high-resolution CT scan approaches 95% with 48 hours of hemorrhage, but may drop to 60% after 5 days. Hyperdense signal in the area of the circle of Willis and the Sylvian fissure is suggestive of aneurysmal origin of SAH. Furthermore, certain distributions of hemorrhage may indicate the location of a ruptured aneurysm in 78% of cases. Blood products primarily in the anterior interhemispheric fissure are suggestive of an ACom aneurysm (Figure 12.4). Sylvian fissure hemorrhage is seen in MCA and PCom aneurysms. Hemorrhage in the prepontine or peduncular cistern suggests basilar tip or superior cerebellar artery aneurysm. Intraventricular hemorrhage involving the third and fourth ventricles can be seen in posterior circulation aneurysms involving the posterior inferior cerebellar artery or vertebral artery dissection. Isolated third ventricular hemorrhage may be caused by a basilar tip aneurysm. The amount of hemorrhage identified on CT may be used as a prognostic indicator for risk of developing vasospasm (see the Fisher grading scheme). CT scanning can provide additional valuable information, including the presence of a subdural or epidural hematoma requiring surgical evacuation. Distal anterior cerebral artery (ACA) aneurysms, as well as PCom aneurysms, have been reported to cause isolated subdural hematoma.

Historically, lumbar puncture (LP) for cerebrospinal fluid analysis was an integral test for evaluation of presence of SAH after negative imaging. While LP still serves to evaluate for the presence of SAH, false positive rates often complicate diagnostic value. Nevertheless, CSF evaluation is recommended when clinical suspicion is high and CT and MRI are negative. An LP may be considered positive when the red blood

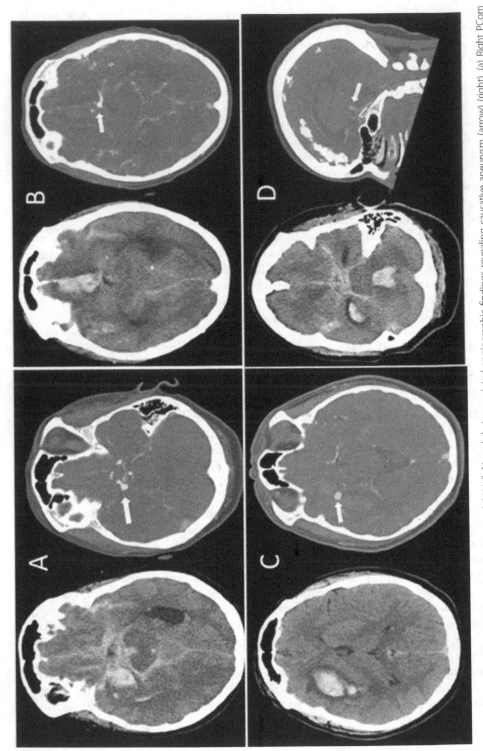

Figure 12.4 Representative CT imaging of aneurysmal SAH (left) and their associated angiographic findings revealing causative aneurysm (arrow) (right). (a) Right PCom aneurysm; (b) ACom aneurysm; (c) right MCA aneurysm; (d) basilar artery tip aneurysm.

cell count is >100,000 with little or no variability between tubes 1–4, opening pressure is elevated, and the supernatant has yellow discoloration, or xanthochromia (100% sensitive 12 hours after the ictus, but decreases to 70% at 3 weeks and 60% at 4 weeks).

Once presence of SAH has been established, or an index of suspicion remains high in the setting of a negative CT, vascular imaging should be obtained. The most sensitive noninvasive test for detection of a cerebral aneurysm remains a contrast-enhanced CT angiogram (CTA). CTA is 95–100% sensitive in identifying aneurysms >5 mm and 64–83% sensitive for aneurysms <5 mm. Magnetic resonance angiography (MRA) offers sensitivity of 85–100% for aneurysms >5 mm and 56% for aneurysms <5 mm, or 74–98% for aneurysms >3 mm. Sensitivity drops significantly for aneurysms <3 mm. While CTA is generally cheaper, more quickly obtained, and provides overall higher sensitivity compared with MRA, renal insufficiency may preclude certain patients from this test. Digital subtraction angiography (DSA) is the most sensitive test and remains the gold standard for imaging of cerebral aneurysms. Furthermore, it allows evaluation of anatomy usable in decision-making for endovascular and surgical therapy.

12.5.4.2 Grading of SAH

The severity of clinical presentation is the most reliable prognostic indicator of aneurysmal SAH. The most commonly used scales are the Hunt and Hess (Table 12.3) and World Federation of Neurological Surgeons (Table 12.4) scales.

Table 12.3 Hunt Hess grading scale (1968)

Grade	Signs and symptoms	Survival
1	Asymptomatic or minimal headache and slight neck stiffness	70%
2	Moderate to severe headache, neck stiffness, no neurologic deficit except cranial nerve palsy	60%
3	Drowsy, minimal neurologic deficit	50%
4	Stuporous, moderate to severe hemiparesis, possibly early decerebrate rigidity	20%
5	Deep coma, decerebrate rigidity, moribund appearance	10%

Table 12.4 World Federation of Neurological Surgeons grading scale (1988)

Grade	GCS score	Focal neurological deficit
1	15	Absent
2	13–14	Absent
3	13–14	Present
4	7–12	Present or absent
5	3–6	Present or absent

12.5.5 Management

Large-scale reviews have shown that the 30-day mortality rate was significantly higher in centers admitting <10 patients with aneurysmal SAH compared to centers that admitted >35 patients per year (39% vs 27%). If possible, patients should be transferred to a center with high cerebrovascular volume, availability of both a cerebrovascular neurosurgeon and a neurovascular interventionalist, and dedicated neurological intensive care services. The greatest threat after aneurysmal SAH is re-rupture. Aneurysm rebleeding is associated with high mortality and poor prognosis for functional recovery. Rate of re-rupture is highest within 2–12 hours of initial rupture, with a rate of 4–13.6% within the first 24 hours. While optimal SBP goals have not been identified, SBP <160 mm Hg is recommended. When definitive securing of the aneurysm is not possible, short-term therapy (<72 hours) with antifibrinolytic therapy using tranexamic acid or aminocaproic acid may reduce the risk of aneurysm rebleeding. The most effective means to reduce the risk of rebleeding is obliteration of the aneurysm using either microsurgical clipping or endovascular embolization.

12.5.6 Management of Complications

12.5.6.1 Rebleeding

The risk of rebleeding is approximately 3–4% in the first 24 hours after aneurysmal SAH. The overall risk of rebleeding during the first 2 weeks is 15–20% and up to 50% if the aneurysm is not repaired. Nonmodifiable risk factors for rebleeding include higher clinical grade at presentation, history of sentinel bleed, size of aneurysm, loss of consciousness during initial hemorrhage, and presence of intraparenchymal or intraventricular hemorrhage. Modifiable risk factors include uncontrolled hypertension with SBP >160 mm Hg, seizures, and elevated ICP. Antifibrinolytic therapy may reduce the risk of rebleeding, but should only be employed when definitive obliteration of aneurysm is not possible. The most effective reduction in risk of rebleeding remains treatment of the aneurysm by endovascular or microsurgical therapy.

12.5.6.2 Hydrocephalus and Elevated Intracranial Pressure

Acute hydrocephalus is found in 15–87% of patients presenting with aneurysm SAH, based on radiographic findings. However, only some of those patients will be symptomatic from hydrocephalus. Hydrocephalus is believed to result from blood obstructing the Sylvian aqueduct, fourth ventricular outlet, or interfering with reabsorption through arachnoid granulations. Acute hydrocephalus should be treated with CSF diversion in the form of an EVD or lumbar drain. It is unclear whether a decision for CSF diversion should be made based on radiographic findings alone or only in the setting of symptomatic hydrocephalus. Of symptomatic patients, 40–80% will experience clinical improvement with CSF diversion. Targeted ICP should be no lower than 15–25 mm Hg in order to avoid rapidly altering transmural pressure of the vasculature and precipitating rebleeding of the aneurysm. Preliminary data suggest CSF diversion may reduce the incidence of vasospasm.

12.5.6.3 Hyponatremia

Electrolyte disturbance is common after aneurysmal SAH, with hyponatremia observed in 10–30% of patients. Data suggests a chronological association of hyponatremia with the onset of sonographic and clinical vasospasm. The two main causes of hyponatremia are cerebral salt wasting, believed to be related to excessive secretion of neural hormonal control of atrial natriuretic factor and brain natriuretic peptide, and the syndrome of inappropriate antidiuretic hormone (SIADH). The two are distinguished by fluid status, the former being a hypovolemic hyponatremia, the latter being an isovolemic hyponatremia. Goals of treatment should include adequate fluid resuscitation and use of hypertonic saline or salt tablets to maintain a physiologic range of serum sodium. Furthermore, use of hypertonic saline has been associated with increased cerebral blood flow, brain tissue oxygen, and pH in patients with high-grade aneurysmal SAH. SIADH not responding to hypertonic saline may require treatment with hydrocortisone or vasopressin.

12.5.6.4 Seizures

The incidence of seizures is 6–18% in acute aneurysmal SAH. Delayed seizures may be seen in 3–7% of patients. Risk factors for development of early seizures include MCA aneurysm location, thick layers of SAH, intracerebral hematoma, rebleeding, infarction, poor clinical grade, microsurgical clipping, and history of hypertension. In the setting of a poor neurologic exam, clinical suspicion for subclinical seizures or nonconvulsive status epilepticus should be high. Current recommendations include routine short-term prophylaxis with antiseizure medication. Long-term treatment with antiseizure medication is not supported in the absence of proven seizure activity.

12.5.6.5 Cardiovascular

Neurogenic stunned myocardium (NSM) is a common systemic complication of aneurysmal SAH believed to be due to a surge of catecholamines as a result of hypothalamic stimulation or injury. It typically occurs between 2 days and 2 weeks after SAH and may manifest as hypotension, congestive heart failure, and arrhythmias, all possibly exacerbating cerebral ischemia. Commonly, NSM resolves spontaneously, but in a small percentage of patients may lead to myocardial infarction. Evaluation with echocardiography is recommended to assess cardiac output. Treatment may necessitate vasopressor support to maintain adequate end-organ perfusion and ionotropic support in case of insufficient cardiac output. Severe congestive heart failure from NSM may complicate aggressive treatment of vasospasm.

12.5.6.6 Fever, Glycemic Control, and Anemia

Central fever is a common complication of aneurysmal SAH associated with severity of cerebral injury, amount of intracranial hemorrhage, and development of vasospasm. Fever is an independent predictor of poor outcome after aneurysmal SAH and should be treated aggressively. Nevertheless, an infectious work-up should be completed to rule out a noncentral origin of fever.

Neurotoxic effects of hyperglycemia have been associated with poor outcome after ischemic brain injury. Conversely, hypoglycemia may lead to a cerebral metabolic crisis, elevate lactate-pyruvate ratios, and also worsen outcomes. Effective glycemic control is recommended, with strict avoidance of hypoglycemia.

Although optimal hemoglobin goals have not been identified, higher hemoglobin values are associated with improved outcomes after aneurysmal SAH. Especially for patients who are at high risk for vasospasm, hemoglobin should remain high and the threshold for transfusion should be low.

12.5.6.7 Vasospasm

Vasospasm is a common, feared complication of aneurysmal rupture. It is defined as narrowing of cerebral vasculature leading to cerebral ischemia and ultimately infarction. Its pathogenesis remains poorly understood. Symptomatic vasospasm, also termed delayed ischemic neurologic deficit, is defined as a clinical deterioration not otherwise attributable to other causes, such as seizure, hydrocephalus, or cerebral edema. Symptomatic vasospasm will affect 20–30% of patients after aneurysmal SAH, whereas angiographic vasospasm might be seen in 30–70% when evaluated on day 7 following SAH. Onset of vasospasm is typically between days 7 and 10 after SAH (almost never before day 3), and resolves spontaneously after 21 days. Severity of vasospasm may vary, with up to 7% of cases resulting in death. Risk factors for the development of vasospasm include poor clinical grade, thick blood on CT, presence of intraparenchymal or intraventricular hemorrhage, history of a sentinel bleed, volume depletion, low cardiac output, and smoking. The Modified Fisher Scale (Table 12.5) may be used to predict the likelihood of development of vasospasm.

The only evidence supporting a prophylactic measure for vasospasm is administration of nimodipine, a calcium channel blocker given at 60 mg every 4 hours for 21 days after aneurysmal SAH (Figure 12.5). A meta-analysis revealed nimodipine improves neurologic outcomes in mechanisms other than improvement of large vessel narrowing. As vasospasm is associated with fever and hypovolemia, aggressive measures should be taken to maintain normothermia, euvolemia, and normal circulating blood volume.

If symptomatic vasospasm is suspected, treatment should commence promptly. Historically, triple-H therapy (hypervolemia, hypertension, hemodilution) has been the mainstay of vasospasm treatment. Induced hypertension appears to be effective in improving outcomes in clinical vasospasm, by increasing cerebral blood flow during autoregulatory dysfunction and increasing transluminal pressure. Elevating the blood pressure to at least 20 mm Hg above baseline to a maximum blood pressure of 220/120 mm Hg is a commonly used goal. Efficacy of hemodilution and hypervolemia remains in question. Current recommendations have shifted from triple-H therapy to induced hypertension with maintenance of euvolemia.

When available, endovascular treatment of vasospasm may reverse symptoms of delayed cerebral ischemia with 30–70% success, especially when initiated within 2 hours. Intervention includes balloon angioplasty for accessible lesions and local infusion of vasodilators, including calcium channel blockers and nitric oxide donors. While randomized trials are lacking, observational and retrospective studies support interventional treatment of vasospasm.

Table 12.5 Modified Fisher Scale

Score	Blood on CT scan	Risk of symptomatic vasospasm
1	Thin SAH, no IVH	24%
2	Thin SAH, IVH present	33%
3	Thick SAH, no IVH	33%
4	Thick SAH, IVH present	40%

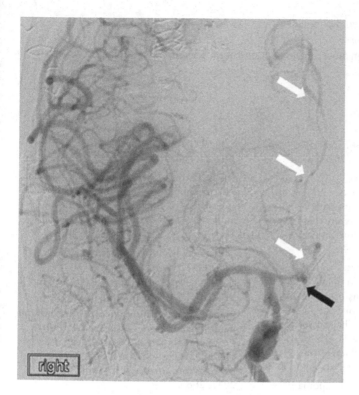

Figure 12.5 Cerebral angiography of right internal carotid artery revealing severe narrowing of right ACA representing vasospasm after aneurysmal SAH (white arrows). Note clip obliteration of ACom aneurysm (black arrow).

12.5.7 Prognosis

Mortality prior to hospital admission is reported to be 12–15%. The overall median mortality of aneurysmal SAH in the United States is 32%. While 65% of patients experience some form of cognitive impairment, functional dependence in survivors is as high as 20%. Recovery from aneurysmal SAH can be protracted, with rehabilitation, and physical and occupational therapy playing increasingly important roles in improving neurologic recovery and overall outcome.

Pearls and Pitfalls

- In ICH patients with SBP of 150–220 mm Hg, it is safe to lower SBP to <140 mm Hg within 1 hour of presentation.
- In warfarin-related ICH, vitamin K should be given to replace vitamin K- dependent clotting factors and FFP or PCC should be given to correct the INR.
- FDA-approved reversal agents, PCC or rFVIIa may be considered in life-threatening NOAC-related ICH. The patient's risk for thromboembolic events must be taken into account on a case-by-case basis.
- In the setting of aneurysmal SAH, transfer to a high-volume center and early neurosurgical consultation are paramount. Lack of SAH in the setting of subdural, epidural, or intraparenchymal hemorrhage does not exclude aneurysmal rupture.
- Hydrocephalus is common and should be treated with CSF diversion (EVD).
- Early blood pressure control (SBP <160), seizure prophylaxis, and nimodipine therapy are recommended.

- Ruptured aneurysm should be secured by endovascular embolization or surgical obliteration when possible.
- Suspicion for vasospasm must remain high, and aggressive treatment initiated when it is identified.

Bibliography

Abraham MK, Chang WTW. Subarachnoid hemorrhage. *Emerg Med Clin* 2016;**34**(4):901–916.

Al-Rawi PG, Tseng MY, Richards HK, et al. Hypertonic saline in patients with poor-grade subarachnoid hemorrhage improves cerebral blood flow, brain tissue oxygen, and pH. *Stroke* 2010;**41**:122–128.

Baharoglu MI, Cordonnier C, Al-Shahi Salman R, et al. Platelet transfusion versus standard care after acute stroke due to spontaneous cerebral hemorrhage associated with antiplatelet therapy (PATCH): a randomized, open-label, phase 3 trial. *Lancet* 2016;**387**(10038):2605–2613.

Connolly ES, Rabinstein AA, Carhuapoma JR, et al. Guidelines for the management of aneurysmal subarachnoid hemorrhage. *Stroke* 2012;**43**:1711–1737.

Dastur CK, Yu W. Current management of spontaneous intracerebral hemorrhage. *Stroke Vasc Neurol* 2017;**2**:21–29.

Dubosh NM, Bellolio, MF, Rabinstein AA, et al. Sensitivity of early brain computed tomography to exclude aneurysmal subarachnoid hemorrhage: a systematic review and meta-analysis. *Stroke* 2016;**47**:750–755.

Frontera JA, Lewin JJ 3rd, Rabinstein AA, et al. Guidelines for reversal of antithrombotics in intracranial hemorrhage: a statement for healthcare professionals from the Neurocritical Care Society and Society of Critical Care Medicine. *Neurocrit Care* 2016;**24**(1):6–46.

Gehrie E, Tormey C. Novel oral anticoagulants: efficacy, laboratory measurement, and approaches to emergency reversal. *Arch Pathol Lab Med* 2015;**139**:687–692.

Heit JJ, Iv M, Wintermark M. Imaging of intracranial hemorrhage. *J Stroke* 2017;**19**(1):11–27.

Hemphill JC 3rd, Greenberg SM, Anderson CS, et al. Guidelines for the management of spontaneous intracerebral hemorrhage: a guideline for healthcare professionals from the American Heart Association/American Stroke Association. *Stroke* 2015;**46**(7):2032–2060.

Panos NG, Cook AM, John S, et al. Factor Xa inhibitor-related intracranial hemorrhage: results from a multicenter, observational cohort receiving prothrombin complex concentrates. *Circulation* 2020;**141**(21):1681–1689.

Qureshi A, Palesch YY, Barsan WG, et al. Intensive blood-pressure lowering in patients with acute cerebral hemorrhage. *N Engl J Med* 2016;**375**(11):1033–1043.

Sarode R, Milling Jr T, Refaai MA, et al. Efficacy and safety of a 4-factor prothrombin complex concentrate in patients on vitamin k antagonist presenting with major bleeding; a randomized, plasma-controlled, phase IIIb study. *Circulation* 2013;**128**:1234–1243.

Chapter 13

Seizures

Kevin M. Kelly, Timothy A. Quezada, and Thomas P. Campbell

13.1 Introduction

There are an estimated 150,000 new cases of epilepsy per year in the United States, with prevalence rates of 7–8 per 1,000 persons. These data, combined with the large number of patients who have seizures from nonepileptic causes, indicate that seizure occurrence is relatively frequent and can result from diverse causes. Although many patients who have a seizure do not need emergency department (ED) care, some present to the ED critically ill and require immediate, definitive management. Advances in the understanding of seizure types and use of new antiseizure medications (ASMs) have enhanced the emergency physician's ability to diagnose the cause of a patient's seizures accurately and to treat both the underlying abnormality and the seizures in a rational and systematic fashion.

13.2 Epileptic Seizures

The International League Against Epilepsy (ILAE) defines a seizure as "a transient occurrence of signs and/or symptoms due to an abnormal excessive or synchronous neuronal activity in the brain." Epilepsy is defined as "a disease characterized by an enduring predisposition to generate epileptic seizures and by the neurobiological, cognitive, psychological, and social consequences of this condition." In other words, seizures are an event; epilepsy is a disease leading to recurrent, unprovoked seizures.

The ILAE classifies seizures based on clinical and electrophysiological properties of the ictal event that categorize it as one of three fundamental groups of seizure: focal onset, generalized onset, or unknown onset. A focal onset seizure has clinical or EEG evidence indicating onset in an area of one cerebral hemisphere. A generalized onset seizure has neither clinical nor EEG evidence of focal onset and appears to begin simultaneously from both cerebral hemispheres on EEG. An unknown onset seizure has no identifying clinical or EEG feature at its initiation (Figure 13.1).

Similar to the different types of seizures, the types of epilepsies are divided into focal epilepsy, generalized epilepsy, combined generalized and focal epilepsy, and unknown epilepsy. For the ED physician, a basic understanding of the types of focal onset and generalized onset seizures is important for the evaluation and treatment of seizures in the ED.

13.2.1 Focal Onset Seizures

Focal onset seizures are subdivided into having either intact or impaired awareness (i.e., focal onset aware or focal onset impaired awareness seizures, respectively). Focal onset seizures are classified by the type of symptoms experienced by the patient and are

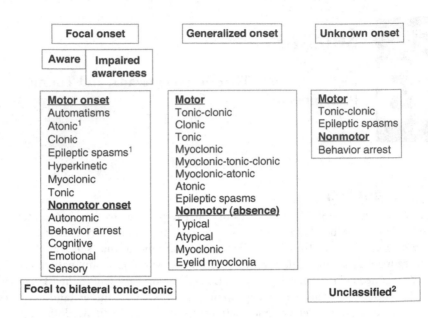

Focal onset	Generalized onset	Unknown onset

Aware	Impaired awareness		

Motor onset
Automatisms
Atonic[1]
Clonic
Epileptic spasms[1]
Hyperkinetic
Myoclonic
Tonic
Nonmotor onset
Autonomic
Behavior arrest
Cognitive
Emotional
Sensory

Motor
Tonic-clonic
Clonic
Tonic
Myoclonic
Myoclonic-tonic-clonic
Myoclonic-atonic
Atonic
Epileptic spasms
Nonmotor (absence)
Typical
Atypical
Myoclonic
Eyelid myoclonia

Motor
Tonic-clonic
Epileptic spasms
Nonmotor
Behavior arrest

Focal to bilateral tonic-clonic		Unclassified[2]

[1]Degree of awareness usually is not specific
[2]Due to inadequate information or ability to place in other categories

Figure 13.1 2017 ILAE classification of seizure types. Adapted from Fisher et al. 2017.

further subdivided as having a motor vs nonmotor onset; the latter include sensory, autonomic, and psychic events. The EEG shows a restricted area of electrical discharge over the contralateral cerebral cortex corresponding to the body area involved. A focal onset seizure with motor signs is a focal motor seizure that can occur in any body area (e.g., clonic activity of digits). If the abnormal electrical discharge causing the seizure spreads to contiguous cortical areas, a sequential involvement of body parts occurs in a "march" (e.g., clonic activity of digits spreading to the wrist and then to the elbow). This type of seizure is known as a Jacksonian seizure. When focal motor seizures are continuous, the condition is known as epilepsia partialis continua, a form of status epilepticus (SE), which is a condition characterized by a seizure that lasts longer than 30 minutes or when a patient has two or more consecutive seizures without regaining consciousness. A focal onset seizure with somatosensory symptoms is a focal sensory seizure, usually consisting of paresthesias (tingling, pins-and-needles sensations) or numbness. These symptoms may also undergo a progression, or march, as in focal motor seizures. A focal onset seizure with special sensory symptoms includes elaborate visual or auditory experiences, olfactory sensations (e.g., unpleasant odor), or gustatory sensations (e.g., metallic taste). A focal onset seizure with autonomic symptoms can include pallor, flushing, diaphoresis, piloerection, and pupil dilatation. A focal onset seizure with psychic symptoms is a disturbance of higher cerebral function usually occurring with impairment of consciousness. The psychic symptoms include distorted memories such as déja vu (the sensation that the present situation has already been experienced) and jamais vu (a familiar visual experience is not recognized). Other symptoms include dreamy states, intense fear or terror, illusions, and structured hallucinations.

The word "aura" has been used traditionally to describe the sensory, autonomic, or psychic symptoms perceived by the patient before the onset of impaired consciousness and/ or a motor seizure. Actually, an aura is itself a focal onset seizure that may or may not progress to another seizure type. Prodromal symptoms of prolonged mood changes, uneasiness, or premonitions are usually not auras. Postictal paralysis (Todd's paralysis) or weakness can occur in muscles involved in a seizure. The paralysis usually resolves within 48 hours, although it may persist for much longer periods. Less commonly, focal sensory seizures that have associated paresthesias may be followed by postictal numbness in the same body distribution. The numbness is the sensory equivalent of a postictal paralysis. The cause of these postictal phenomena is thought to be transient, reversible biochemical alterations in the neurons involved in the seizure activity.

A focal aware seizure (motor or nonmotor) may progress to a focal impaired awareness seizure, which also can occur spontaneously. A focal impaired awareness seizure includes impairment of consciousness, which refers to the patient's abnormal awareness and responsiveness to environmental stimuli. The initial features of the seizure often include an arrest reaction or motionless stare, usually followed by automatisms, which are relatively coordinated motor activities occurring during the period of impaired consciousness. The automatism may be a continuation of motor activity that was present at the time of seizure onset (e.g., continuing to drive a car) or an apparently purposeful activity such as scratching, lip smacking, or fumbling with clothing. The seizure is usually brief, lasting from seconds to minutes, and there is a period of postictal confusion. Focal impaired awareness SE is a series of these seizures without an intervening return to full responsiveness. A focal onset seizure, aware or with impaired awareness, can evolve into a bilateral tonic-clonic seizure and is then referred to as a "focal to bilateral tonic-clonic seizure."

13.2.2 Generalized Seizures

Generalized onset seizures are divided into motor or nonconvulsive nonmotor (absence) types. Generalized motor seizures include tonic, clonic, myoclonic, and tonic-clonic types, among others. Generalized tonic seizures typically occur in childhood and generally include impaired consciousness, muscle contraction of the face and trunk, flexion of the upper extremities, flexion or extension of the lower extremities, and postictal confusion. Generalized clonic seizures usually begin in childhood and include impaired consciousness, bilateral limb jerking, and postictal confusion. Generalized tonic-clonic seizures, commonly referred to as "grand mal" seizures, are characterized by a sudden loss of consciousness and tonic and clonic phases. The tonic phase lasts 10–20 seconds and begins with brief flexion, eyelid opening, upward movement of the eyes, and elevation and external rotation of the arms. More prolonged extension follows involving the back and neck, a cry may occur, the arms extend, and the legs extend and rotate externally. At this point the patient becomes apneic. The clonic phase lasts about 30 seconds and begins by brief, repetitive relaxations of the tonic rigidity, creating pronounced flexor spasms of the face, trunk, and limbs. This clonic jerking gradually decreases in rate until it ceases. Following this, there is muscular flaccidity, respirations resume, and there may be incontinence. Consciousness returns gradually and the patient awakens in a confused state. Fatigue and headache are common.

Generalized myoclonic seizures are bilaterally synchronous jerks that can be single or repeated in trains. The muscles involved may be few and restricted to a body part (e.g., the face) or extensive, involving all limbs. Most myoclonic seizures occur with no impairment of consciousness. Generalized tonic seizures that are brief are considered nonconvulsive, in contrast to the longer generalized tonic seizures, which are classified as convulsive. Generalized atonic seizures, commonly referred to as drop attacks, consist of a sudden loss of tone in postural muscles, often resulting in a fall. There is brief, mild impairment of consciousness and little postictal confusion.

Generalized nonmotor seizures include typical, atypical, myoclonic, and eyelid myoclonia subtypes of absence seizures. Generalized absence seizures, commonly referred to as "petit mal" seizures, typically are 5–10 second episodes of impaired consciousness characterized by staring and unresponsiveness. Although classified as "nonmotor," clonic movements, changes in postural tone, automatisms, and autonomic phenomena commonly accompany absence seizures. The patient quickly resumes normal consciousness, has no postictal confusion, and is generally unaware of the episode. Continuous absence seizures are known as absence SE.

13.2.3 Pre-hospital Care

Most seizures that occur in an out-of-hospital setting do not result in the patient going to the ED for evaluation. This is because most seizures occur in patients with epilepsy who recognize that their seizures are usually self-limited and do not require immediate evaluation. However, some seizures are severe or life-threatening and require immediate evaluation and management. Management of airway, breathing, and circulation is addressed first with concern for head and neck injury using cervical spine precautions if there is evidence of or a witnessed fall. Management of SE by EMS personnel essentially follows the same guidelines as in the ED. When EMS personnel are called for a patient who has had a seizure, information obtained in the field is frequently important for establishing a diagnosis and a treatment plan, especially if there is any evidence of intoxication or the result of blood glucose evaluation. The patient is usually transported to the ED for evaluation, and the emergency physician is updated as needed. Conditions that can require transport to the hospital include seizures that last for several minutes without evidence of abatement, failure to regain consciousness after a seizure, serial seizures, seizures resulting in significant injury, new or severe seizures in pregnancy, medical conditions such as diabetes, or seizures occurring at the extremes of age.

13.2.4 ED Evaluation

13.2.4.1 History

Patients assessed in the ED can be postictal or experiencing a recurrent seizure. It is the responsibility of the emergency physician to evaluate the seizure by obtaining pertinent information regarding the patient's medical, surgical, neurological, and psychiatric history. This information is obtained from all available sources including patient, family, friends, witnesses to the seizure, EMS personnel, the patient's physician, and hospital records. A history of a seizure disorder is especially important and ideally provides information regarding the patient's age at seizure onset, the cause and type of the seizure(s), the frequency of seizures, the last known seizure occurrence, and the use of ASMs. When little information is available about the patient, descriptions of the seizure and the circumstances of its occurrence are extremely important in determining the cerebral localization of the epileptogenic lesion, the seizure type, and its potential cause; however, the seizure may not have been witnessed, and the patient may be unable to provide information. Important information includes whether the seizure is nocturnal only, diurnal/nocturnal, or during wakefulness only; the occurrence of a prodrome or aura; the features of the clinical seizure (e.g., autonomic changes, alteration of consciousness, arrested body movements, automatisms, the temporal sequence of tonic and/or clonic movements affecting one or both sides of the body, tongue biting, incontinence), and postictal symptoms. When ASMs are used, recent drug or dosage changes and the patient's compliance with medication-taking should be determined. Associated factors that may be important include chronic disease states, intercurrent illness, stress, sleep deprivation, menses, pregnancy, the use of other medications, alcohol or drug ingestion, or withdrawal.

13.2.4.2 General Physical Examination

A careful general physical examination is performed to assess the condition of the patient with protection of the cervical spine if there is any evidence or history of head trauma in order to ascertain any physical signs that may be related to the underlying cause of the seizure and to possible resultant trauma. Vital signs can give evidence of infection, hypotension or hypertension, arrhythmias, and respiratory or metabolic disturbances. The skin may reveal decreased turgor with dehydration, a rash with infection or connective tissue disorders, cyanosis with hypoxemia, hirsutism with chronic phenytoin therapy, contusions, lacerations, scarring from seizure-related injury, characteristic abnormalities of the phakomatoses, or congenital ectodermal disorders. These include axillary freckling, café-au-lait spots, and neurofibromas associated with neurofibromatosis; facial sebaceous adenoma, ash leaf spots, and shagreen patches associated with tuberous sclerosis; and port wine stain of the face associated with Sturge–Weber syndrome. The head may reveal microcephaly, macrocephaly, or facial asymmetry, suggesting abnormal cerebral development or injury. A tense fontanelle can be seen in infection or hydrocephalus. There may be evidence of trauma or previous neurological surgery such as craniectomy for tumor or arteriovenous malformation (AVM) removal or aneurysm clipping, or placement of a ventriculoperitoneal shunt for hydrocephalus. The sinuses may be tender to tap and the tympanic membranes or oropharynx may be red – findings associated with infection. The mouth may reveal gingival hypertrophy with chronic phenytoin therapy, lacerations or scarring of the tongue and buccal mucosa, or a smell of alcohol. The neck may be stiff, and a positive Brudzinski or Kernig sign suggests meningeal irritation from infection or subarachnoid hemorrhage. The limbs may be asymmetrical, suggesting lateralized cerebral injury. Auscultation of the heart may reveal arrhythmia or murmurs of acquired heart disease underlying inadequate cerebral perfusion and hypoxia or embolism. Auscultation of the lungs may reveal decreased ventilation in several disease states, including exacerbations of chronic obstructive pulmonary disease and asthma resulting in cerebral hypoxia, infection resulting in cerebral abscess, and tumor resulting in cerebral metastasis. The abdomen may be rigid with infection or hemorrhage, resulting in hypotension or shock. Hepatomegaly may be associated with liver insufficiency and an encephalopathic state. There may be urinary or fecal incontinence.

13.2.4.3 Neurological Examination

A focused neurological examination assesses mental status, functioning of the cranial nerves, motor and sensory systems, and deep tendon reflexes. Abnormal findings may be from ictal or postictal states of focal impaired awareness or generalized seizures, the patient's interictal condition, toxic or metabolic encephalopathies, or intracranial injury. Prolonged bizarre behavior with alteration of consciousness may represent nonconvulsive status epilepticus (NCSE) and not delirium or a psychotic event. Prolonged lethargy and decreased mental status may represent absence SE rather than a postictal state. Reversible memory impairment occurs frequently with focal impaired awareness and bilateral tonic clonic seizures.

Cranial nerve examination is focused. The optic nerve may show papilledema, suggesting increased intracranial pressure. Abnormalities of pupil size may suggest focal impairments (e.g., a nonreactive dilated pupil in transtentorial herniation) or generalized effects (e.g., bilateral miosis or mydriasis from drug effect). Seizures can have a direct effect on pupillary size, such as causing mydriasis. Tonic deviation of the eyes may represent an ictal event and can localize the abnormality (e.g., a right hemisphere seizure tonically drives the eyes to the left). Importantly, the direction of gaze in relation to hemiparesis and other examination findings can be very helpful in distinguishing a seizure from a postictal state or stroke. Nystagmus may be due to ASM intoxication. A central facial paresis is caused by a contralateral cerebral hemisphere abnormality and may represent a postictal paralysis.

Motor function should be assessed initially by inspection of the patient. An externally rotated lower extremity suggests focal weakness that may be related to stroke in the contralateral cerebral hemisphere or to postictal paralysis. Tremors may be related to alcohol withdrawal states, and fasciculations can occur in severe dehydration. Myoclonus may be caused by toxic, metabolic, or infectious disturbances. Tonic rigidity or clonic movements occur with ongoing seizure activity.

Sensory function impairments such as paresthesias or numbness may result in abnormal responses to testing by light touch or pinprick. When focal, these abnormalities suggest ipsilateral mononeuropathy, plexopathy, radiculopathy, or contralateral brain impairment, including ongoing simple focal onset seizure activity or a postictal equivalent.

Muscle stretch reflexes may be decreased in postictal paralysis or increased because of contralateral upper motorneuron impairment, which also underlies a plantar extensor response. A decreased rate of reflex relaxation (a "hung-up" reflex) suggests hypothyroidism.

13.3 Differential Diagnosis

13.3.1 Epileptic Seizures

The ED evaluation of a seizure is directed toward determining whether the seizure is due to epilepsy or nonepileptic causes. When a seizure has the characteristics of a focal onset or generalized seizure, represents a chronic condition, and has no identifiable cause or a cause that cannot be cured by specific treatment, the seizure is caused by epilepsy. This distinguishes provoked seizures, due to a transient reversible insult (e.g., minor head trauma), from recurrent provoked seizures, which potentially can be cured by definitive therapy of an underlying disease state (e.g., resection of a brain tumor, hypoglycemia). The causes of epileptic seizures are numerous and diverse. Table 13.1 provides of causes of epileptic seizures and representative examples.

13.3.2 Nonepileptic Paroxysmal Events

Paroxysmal events from nonepileptic causes are frequently confused with epileptic seizures, and their accurate identification is important for appropriate management. Nonepileptic paroxysmal events that cannot be distinguished from epileptic seizures on clinical features alone are studied by appropriate tests, including EEG. Nonepileptic paroxysmal events have

Table 13.1 Causes of epileptic seizures and representative examples

Structural

Mesial temporal sclerosis

Hypothalamic hematoma

Rasmussen syndrome

Genetic

Inferred – family history of an autosomal disorder

  Benign familial neonatal epilepsy

  Autosomal dominant nocturnal frontal lobe epilepsy

Suggested – populations with the same syndrome

  Childhood absence epilepsy

  Juvenile myoclonic epilepsy

Identified molecular basis

  Dravet syndrome

  Genetic epilepsy with febrile seizures plus (GEFS+)

Infectious

Neurocysticercosis

HIV

Tuberculosis

Subacute sclerosing panencephalitis

Cerebral toxoplasmosis

Congenital infections

Metabolic

Porphyria

Amino acidopathies

Pyridoxine-dependent

Immune

Anti-NMDA receptor encephalitis

Anti-LG1 encephalitis

Unknown

Frontal lobe epilepsy

Adapted from Scheffer et al. 2017

been classified as being inducible by systemic, neurological, or psychiatric disorders. Examples of these disorders, which occur commonly in the ED, are listed in Table 13.2 and described below.

Table 13.2 Nonepileptic paroxysmal
events

Systemic disorders

Syncope

Breath-holding

Hyperventilation

Toxic and metabolic disturbances

Alcohol and drug withdrawal

Hepatic and renal failure

Neurologic disorders

Cerebrovascular disorders

Migraine

    Classical

    Complicated

    Equivalent

Transient global amnesia

Narcolepsy

Movement disorders

Paroxysmal dyskinesias

Hemifacial spasm

Sensory disorders

Trigeminal neuralgia

Positional vertigo

Acute labyrinthitis

Meniere's disease

Psychiatric disorders

Psychogenic seizures

Intermittent explosive disorders

Dissociative states

Fugue states

Systemic Disorders. Systemic disturbances include syncope, breath-holding, hyperventilation, and toxic and metabolic disturbances. Syncope is a relatively frequent event and is related to a sudden decrease in cerebral blood flow. After a syncopal episode, the patient usually falls to the ground, can display tonic and clonic movements lasting only a few seconds, and has a prompt return to consciousness. These brief tonic and clonic movements reflect decerebrate rigidity and are commonly called syncopal seizures or convulsive syncope. They can occur with prodromal diaphoresis and vertigo, are frequently associated with stress (such as the death of a relative), and do not require treatment.

Breath-holding in infants and children can also result in syncope and is common between 6 and 18 months of age. It is often precipitated by frustration, fear, or surprise followed by autonomic phenomena and loss of consciousness. Brief syncopal seizures may follow and do not require treatment.

Hyperventilation occurs most frequently in adolescents and adults and is usually precipitated by anxiety or stress. Typical symptoms include shortness of breath, lightheadedness, and perioral and phalangeal tingling. Carpopedal spasm and loss of consciousness may occur. Seizures are infrequent but can occur in susceptible patients or those with a history of epilepsy. Treatment of hyperventilation consists of rebreathing expired air, calm reassurance of the patient, and sedation when indicated.

Toxic and metabolic disturbances can result in transient neurological dysfunction that may be difficult to distinguish from some features of seizure activity. Toxic disturbances that are frequently seen in the ED are caused by alcohol and psychomimetic drugs. Delirium tremens (DTs) occurs within 48 hours of cessation of drinking and is characterized by confusion, hallucinations, tremor, and autonomic changes. Psychomimetic drugs can cause altered awareness and responsiveness, hallucinations, and autonomic changes. Aspects of DTs and drug intoxication can resemble features of focal impaired awareness seizures. Metabolic disturbances such as hepatic and renal failure can create lethargy and confusion, which may be mistaken for ictal or postictal phenomena.

Neurological disturbances include cerebrovascular, sleep, movement, and sensory disorders. Cerebrovascular disorders include transient ischemic attacks (TIAs), stroke, migraine, and transient global amnesia. Stroke can be the reason for a provoked seizure (secondary to ischemia-related physiological derangement) and epileptic seizures (secondary to scar formation in the area of stroke). Complicated migraine is migraine headache followed by prolonged neurological deficits including mental aberrations. These impairments can be difficult to distinguish from those related to focal onset seizures or TIAs. Transient global amnesia is an episode lasting approximately 20 minutes to several hours characterized by a sudden loss of memory and apparent confusion with repetitive questions. After the episode there is permanent amnesia concerning the event. This constellation of symptoms can suggest a postictal state following a focal impaired awareness seizure.

Movement disorders that occur as paroxysmal events can resemble epileptic seizures. Paroxysmal dyskinesias include familial and acquired types. Hemifacial spasm consists of irregular contractions of one side of the face, including blinking, and is related to facial nerve pathology. Although hemifacial spasm may resemble a focal onset motor seizure clinically, the EEG is normal.

Sensory disorders with paroxysmal features include those that are characterized by pain (e.g., trigeminal neuralgia) and vertigo (e.g., positional vertigo, acute labyrinthitis, and Meniere's disease). The specific symptoms and precipitants of these sensory disorders generally distinguish them as nonepileptic paroxysmal events.

Psychiatric Disorders. Psychogenic disturbances include psychogenic nonepileptic seizures (PNES), intermittent explosive disorders, and dissociative states. PNES (often inappropriately termed "pseudoseizures") are nonepileptic behavioral events that can mimic different seizure types, usually convulsive. Clinical clues of PNES include: (1) retained consciousness: movement of all extremities with preservation of consciousness (e.g., speaking or following commands) and responsiveness to noxious stimuli; (2) unusual movements: out-of-phase movement of limbs (in a true generalized seizure the limbs generally move relatively synchronously), pelvic thrusting, and side-to-side head movements; (3) ocular findings: eyes that are squeezed shut (in a true generalized seizure the patient should be unconscious and not resist eyelid raising), irregular eye movements (unlike consistent gaze deviation that may be seen in seizure), and optokinetic nystagmus when viewing an optokinetic strip or drum; (4) lack of a postictal period. Intermittent explosive disorders (episodic dyscontrol) are episodic or impulsive violent behaviors resulting in personal assault or destruction of property without significant precipitating psychosocial stress. The directed aggression of these episodes distinguishes them from stereotyped, aggressive epileptic ictal behavior, which is relatively rare. Dissociative states include fugue states, psychogenic amnesia, and depersonalization disorders. Features of these disorders can resemble some of the cognitive features of focal impaired awareness SE, particularly memory loss. The specific nature of the abnormality seen in dissociative states generally distinguishes them from epileptic seizures. However, EEG may be required for definitive diagnosis.

13.3.3 Laboratory Studies and Procedures

Patients with a new-onset seizure are assessed for underlying systemic abnormalities that can cause or predispose to the occurrence of a seizure. Seizures can produce a serum leukocytosis due to demargination of white blood cells. When ordering a CBC, it is important to include a differential, as a postictal leukocytosis will not produce a "left shift." Consequently, if there are abnormal levels of immature white cells in the setting of a leukocytosis, a systemic infection should be considered as a possible cause, rather than the seizure. Chemistries include a capillary blood sugar level upon arrival in the ED, followed by serum sodium, potassium, chloride, bicarbonate, calcium, magnesium, and glucose levels. Blood urea nitrogen, creatinine, serum glutamic-oxaloacetic transaminase, alkaline phosphatase, total bilirubin, and ethanol levels can be helpful. Prolactin levels can be obtained but it is important to recognize that many conditions can cause elevated levels; in an appropriate clinical setting it may assist in deciding whether a seizure occurred. ASM levels can be useful to obtain (e.g., phenytoin and divalproex), with the understanding that many of the commonly used ASMs (e.g., levetiracetam and lacosamide) take days to result. When indicated, urine is obtained for routine and microscopic tests and for a toxicology screen. An electrocardiogram can be helpful with cardiac disease, and a chest radiograph can be obtained when infection is suspected. Patients with known seizure disorders who have had an isolated seizure followed by rapid and complete recovery and a normal neurological examination may not require laboratory studies other than serum ASM levels, especially when medication noncompliance is suspected.

Computerized tomography (CT) of the brain is available in most hospitals, and its judicious use is important in seizures associated with neurodegenerative disease, major brain malformations, intracranial hemorrhage, space-occupying lesions, or head trauma. CT scanning with bone windows can be indicated to assess for penetrating wounds or depressed skull fractures, and has largely replaced the need for skull radiographs. Magnetic resonance imaging (MRI) of the brain is available in many hospitals and has greater sensitivity than CT in demonstrating certain types of abnormalities (e.g., temporal lobe abnormalities in patients with focal onset seizures). The use of MRI is usually not helpful during the ED evaluation of a seizure. However, the patient with a first-time or previously not evaluated unprovoked seizure should be discharged with a prescription for an MRI of the brain to be performed with epilepsy protocol software where available. The EEG is the single most useful study in assessing the cause of seizures. Although its use is also limited in the ED, it should be considered in patients with an unexplained and prolonged impaired level of consciousness.

Lumbar puncture is performed when CNS infection is suspected and there are no signs of increased intracranial pressure. An opening pressure is recorded and CSF is obtained for blood counts, including a WBC differential count, protein, glucose, Gram stain, acid-fast bacilli, cryptococcal antigen, Venereal Disease Research Laboratory test (VDRL), bacterial cultures, and counterimmunoelectrophoresis or agglutination assays for bacterial antigens. Treatment of suspected meningitis or encephalitis is instituted immediately. It is important to note that the CSF may reveal pleocytosis after a single focal onset seizure, a bilateral tonic-clonic seizure, or SE. Treatment of suspected CNS infection is not withheld because of the possibility that the observed pleocytosis is simply due to seizure occurrence.

13.4 Management

The ED management of a patient with a seizure is commonly determined by the cause, type, severity, and frequency of the seizure. At times, treatment of the seizure precedes diagnosis of its cause. When identified, the underlying cause of seizures is treated, and ASMs are used when indicated. ASMs are chosen on the basis of their clinical effectiveness in treating specific epileptic syndromes or seizure types. Treatment of a seizure in the ED may warrant IV treatment, such as a patient who presents having experienced multiple seizures that day but does not meet the definition of SE, and may be best served by the administration of an intravenous "load" of an ASM before discharge. For example, a patient maintained on phenytoin who experiences a seizure is brought to the ED, returns to baseline, and has an unrevealing work-up except for a free phenytoin level of 0.6 µg/mL, should be given an IV load to reach a "therapeutic" level of 1-2 µg/mL prior to discharge. Commonly prescribed ASMs and their associated clinical indications, dosing requirements, and therapeutic serum concentrations are given in Table 13.3.

13.4.1 Status Epilepticus

SE can be nonconvulsive or convulsive. Nonconvulsive SE includes absence SE, focal aware SE, and focal impaired awareness SE. These conditions are encountered relatively infrequently in the ED and are not as immediately serious as convulsive (bilateral tonic-clonic) SE. The diagnosis of NCSE is often difficult to make unless the patient has a history of such episodes. EEG may be necessary to confirm the diagnosis. Absence SE is treated with diazepam, 0.3 mg/kg given intravenously (<5 mg per minute), followed by an initial dose of ethosuximide or valproic acid, 20 mg/kg per day, in three divided doses. Focal aware SE and focal impaired awareness SE can be treated with the same ASM regimens as in convulsive SE, but aggressive treatment is usually not necessary or warranted.

Convulsive SE is a medical emergency requiring prompt and focused treatment. Treatment of convulsive SE must be aimed at controlling the seizures while proceeding with the evaluation to establish their cause. Failure to stop the seizures of convulsive SE can cause significant morbidity or mortality, which is directly related to the duration of ongoing seizure activity. Descriptive details of management of convulsive SE are given below and summarized in Table 13.4. Management of convulsive SE begins by placing the patient in

Table 13.3 Antiseizure medications, clinical indications, adult dosing requirements, and therapeutic serum concentrations

Drug	Seizure types	Daily dosing	Therapeutic levels
Phenytoin	Focal, tonic-clonic	4–7 mg/kg	10–20 µg/mL
Carbamazepine	Focal, tonic-clonic	8–20 mg/kg	4–12 µg/mL
Phenobarbital	Focal, tonic-clonic	1–3 mg/kg	15–40 µg/mL
Primidone	Tonic-clonic, focal	750–2,000 mg	5–12 µg/mL
Valproic acid	Tonic-clonic, myoclonic absence, focal	15–60 mg/kg	50–100 µg/mL
Ethosuximide	Absence	500–1,500 mg	40–100 µg/mL
Clonazepam	Focal, generalized (Lennox–Gastaut)	2–20 mg	20–80 ng/mL
Felbamate	Focal, generalized	1,200–3,600 mg	Not defined
Gabapentin	Focal	900–4,800 mg not defined	
Lamotrigine	Focal, tonic-clonic, absence, myoclonic, generalized szs in Lennox–Gastaut (with VPA)	300–500 mg 100–400 mg	3–14 µg/mL
Topiramate	Focal, tonic-clonic, generalized szs in Lennox–Gastaut	200–600 mg	Not defined
Levetiracetam	Focal, tonic-clonic	1–3 g	3–14 µg/mL
Oxcarbazepine	Focal, tonic-clonic	1,200–2,400 mg	12–30 µg/mL
Zonisamide	Focal, tonic, myoclonic	200–600 mg	10–30 µg/mL
Rufinamide	Focal, tonic-clonic, generalized szs in Lennox–Gastaut	400–3,200 mg	10–40 µg/mL
Lacosamide	Focal	100–400 mg	10–20 µg/mL
Clobazam	Focal, tonic-clonic, generalized szs in Lennox–Gastaut	10–40 mg	0.03–0.3 µg/mL
Brivaracetam	Focal, tonic-clonic	50–200 mg	
Eslicarbazepine	Focal	400–1,600 mg	3–35 µg/mL
Perampanel	Focal, generalized	4–12 mg	0.05–0.4 µg/mL

Table 13.3 (cont.)

Drug	Seizure types	Daily dosing	Therapeutic levels
Pregabalin	Focal	150–600 mg	Not defined
Vigabatrin	Focal, tonic-clonic, generalized	1–3 g	0.8–36 µg/mL
Cenobamate	Focal	50–400 mg	30–60 µg/mL

Table 13.4 Treatment protocol for convulsive status epilepticus in adults

Time (min)	Management
0	Place patient on left side to prevent aspiration. Establish airway and administer oxygen. Obtain blood pressure and begin ECG monitoring. Establish a peripheral IV line with isotonic saline in the right arm. Place a nasogastric tube for persistent vomiting. Obtain EEG where available. Obtain blood for laboratory tests, including a capillary blood glucose level. Consider thiamine, 100 mg IV, followed by glucose, 50 g IV.
5	Give lorazepam, not to exceed 2 mg/min IV, until seizures cease or a total dose of 8 mg. or diazepam, not to exceed 2 mg/min IV, until seizures cease or a total dose of 30 mg; if no IV access midazolam 10 mg IM.
10–20	If seizures continue, ASMs can be given in combination: levetiracetam 60 mg/kg IV up to 4,500 mg. or phenytoin 20 mg/kg IV (<50 mg/min) and continuous blood pressure monitoring and ECG or fosphenytoin, 20 mg PE/kg IV (150 mg PE/min), with continuous monitoring of blood pressure and ECG. If seizures continue give an additional dose of phenytoin 5 mg/kg (fosphenytoin 5 mg PE/kg) and, if necessary, repeat the dose to a maximum of 30 mg/kg (fosphenytoin 30 mg PE/kg) or valproate sodium 20–40 mg/kg over 10 minutes at 10 mg/kg/min

Table 13.4 (cont.)

Time (min)	Management
	or
	phenobarbital 15–20 mg/kg over 10 minutes
	or
	lacosamide 200–400 mg IV
	or
	ketamine 1–2 mg/kg every 5 minutes in successive boluses up to a total of ~5 mg/kg. If seizures continue, maintain an infusion rate of 1–7.5 mg/kg/h.
30	If seizures continue, prepare for intubation. Use induction regimen of 1.5 mg/kg propofol, 2 mg/kg ketamine, and a paralytic. Maintain continuous monitoring of vital signs, especially blood pressure, until seizures cease.
	If seizures continue, induce general anesthesia with propofol maintaining a rate of 3–5 mg/kg/h to achieve suppression of all EEG epileptiform activity, followed by 0.5–5.0 mg/kg/h to maintain suppression
	or
	midazolam 0.2 mg/kg IV bolus, then 0.05–0.5 mg/kg/h.

a left lateral decubitus position in the middle of a gurney. The head is supported and protected from injury during convulsions. An adequate airway is established immediately. When the teeth are not clenched, the oropharynx is suctioned and an oral airway inserted. Insertion of other hard objects between the teeth, including a padded tongue blade, is not advised because of potential dislodgement and local trauma. Oxygen can be administered by nasal cannula or face mask. A nasogastric tube can be placed for continuous vomiting. Endotracheal intubation is considered when there is evidence of compromised ventilation despite implementation of these procedures. Rapid sequence intubation usually can be performed with standard methods using direct or video-directed intubation, but for severe, uncontrolled seizures the nasotracheal route can be attempted.

While the patient's airway is being secured, blood pressure is measured and EKG monitoring begun. A peripheral intravenous line is established with plastic catheters and is protected against movement and subcutaneous infiltration during clonic motor activity. Blood is drawn for a capillary blood sugar; complete blood count; serum electrolytes including Na^+, Ca^{2+}, and Mg^{2+}; serum glucose, urea nitrogen, and creatinine; serum ASMs or other potentially neuroactive medications; and a toxicology screen. After blood drawing is complete, the intravenous line is kept open with isotonic saline. Thiamine, 100 mg by intravenous push, is given to protect patients with thiamine deficiency against a possible exacerbation of Wernicke's encephalopathy precipitated by administration of glucose. Wernicke's encephalopathy occurs in chronic alcoholics or patients with chronic malnutrition and is relatively common among patients with SE. Glucose, 50 g (50 mL of 50% dextrose in water), by intravenous push, can be given for treatment of potential hypoglycemia. Only rarely does hypoglycemia cause SE. Administration of thiamine and glucose does not pose a risk to patients who are not deficient in them.

13.4.1.1 Use of Medications in Status Epilepticus

Medications to treat SE are typically given sequentially until seizure control is achieved. ASMs within a class of agents are selected based on efficacy, availability, and the practitioner's familiarity with their use (Table 13.4). A benzodiazepine is a first-line class of drug to be administered in treating SE. The available benzodiazepines for initial intravenous treatment of SE are lorazepam and diazepam; midazolam can be considered for IM use when IV access is not obtainable. Sedation, hypotension, and respiratory depression can occur with their use. If initial use of an appropriate dose of a benzodiazepine has not terminated SE, second-line use of select maintenance ASMs is indicated. A pivotal study demonstrated equivalent efficacy of levetiracetam, fosphenytoin, and valproate in seizure cessation with benzodiazepine-refractory SE. If one or more second-line agents is ineffective in terminating SE, use of a sedative anesthetic such as propofol or midazolam is indicated to achieve EEG burst suppression.

Levetiracetam is given as a rapid intravenous infusion and is safe and well-tolerated. It is increasingly used as the initial second-line ASM due to its several favorable characteristics, including lack of hepatic metabolism, not inhibiting or inducing hepatic enzymes, minimal protein binding, and lack of interaction with other drugs. It can be used for patients already receiving it as maintenance therapy, and it is the preferred agent for those with liver failure.

Phenytoin is given by intravenous push with continuous monitoring of ECG and blood pressure because of the potential for cardiac arrhythmias and hypotension, respectively. Cardiac arrhythmias and hypotension occur largely due to the effects on the atrioventricular conduction system by propylene glycol, the diluent for phenytoin. Therefore, the use of phenytoin is relatively contraindicated in patients with known cardiac conduction abnormalities; fosphenytoin (see below) should be used instead when available. Cardiac arrhythmias and hypotension can often be corrected by decreasing the rate of phenytoin infusion. Phenytoin usually can be given safely to patients who have been on maintenance phenytoin therapy before a serum phenytoin level is available.

Fosphenytoin is a phosphorylated pro-drug of phenytoin, which is cleaved by tissue phosphatases into phenytoin. Fosphenytoin is water-soluble and, therefore, does not need to be diluted with propylene glycol. Rates of infusion of the drug can be approximately three times faster than that of phenytoin. Therefore, it takes approximately 10 minutes to infuse 1,500 mg of fosphenytoin (expressed as 1,500 mg of phenytoin equivalents (PE) when ordering fosphenytoin) at a rate of 150 mg PE/min. However, it takes approximately 10–15 minutes for the full *in vivo* conversion of fosphenytoin to phenytoin. Comparing this to the expected 30 minute loading time for 1500 mg of phenytoin given intravenously at 50 mg per minute, there is marginal savings in time with use of fosphenytoin. However, phenytoin is frequently given more slowly than 50 mg per minute, thus increasing the time saved by using fosphenytoin.

Valproate is given as an intravenous infusion and should be used advisedly in patients with hepatic disease. It is nearly fully metabolized in the liver, involving several cytochrome P450 enzyme systems. Its multiple metabolites can contribute to its efficacy, drug–drug interactions, and toxicity when given in high doses for treatment of SE.

Phenobarbital, a barbiturate, can be given when phenytoin or fosphenytoin has not been effective after 25–30 minutes. Severe respiratory depression and hypotension can occur with high doses of phenobarbital, requiring continuous monitoring of vital signs. When seizures have not stopped after the use of phenobarbital, pentobarbital can be used to induce coma. This step involves EEG monitoring to assess the desired aim of burst suppression or EEG silence. The patient can be kept in an EEG burst suppression pattern for days, when necessary, and the rate of pentobarbital infusion lowered every 2–4 hours to determine when seizure activity has ended. The major side effect of pentobarbital is hypotension, which can be reversed with saline infusion or pressors.

Lacosamide has proven to be a safe and effective ASM in refractory SE. It can cause hypotension and is contraindicated in patients with heart block or conduction system defects. Its use is associated with several drug–drug interactions and dosing should be reduced in patients with hepatic or renal failure.

Ketamine, a dissociative anesthetic, increasingly has been used in refractory SE as an effective ASM. It can be used in conjunction with phenobarbital, propofol, or midazolam (see below), has a short half-life, is hemodynamically stable, and can be titrated rapidly. Because it is hepatically metabolized, dosing is adjusted in hepatically impaired patients. It can increase blood pressure and heart rate, and cause hypersalivation.

Propofol is a sedative anesthetic that is increasingly used in the treatment of refractory SE. As with other anesthetics used in treating SE, the dose is titrated using EEG monitoring to ensure suppression of all ictal activity and maintenance of a burst suppression pattern. Propofol has the advantage of a very short half-life, and patients can recover more quickly from prolonged intravenous infusions than with benzodiazepines or barbiturates. Hypotension is common with infusion, so blood pressure is supported as required.

Midazolam also can be used in cases of refractory SE and titrated to EEG burst suppression. Mild to moderate hypotension can be associated with its use, and can be treated with fluid or pressors as needed.

13.4.2 Alcohol Withdrawal Seizures

Alcohol withdrawal seizures are generalized tonic-clonic convulsions that usually occur within 48 hours after cessation of ethanol ingestion, with a peak incidence between 13 and 24 hours. The seizures are usually brief, occur as a single episode or in bursts of two or more, and can evolve into SE. These seizures typically occur in chronic alcoholics or after episodes of binge drinking. Other causes of generalized seizures that may occur during alcohol withdrawal include head trauma, subdural hematoma, meningitis, and metabolic derangements, which should be evaluated as indicated. Focal onset seizures that occur during the withdrawal period suggest focal brain injury – old or new – and require evaluation.

The standard treatment of alcohol withdrawal seizures is based on the principle of providing a medication with cross-tolerance to alcohol. Because these seizures are usually brief and limited in number, a benzodiazepine such as chlordiazepoxide (Librium), 50–100 mg IV, or diazepam, 5–10 mg IV, can be administered to treat an ongoing seizure. These medications can be repeated at regular intervals (chlordiazepoxide every 1–2 hours orally or intravenously, diazepam every 15–20 minutes orally or intravenously) as indicated to suppress other withdrawal symptoms and continued for several days on a tapering schedule. Patients are assessed carefully for hypotension and respiratory depression. In addition, thiamine 300–500 mg/day can be administered. Patients who have a history of epileptic seizures should have serum levels obtained for their prescribed ASMs and supplemented as needed to achieve therapeutic serum concentrations. Patients with seizures refractory to benzodiazepine treatment or those with a history of epileptic seizures not currently treated can be given a loading dose of phenytoin, 15–18 mg/kg IV (50 mg per minute with ECG monitoring) or orally (2–3 split doses over 6 hours), respectively. Alcohol withdrawal seizures that evolve into SE should be treated as described previously.

13.4.3 Disposition of Patients Following a Seizure

The disposition of a patient who has experienced a seizure is largely based on the cause and the severity of the seizure. New-onset seizures may or may not require treatment with an ASM. A decision to treat with an ASM is best made after discussing the patient's case with his or her primary care physician or a neurologist. Usually, patients can be discharged safely when the seizure is brief, nonfocal, and uncomplicated, the neurological examination is normal, and the diagnostic evaluation is unremarkable. Patients who have experienced bilateral tonic-clonic seizures, especially those occurring nocturnally, should be aware of the relatively rare risk of sudden unexplained death in epilepsy (SUDEP) and advised accordingly. Patients are admitted to the hospital for further evaluation and management when there has been SE, trauma-induced seizures, identification of a space-occupying CNS lesion or infection, anoxia, or a serious toxic or metabolic derangement. Typically, patients admitted to the hospital are started and maintained on an ASM during their hospitalization.

13.5 Medicolegal Issues

A patient who has experienced a seizure must be informed of the cause of the seizure, the determined need for ASMs and their potential side effects, reasonable restrictions on activities of daily living, and the state's law regarding restriction of driving privileges. This information is documented clearly in the medical record for potential medicolegal issues.

For patients with seizures, there are no uniform restrictions on activities of daily living that might be of potential harm to them or others. The range of activities must be determined for each patient based on the type of seizures experienced, the associated functional impairment, and the degree of seizure control achieved with ASMs. In general, patients with seizures are encouraged to lead full and active lives. They are advised to develop regular routines for sleeping, eating, working, and medication-taking, and to avoid excessive exertion, sleep deprivation, excessive use of alcohol and caffeine, and undue stress. Excessive use of alcohol can increase the risk of seizure recurrence during a withdrawal period. Excessive use of caffeine can make seizures more difficult to control. Common sense and good judgment should dictate avoidance of certain activities that may pose substantial risk to the patient or others. These include driving, swimming, bathing, and working at heights or with heavy machinery or power tools. Patients with seizures may be able to swim but should never swim alone. High-risk sports such as sky diving, hang gliding, or rock climbing should probably be avoided.

The laws for restriction of driving privileges after a seizure with impairment of consciousness vary between states. It is important that the emergency physician know the laws of the state so that the patient can be informed accurately. Generally, patients who experience a seizure are not permitted to drive for 6–12 months. Most neurologists consider a patient capable of driving without serious risk posed to the patient or others when the patient is seizure-free for 1 year and compliant with the prescribed AEDs. In patients with seizures who have no history of seizures associated with impairment in awareness or significant motor dysfunction (e.g., minor focal aware motor seizures), driving may be considered safe when the patient can drive without difficulty during a seizure. Patients experiencing only nocturnal seizures may not need to have their licenses suspended. When seizures have been well controlled on an ASM regimen and drug withdrawal is undertaken, it is reasonable to recommend against driving during the withdrawal period or for 6 months, whichever is longer.

Some states require that the physician responsible for treating the seizures report that information to the agency responsible for issuing drivers' licenses. Most states hold the patient responsible for providing information about his or her condition to the appropriate authority when applying for a driver's license. Specific information regarding driver's license restrictions can be obtained from each state's Department of Motor Vehicles.

Documentation on the ED medical record of the patient who has had a seizure includes common side effects of ASMs, informing the patient of the state laws regarding driving restrictions, and potential risks. When an ASM is not initiated in the ED, or is delayed, the reasons are documented. For example, when the seizure has been a single, isolated event, treatment with an ASM may not be initiated. This decision is made with the patient's physician, and appropriate follow-up determined.

Pearls and Pitfalls

- Patients evaluated in the ED following a seizure may be postictal, normal, or experiencing a recurrent seizure.
- Patients who appear confused or postictal may be experiencing absence or focal impaired awareness SE.
- Convulsive SE is a medical emergency associated with high morbidity and mortality.
- Although used infrequently in the ED, an EEG can diagnose ongoing seizure activity in a patient with a prolonged period of impaired consciousness.
- Syncope can be difficult to distinguish from seizure.
- The diagnosis of PNES is made cautiously after a thorough neurological examination and focused diagnostic evaluation are normal; many patients with psychogenic seizures have epilepsy.
- It is important that the emergency physician knows the state's laws regarding restriction of driving privileges for patients who have experienced a seizure.

Bibliography

Ameli PA, Ammar AA, Owusu KA, Maciel CB. Evaluation and management of seizures and status epilepticus. *Neurol Clin* 2021; 39(2):513–544.

Farkas J. Status Epilepticus. In *The Internet Book of Critical Care*. 2021. Available at: https://emcrit.org/ibcc/sz.

Fisher RS, Cross JH, D'Souza C, et al. Instruction manual for the ILAE 2017 operational classification of seizure types. *Epilepsia* 2017;58(4):531–542.

Kapur J, Elm J, Chamberlain JM, et al. Randomized trial of three anticonvulsant medications for status epilepticus. *N Engl J Med* 2019;381(22):2103–2113.

Rossetti AO, Alvarez V. Update on the management of status epilepticus. *Curr Opin Neurol* 2021;34(2):172–181.

Scheffer IE, Berkovic S, Capovilla G, et al. ILAE classification of the epilepsies position paper of the ILAE Commission for Classification and Terminology. *Epilepsia* 2017;58(4):512–521.

Chapter

14

Infections of the Central Nervous System

Zaw Min, Richard M. Kaplan, Kate DeAntonis, and Evelina Krieger

14.1 Introduction

Central nervous system (CNS) infections are typically transmitted hematologically or by contiguous spread. Frequently, there is colonization of the upper respiratory tract, invasion across the epithelium, and then activation of the complement cascade. Polymorphonuclear leukocytes and the cytokines reduce the blood–brain barrier (BBB) integrity and the host defenses. Pathogens invade the meninges, resulting in inflammation and an increased BBB permeability. A subsequent inflammatory response by neutrophils creates edema and increased intracranial pressure, CNS tissue ischemia, and hydrocephalus. Clinical features of meningitis depend upon the age and health status of the patient, the specific pathogen, and the duration of illness. Diagnosing a CNS infection in infants and young children or in patients with nonspecific signs and symptoms is a challenge in the emergency department (ED). A thorough history and physical examination should help lead to a clinical suspicion of a CNS infection. In this chapter, we focus on ED management of CNS infections in adults and children. We review community-acquired, post-traumatic, healthcare-associated bacterial meningitis, and aseptic meningitis.

14.2 Prevention

CNS infections that are vaccine-preventable include *Streptococcus pneumoniae*, *Haemophilus influenzae* type b, and *Neisseria meningitidis*. Available vaccines may be accessed at www .cdc.gov/vaccines/schedules/easy-to-read.

Preventive measures for pregnant women include screening for group B *Streptococcus* (GBS) at 36 weeks of gestation. For women who have a primary outbreak of genital herpes simplex virus (HSV) lesions at the time of delivery, cesarean section is indicated. Pregnant women with a history of genital HSV before 36 weeks of gestation are treated with antiviral suppressive therapy starting from 36 weeks of gestation through delivery.

14.3 Approach to the Patient with a Possible CNS Infection

14.3.1 History

History and physical examination remain the essential factors in developing the index of suspicion to discover a CNS infection in children and adults. A birth history is pertinent in infants and young children and should include maternal GBS status, prenatal HSV status, prematurity, and complications during pregnancy. Vaccination status is an essential component of the history, as well as sick contacts, group settings such as childcare or group-living situations, and travel to endemic areas or vector-heavy regions. Past medical history should include specific inquiries about asplenia, immunosuppression, and recent illness or antibiotic use.

Identification of risk factors may aid in the early diagnosis of meningitis (Table 14.1). Most risk factors can be identified with the six Is:

- infection (upper or lower respiratory tract infection, sinusitis, otitis)
- immunosuppression (splenectomy, sickle cell disease, corticosteroids, Hodgkin disease, myeloma, organ transplant, HIV)
- injury (head trauma, neurologic or ENT (ear, nose, throat) procedures)
- indwelling (catheters, shunts, ventricular reservoirs)
- imbiber (alcoholic)
- identification (close contacts)

14.3.2 Physical Examination

Fever, a change in mental status, and/or nuchal rigidity should prompt serious consideration of the diagnosis of meningitis. Nuchal rigidity is characterized by neck stiffness and the inability to passively flex and extend the head in a normal manner. Meningeal irritation may be characterized by classic Kernig or Brudzinski signs. The Brudzinski sign occurs when flexion of the neck results in spontaneous flexion of the knees and hips. The Kernig sign refers to the resistance to extension of the lower leg with the hip flexed at 90 degrees, by stretching of the lumbar roots causing pain in the hamstring and paraspinal muscles. The jolt accentuation test, the horizontal movement of the head at a frequency of 2–3 rotations/second, has also been recommended to assess for the possibility of meningitis. A positive test is a worsening of the baseline headache.

Poorly reactive pupils, a bulging fontanel (in upright position), and papilledema are signs of increased intracranial pressure. For infants it has been recommended to measure head circumference. The patient should be examined for HEENT (head, eyes, ears, nose, and throat) infections and focal neurologic signs, as well as subtle signs of a seizure. The skin examination may reveal erythema migrans (neuroborreliosis), petechiae or purpura (invasive streptococcal or meningococcal disease), or vesicles (HSV).

Physical findings in infants and toddlers may be difficult to interpret. Healthy infants sleep much more than older children and lethargy may go unnoticed. Toddlers are inherently labile and frequently protest examination or interaction in the medical setting, making irritability more difficult to discern. Altered level of consciousness may exist as any of these findings, or as a patternless intermittent symptom. Nuchal rigidity is not consistently found in children under 2 years of age. Mottling or other signs of poor perfusion in a child may be the first notable sign of critical illness. In short, a toxic appearance in a child warrants evaluation and empiric treatment for a CNS infection.

14.4 Differential Diagnosis

The differential diagnosis of a CNS infection includes neurologic, toxicologic, metabolic, oncologic, environmental, and behavioral disorders. A wide range of other diagnoses, from a nonspecific viral syndrome to a new-onset seizure disorder, are within the differential diagnosis. Evaluation for CNS infection is important in any patient who has fever without source, particularly in infants less than 2 months of age and immunosuppressed patients.

Table 14.1 Risk factor and CNS infections

Patient characteristic	Type of infection	Likely organism
Age of patient		
Neonatal	Congenital Meningitis	*Escherichia coli* *Streptococcus agalactiae* (GBS) *Listeria monocytogenes*
Elderly	Community acquired	*Streptococcus agalactiae* (GBS) *Listeria monocytogenes*
Unvaccinated status	Community acquired	*Streptococcus pneumoniae* *Haemophilus influenzae* type b (Hib) *Neisseria meningitidis*
Immunocompromised		
HIV+	Community acquired	*Streptococcus pneumoniae* *Neisseria meningitidis* *Listeria monocytogenes*
Primary immunodeficiency, asplenia (functional or anatomical), chronic steroid use, or chronic immunosuppressive therapy	Community acquired	*Streptococcus pneumoniae* *Neisseria meningitides* *Haemophilus influenzae* *Listeria monocytogenes*
ENT conditions Otitis media, sinusitis, mastoiditis	Community acquired	*Streptococcus pneumoniae*
Traumatic basilar skull fracture	Community acquired	*Streptococcus pneumoniae** *Haemophilus influenza* Group A β-hemolytic streptococci
Healthcare associated		
ENT procedures	Nosocomial meningitis	*Streptococcus pneumoniae*
Neurosurgical procedures	Nosocomial meningitis	*Staphylococcus* species (*S. aureus*, coagulase-negative staphylococci), Gram-negative bacilli (including *Pseudomonas aeruginosa*), and *Propionibacterium acnes*
Social conditions		
Group housing or overcrowding (college students, military)	Community acquired	*Neisseria meningitides*

Table 14.1 (cont.)

Patient characteristic	Type of infection	Likely organism
Dietary practices – consumption of uncooked meats, soft cheeses, cold cuts	Community acquired	*Listeria monocytogenes*
Chronic liver disease, alcoholism, substance abuse	Community acquired	*Listeria monocytogenes*

14.5 Diagnostic Testing

14.5.1 Bloodwork

The laboratory evaluation of a patient suspected of a CNS infection should include a complete blood count with differential, blood culture, basic metabolic panel, and coagulation studies. Leukocytosis, leukopenia, thrombocytopenia, and coagulopathy may be present. Electrolytes may be altered if syndrome of inappropriate antidiuretic hormone secretion (SIADH) accompanies increased intracranial pressure, and the serum glucose is necessary to compare with the glucose level in the CSF. Blood cultures should be drawn prior to the administration of antibiotics.

14.5.2 Imaging

The CT scan is the primary imaging technique in the ED. If a patient has suspected cerebral mass, focal neurologic findings, a prolonged or deteriorating course, or papilledema, a CT of the head should be performed (Table 14.2). A CT scan may show meningeal inflammation as well as involvement of the cerebral cortex and ventricles.

14.5.3 CSF Examination

CSF evaluation may include a cell count and differential, Gram stain and culture, protein, glucose, and lactate level, along with possible bacterial antigen and polymerase chain reaction (PCR) testing (Table 14.3).

The Gram stain is extremely helpful when it is immediately positive. Its reported sensitivity is up to more than 90% in pneumococcal and meningococcal meningitis. A negative Gram stain does not rule out the possibility of bacterial meningitis.

Antigen, PCR, and antibody testing is a useful adjunct to CSF testing. CSF bacterial antigen studies are available for *H. influenzae* type b, *N. meningitidis* A, B, C, Y, W-135, *Streptococcus agalactiae* (GBS), *Streptococcus pneumoniae*, and *Escherichia coli*. These antigen studies may identify an organism when the Gram stain is negative. After antibiotic therapy, bacterial antigens may persist in the CSF for several days and this test may be useful when the patient has been treated with antibiotics prior to lumbar puncture (LP). A CSF multiplex PCR assay is commercially available for *Escherichia coli* K1, *Haemophilus influenzae*, *Listeria monocytogenes*, *Neisseria meningitidis*, *Streptococcus agalactiae*, *Streptococcus pneumoniae*, cytomegalovirus,

Table 14.2 Patients with suspected CNS infection who should undergo CT head scan prior to lumbar puncture

Abnormal level of consciousness	Focal neurologic deficit
History of CNS disease	Dilated nonreactive pupil
Mass lesion	Visual gaze palsy
Stroke	Arm or leg drift
New-onset seizure	Immunocompromised state
Seizure activity in prior week	HIV infection
Signs of increased intracranial pressure	Immunosuppressive therapy
Papilledema	Cancer patients
Hypertension with bradycardia	Hematopoietic stem cell transplantation

enterovirus, herpes simplex virus 1 and 2, human parechovirus, varicella zoster virus, human herpes virus 6, and *Cryptococcus* neoformans/gattii. In patients suspected of cryptococcal meningitis, CSF cryptococcal antigen is recommended to be added due to cases of cryptococcal meninigits in which CSF multiplex PCR test was negative for *Cryptococcus neoformans* or *Cryptococcus gatti*, whereas CSF cryptococcal antigen was positive. In addition, IgM antibody in the CSF may be detected within 8 days of symptoms in patients with West Nile virus meningoencephalitis.

CSF culture is the gold standard for diagnosis of bacterial meningitis. In the absence of antibiotics, culture results were reported as positive in 80–90% of patients with acute community-acquired bacterial meningitis. The yield of both CSF Gram stain and culture is reduced by prior antibiotic therapy. There are limited studies evaluating the effects of antibiotics on CSF parameters.

14.5.4 Other Cultures

Wound cultures, skin lesions, operative site cultures, and sputum cultures may all reveal the causative agent, especially for brain abscesses.

14.6 Diagnosis and Treatment

14.6.1 Meningitis

Meningitis is inflammation of the leptomeninges of the brain and spinal cord. The leptomeninges are composed of the arachnoid and the pia mater, between which the CSF circulates in the subarachnoid space. CSF analysis and cultures are needed to establish the diagnosis of meningitis.

14.6.2 Bacterial Meningitis

14.6.2.1 Community-Acquired Bacterial Meningitis

The annual incidence of acute community-acquired bacterial meningitis ranges from 1.3 to 6 cases per 100,000 adults in the United States to 500 cases per 100,000 in the "meningitis belt"

Table 14.3 CSF findings in patients with CNS infections (meningitis)

CNS infection	Cell count and differential	Glucose (mg/dL)	Protein (mg/dL)	Gram stain	Lactic acid	Pathogen recovery
No infection	<5 WBC mm³, all lymphocytes	Comparable to serum level, or a CSF to serum glucose ratio of at least 0.6	15–45	Negative		None
Bacterial	100–10,000 WBC/mm³, neutrophil predominance	<50 mg/dL or a CSF serum to glucose ratio of <0.5	>100	See Table 14.4	May be elevated	Aerobic or anaerobic culture, bacterial antigen testing, multiplex PCR
Viral	10–1,000 WBC/mm³, monocytes predominance; Elevated RBC or xanthochromia in HSV	Normal/comparable to serum level	<200	No organism	Usually normal	Multiplex PCR or virus-specific IgM
Neurosyphilis	>5 WBC/mm³, lymphocyte predominance	>45	>45			CSF VRDL
Tuberculous	50–300 WBC/mm³, monocyte predominance	<45	50–300	Acid-fast smear		Mycobacterial culture, PCR
Lyme	160 WBC/mm³, lymphocyte predominance	>45	200–300			CSF:Serum Lyme antibody index
Cryptococcal	20–500 WBC/mm³, monocyte predominance	Normal/comparable to serum level or decreased	>100 mg/dL	India ink prep	May be elevate	Fungal culture, antigen testing, multiplex PCR

A traumatic LP increases 1 WBC for every 700–1,000 RBC, and protein increases 1 mg/dL for every 1,000 RBC. Hemorrhagic lesions of herpes encephalitis may lead to elevated RBC in CSF or xanthochromia, and must be considered.

of Africa. The median age of bacterial meningitis in the United States is 41, with an overall mortality of 15%. The major causes of this type of bacterial meningitis include *Streptococcus pneumoniae* (58%), *Streptococcus agalactiae* (GBS) (18.1%), *Neisseria meningitidis* (13.9%), *Haemophilus influenzae* type b (6.7%), and *Listeria monocytogenes* (3.4%).

Antibiotic therapy should be started immediately. Empiric antibiotic therapy for community-acquired bacterial meningitis in adults is recommended to cover *S. pneumoniae*, *N. meningitidis*, and *H. influenzae*. Added antibiotic coverage is recommended for *L. monocytogenes* in adults older than 50 years of age and in children younger than 3 months of age (Tables 14.4 and 14.5). Vancomycin is added to ceftriaxone in patients with suspected pneumococcal meningitis to cover cephalosporin-resistant pneumococci strains. The intravenous antibiotic doses used in CNS infections are higher for better CSF penetration (Table 14.5). Adjunctive intravenous dexamethasone use (10 mg every 6 hours) is recommended in all adult patients with suspected pneumococcal meningitis to minimize hearing loss or other neurologic complications. Dexamethasone may be given 10–20 minutes before or with the first dose of antibiotic, and it is continued for the first 4 days of antibiotic treatment when blood or CSF cultures are positive for *S. pneumoniae*. For infants and children older than 2 months of age, dexamethasone may be given as 0.6 mg/kg/day IV divided every 6 hours for the first 4 days of antibiotic treatment.

14.6.2.2 Chemoprophylaxis in Community-Acquired Bacterial Meningitis

Antimicrobial chemoprophylaxis is indicated in close contacts of patients with meningococcal or *H. influenzae* type b infection. Chemoprophylaxis should be administered within 24 hours of exposure.

Close contacts of patients with meningococcal meningitis have an increased risk (400- to 800-fold) of contracting the disease. Five to ten percent of adults are asymptomatic nasopharyngeal carriers of *N. meningitidis*, and most are not pathogenic. Asymptomatic nasopharyngeal carriers are not treated. Oropharyngeal or nasopharyngeal cultures are not helpful in determining chemoprophylaxis. "Close contacts" in cases of meningococcal infection are generally defined as:

- household members, roommates, intimate contacts, contacts at a childcare center, young adults exposed in dormitories, military recruits exposed in training centers;
- long-flight travelers (i.e., one lasting ≥8 hours) who were seated directly next to an index patient; and
- individuals who have been exposed to oral secretions (e.g., intimate kissing, mouth-to-mouth resuscitation, endotracheal intubation, or endotracheal tube management).

Table 14.4 Microorganisms of acute community-acquired bacterial meningitis based on the characteristics of CSF Gram stain

CSF Gram stain	Suspected microorganism
Gram-positive diplococci	*Streptococcus pneumonia*
Gram-negative diplococci	*Neisseria meningitides*
Gram-positive rods/coccobacilli	*Listeria monocytogenes*
Gram-negative small pleomorphic coccobacilli	*Haemophilus influenza*

Table 14.5 Recommendations for empiric antimicrobial therapy in patients with community-acquired bacterial meningitis

Patient	Microorganism	First-line therapy	Alternative therapy for serious penicillin allergy
0–1 months	GBS, Listeria monocytogenes, Escherichia coli, Herpes simplex virus	IV ampicillin 300 mg/kg/day divided q 6 h and either IV gentamicin; 0–7 days: 4 mg/kg/24 h q 24 h >7 days: 4 mg/kg/24 h divided 12–18 h OR IV cefotaxime 300 mg/kg/day divided q 6 h Acyclovir IV 60 mg/kg/24 h (Q 8 h IV × 14–21 days)	
1 month to 24 months	Streptococcus pneumoniae, Haemophilus influenzae type b, Neisseria meningitidis	Vancomycin 15 mg/kg LD (60 mg/kg/day q 6 h) (max 4 g/day) + IV cefotaxime 100 mg/kg IV LD or IV ceftriaxone 50 mg/kg IV LD	For serious penicillin allergy, IV meropenem 120 mg/kg/day divided q 8 h (max 6 g/day)
Children and adolescents	Streptococcus pneumoniae, Neisseria meningitidis	IV vancomycin + 1–12 yr: 20 mg/kg divided q 6 h >12 yr: 20 mg/kg divided q 6–8 h IV cefotaxime 100 mg/kg IV LD If >12 yr or >50 kg: 2 g cefotaxime q 4–6 h OR IV ceftriaxone 50 mg/kg IV LD, max of 2 g LD	For serious penicillin allergy, IV meropenem 120 mg/kg/day divided q 8 h (max 6 g/day)
Immunocompetent, age <50 years	Streptococcus pneumoniae, Haemophilus influenzae, Neisseria meningitidis	IV ceftriaxone 2 g q 12 h + IV vancomycin load with 25–35 mg/kg, then 15–20 mg/kg q 8–12 h	IV moxifloxacin[a] 400 mg q 24 h + IV vancomycin load with 25–35 mg/kg, then 15–20 mg/kg q 8–12 h

Immunocompetent, age >50 years	Streptococcus pneumoniae, Haemophilus influenzae, Neisseria meningitidis, Listeria monocytogenes, Streptococcus agalactiae (GBS)	IV ceftriaxone 2 g q 12 h + IV vancomycin load with 25–35 mg/kg, then 15–20 mg/kg q 8–12 h + IV ampicillin 2 g q 4 h	IV moxifloxacin 400 mg q 24 h+ IV vancomycin load with 25–35 mg/kg, then 15–20 mg/kg q 8–12 h+ IV TMP-SMX[b] 5 mg/kg (TMP component) q 6 h
Immunocompromised[e]	Streptococcus pneumoniae, Haemophilus influenzae, Neisseria meningitidis, Listeria monocytogenes, Gram-negatives	IV cefepime[c] 2 g q 8 h + IV vancomycin load with 25–35 mg/kg, then 15–20 mg/kg q 8–12 h + IV ampicillin 2 g q 4 h	IV aztreonam[d] 2 g q 4 h + IV vancomycin load with 25–35 mg/kg, then 15–20 mg/kg q 8–12 h + IV TMP-SMX[b] 5 mg/kg (TMP component) q 6 h

[a] IV levofloxacin 500 mg q 12 h is an acceptable alternative if moxifloxacin is not available.

[b] IV meropenem 2 g q 8 h for suspected L. monocytogenes meningitis in severe penicillin and sulfa-allergic patients.

[c] IV ceftazidime 2 g q 8 h is an alternative. Use IV meropenem 2 g q 8 h if multi-drug resistant organism is suspected.

[d] IV ciprofloxacin 400 mg q 8 h can substitute for aztreonam.

[e] Patients on immunosuppressive therapy, HIV infection, organ transplantation.

TMP-SMX – trimethoprim-sulfamethoxazole, LD – loading dose.

Table 14.6 Recommended antibiotic regimens for chemoprophylaxis in meningococcal infection

Drug	Age	Dosage	Duration and route
Rifampin	<1 month	5 mg/kg every 12 hours	2 days, oral
	≥1 month	10 mg/kg every 12 hours	2 days, oral
	Adults, and pregnant women	600 mg every 12 hours	2 days, oral
Ciprofloxacin	Adults (not pregnant)	500 mg	One-time dose, oral
Ceftriaxone	Age <15 years	125 mg	One-time dose, IM
Ceftriaxone	Adults	250 mg	One-time dose, IM
Azithromycin*	Age <15 years	10 mg/kg	One-time dose, oral
Azithromycin*	Adults	500 mg	One-time dose, oral

* Zithromycin is **not** the first-line agent for chemoprophylaxis, and is only reserved for patients who have a serious allergy to rifampin or ceftriaxone, and when ciprofloxacin-resistant *N. meningitidis* is a concern.

Definition of "close contacts" in patients with *H. influenzae* type b infection is different from that of meningococcal infection. Chemoprophylaxis is not indicated for contacts of people with invasive disease caused by non-type b strains of *H. influenzae*. The antibiotic prophylaxis is recommended for the following close household contacts with *H. influenzae* type b infection:

- persons who live with the index patient;
- persons who spent >4 hours with the index patient;
- persons who spent time with the index patient for at least 5 days before hospital admission;
- persons aged <4 years who have not received an age-appropriate number of doses of Hib conjugate vaccine;
- persons aged <12 months who have not completed the primary Hib series; and
- persons who are immunocompromised and aged <18 years, regardless of that child's Hib immunization status.

Rifampin is the only recommended antimicrobial chemoprophylaxis agent for children, adults, and pregnant women who have close contacts with *H. influenzae* type b meningitis. The suggested dose of rifampin is 20 mg/kg/day orally (maximum 600 mg/day) for 4 days.

14.6.2.3 Other Etiologies for Bacterial Meningitis

Healthcare-Associated or Nosocomial Meningitis. Healthcare-associated meningitis is defined as meningitis that developed more than 48 hours after hospitalization or within one week of hospital discharge. Nosocomial meningitis usually results from invasive neurosurgical procedures (craniotomy, ventricular catheters, lumbar drains, intrathecal infusions, or spinal anesthesia), or post-ENT procedures. *Streptococcus pneumoniae* is responsible for the majority of cases of meningitis following ENT surgeries. Pathogens that cause nosocomial meningitis post-neurosurgical procedures include *Staphylococcus* species (*S. aureus*, coagulase-negative staphylococci), streptococci, Gram-negative Enterobacteriaceae (including *Pseudomonas aeruginosa*), and *Propionibacterium acnes*. Infections from CSF shunts may cause only low-grade fever or malaise and signs of meningeal irritation may be seen in fewer than 50% of these patients.

Post-traumatic Meningitis. The incidence of meningitis following moderate or severe head trauma has been estimated at 1.4%. The rate of meningitis may increase to 2–11% following open compound cranial fractures. Following basilar skull fractures, the median onset for meningitis is 11 days, and infection rates may reach 25%. *Streptococcus pneumoniae* is responsible for the majority of cases of meningitis following basilar skull fractures. Other pathogens that could cause meningitis in patients with cranial or facial trauma include *H. influenzae* and Group A β-hemolytic streptococci because these organisms colonize the nasopharynx. In patients with a basilar skull fracture, clear rhinorrhea or otorrhea are risk factors for post-traumatic meningitis.

Table 14.7 lists empiric antimicrobial therapy for bacterial meningitis by the predisposing conditions.

Table 14.7 Empiric antimicrobial therapy for bacterial meningitis by the predisposing conditions

Predisposing conditions	Bacterial pathogens	Empirical therapy
Basilar skull fracture	*Streptococcus pneumoniae,** *Haemophilus influenzae,* group A β-hemolytic streptococci	IV ceftriaxone 2 g q 12 h + IV vancomycin load with 25–35 mg/kg × one time, then 15–20 mg/kg q 8 h–12 h
Craniotomy, ventriculo-peritoneal or pleural shunts, lumbar drains, external ventricular drainage catheter, lumbar drains, other post-neurosurgery, penetrating trauma	*Staphylococcus* species (*S. aureus*, coagulase-negative staphylococci), Gram-negative bacilli (including *Pseudomonas aeruginosa*), and *Propionibacterium acnes*	IV cefepime 2 g q 8 h, OR IV ceftazidime 2 g q 8 h + IV vancomycin load with 25–35 mg/kg, then 15–20 mg/kg q 8–12 h

* Adjunctive dexamethasone therapy is not formally recommended in patients with nosocomial bacterial meningitis caused by *S. pneumoniae*. It may be reasonable to initiate dexamethasone treatment until the CSF culture is negative for *S. pneumoniae*.

14.6.3 Aseptic Meningitis

Aseptic meningitis is defined as patients with clinical and CSF evidence of meningeal inflammation with negative bacterial cultures. It is primarily of viral causes, and other major etiologies of aseptic meningitis include neurosyphilis, neuroborreliosis, tuberculous (TB) meningitis, and cryptococcal meningoencephalitis.

14.6.4 Viral Meningitis

Viral meningitis is generally a self-limited symptom complex of fever, headache, photophobia, and neck stiffness. Enterovirus is the most common cause of aseptic meningitis. HSV-2 is responsible for HSV meningitis. HSV encephalitis is almost exclusively due to HSV-1. Another important cause of viral meningitis is acute HIV infection presenting with a mononucleosis-like syndrome. Other viruses that cause aseptic meningitis include varicella zoster virus (VZV) and West Nile virus (WNV).

Diagnosis of viral meningitis is usually achieved by the commercially available multiplex PCR assay that detects CMV, enterovirus, HSV-1 and HSV-2, VZV, human parechovirus, and HHV-6 in the CSF. For HIV meningitis in an acute retroviral syndrome, PCR is the test of choice to detect HIV viremia since HIV antibody is usually undetectable during the acute HIV infection stage. WNV serology for IgG and IgM in the CSF or serum is the diagnostic test for WNV meningitis. When the clinical manifestations of WNV meningitis develop, WNV viremia is no longer present, and thus WNV PCR is not useful to aid in the diagnosis of WNV meningitis.

Other than in neonates, viral meningitis from enterovirus, HSV, VZV, and WNV is self-limited and antiviral therapy is not recommended. The initiation of antiretroviral therapy is strongly recommended in patients with HIV aseptic meningitis.

For newborns, HSV meningitis is an important pathogen. Symptoms are similar to bacterial sepsis and usually occur in the first 1–2 weeks of life. Neonates with HSV meningitis may have vesicular lesions, seizures, generalized lethargy, or irritability. A maternal history of HSV is important, but not necessary for the diagnosis. Diagnosis is made by viral culture of vesicular lesions or HSV PCR of the CSF. Neonatal HSV is treated empirically with acyclovir.

14.6.5 Neurosyphilis

Treponema pallidum, a spirochete, is the causative agent of neurosyphilis. Neurosyphilis can occur at any time from the initial infection, most commonly in the secondary syphilis. Current high risk factors for neurosyphilis include patients with HIV infection and men who have sex with men. Clinical symptoms include headache, confusion, neck stiffness, or nausea. Skin rash would be a prominent finding if associated with secondary syphilis. Fever is typically absent in neurosyphilis. Serum RPR/VDRL and CSF VDRL are almost always positive. In all patients with neurosyphilis, screening for HIV, hepatitis B and C, gonorrhea, and *Chlamydia* infection is recommended. Neurosyphilis is treated with IV penicillin or ceftriaxone.

14.6.6 Tuberculous Meningitis

Tuberculous meningitis accounts for only 1% of all cases of tuberculosis. Predisposing factors of TB meningitis include advanced age, alcoholism, malnutrition, malignancy, HIV infection, and patients being treated with tumor necrosis factor-alpha blockers. Clinical manifestations are subacute or chronic and usually start with protracted headache, malaise, low-grade fever, and confusion. Late symptoms may include altered mental status, headache, or cranial nerve palsies.

CSF acid-fast bacteria (AFB) smear is usually negative. The CSF nucleic acid amplification test (NAAT) PCR detects *Mycobacterium tuberculosis* and is particularly helpful in the setting of negative CSF AFB staining. CSF mycobacterial culture results may not be available for at least 4–6 weeks. The characteristic CT/MRI brain findings of TB meningitis are basilar meningeal enhancement with hydrocephalus.

Adjunctive dexamethasone therapy in patients with TB meningitis improves both survival and morbidity. Dexamethasone reduces mortality and neurological deficits from TB meningitis by 30%. The recommended dosing of dexamethasone for adults is 0.4 mg/kg/day for the first two weeks, then 0.2 mg/kg/day for week 3, then 0.1 mg/kg/day for week 4, then 4 mg per day and taper 1 mg off the daily dose each week. The total duration of dexamethasone therapy is approximately 8 weeks.

14.6.7 Lyme Meningitis

Lyme meningitis is the infection of the nervous system, secondary to the spirochete, *Borrelia burgdorferi*. Lyme meningitis is a tick-borne illness from the bites of the deer tick, *Ixodes scapularis*. More than 90% of cases of Lyme disease in the United States have been reported from ten states: Massachusetts, Connecticut, Rhode Island, New York, New Jersey, Pennsylvania, Delaware, Maryland, Minnesota, and Wisconsin. It typically occurs in the late summer and early fall of the season. The typical bull's-eye skin rash, erythema migrans, may or may not be present. Many patients do not recall a tick bite or the presence of skin rash. The United States Centers for Disease Control and Prevention (CDC) recommends the standard two-tiered testing (STTT) for the diagnosis of Lyme disease: enzyme-linked immunosorbent assay (ELISA), then a Western blot if the ELISA is positive. The CDC has updated their recommendation to utilize the second EIA assay in place of a Western blot, modified two-tier testing (MOTT), because MOTT is more sensitive than STTT for detecting Lyme disease. In the diagnosis of Lyme meningitis, it is recommended to obtain simultaneous samples of CSF and serum for Lyme antibody levels to determine the CSF:Serum Lyme antibody index after adjusting for total immunoglobulin concentration in the two fluids. The CSF: Serum Lyme antibody index above 1 is highly suggestive of neuroborreliosis.

Treatment of Lyme meningitis includes intravenous ceftriaxone 2 g every 24 hours for 28 days. In Europe, high-dose oral doxycycline 200 mg every 12 hours (maximum 400 mg/day) has been used for treating Lyme meningitis. In the United States the use of oral doxycycline (100 mg every 12 hours) for the treatment of Lyme meningitis is a recommended alternative therapy for patients who cannot be given parenteral ceftriaxone.

14.6.8 Cryptococcal Meningoencephalitis

Cryptococcal meningoencephalitis, secondary to *Cryptococcus neoformans*, is an opportunistic infection. It is most frequently encountered in patients with advanced HIV infection (CD4 <100 cells/µL) and/or patients on immunosuppressive therapy. Clinical symptoms usually occur over 1–2 weeks and include fever, malaise, headache, nuchal rigidity, and photophobia. Frequently there are associated multiple umbilicated cutaneous papules similar to molluscum contagiosum.

Table 14.8 Recommended initial therapy for HSV, tuberculous, Lyme and cryptococcal meningitis

Pathogen	Drug dose, frequency, and route of administration
HSV in neonates	IV acyclovir 60 mg/kg/24 h ÷ q8 h IV × 14–21 days Oral therapy after treatment with IV acyclovir for 14–21 days: 300 mg/m^2/dose q 8 h PO × 6 months
Neurosyphilis	IV penicillin G 4 million units q 4 h for 2 weeks, OR IV ceftriaxone 2 g every 24 h for 2 weeks Penicillin desensitization is recommended
Tuberculous meningitis	Isoniazid 5 mg/kg (maximum 300 mg) daily Rifampin 10 mg/kg (maximum 600 mg) daily Pyrazinamide 20–25 mg/kg (maximum 2,000 mg) daily Ethambutol 15 mg/kg (maximum 1,600 mg) daily
Lyme meningitis (neuroborreliosis)	IV ceftriaxone 2 g every 24 h × 4 weeks PO doxycycline 100 mg q 12 h × 4 weeks
Cryptococcal meningitis	IV amphotericin B deoxycholate 0.3–1 mg/kg q 24 h OR IV liposomal amphotericin B 3–5 mg/kg q 24 h OR Amphotericin B lipid complex 5 mg/kg q 24 h PLUS Flucytosine oral 25 mg/kg q 6 h

In the ED, a high index of clinical suspicion is needed to diagnose cryptococcal meningoencephalitis. Controlling high CSF opening pressure to below 200 mmH$_2$O plays a major role in treatment of cryptococcal meningoencephalitis. India ink staining of CSF should be performed for a rapid diagnosis of cryptococcal infection, and is positive in 88% of the patients with advanced HIV/AIDS. The CSF multiplex PCR assays offers detection of Cryptococcus neoformans or Cryptococcus gattii. However, a negative CSF crytococcal PCR does not rule out cryptococcal meningitis, and CSF cryptococcal antigen and CSF fungal cultures are recommended in patients with suspected cryptococcal meningitis. Table 14.8 summarizes the recommended therapies.

14.7 Encephalitis

Encephalitis is defined as the inflammation of brain parenchyma with neurologic dysfunction. The majority of cases of encephalitis are caused by viruses. Post-immunization encephalitis may occur shortly (usually 1–14 days) after vaccination for anthrax, Japanese encephalitis, yellow fever, influenza, measles, smallpox, or rabies viruses. Postinfectious encephalitis has been observed in a number of viral infections, typically ≤1 week after the appearance of rash; they include measles, mumps, rubella, varicella zoster, Epstein–Barr virus, cytomegalovirus, hepatitis A, influenza, and enterovirus. Post-immunization or postinfectious encephalitis is known as acute disseminated encephalomyelitis (ADEM), and it is thought to be secondary to an autoimmune response to a preceding antigenic stimulus.

The diagnosis of viral encephalitis should be considered in patients who present with fever, headache, nuchal rigidity, altered mental status, seizures, or focal neurologic signs. In the United States the most common causes of acute encephalitis include HSV-1 and HSV-2, arboviruses, and enteroviruses. The arboviruses are arthropod-borne viruses, and mosquitoes or ticks are the most common vectors. The important arboviruses that transmit by mosquito vector in the United States include WNV, St Louis encephalitis virus, Western equine encephalitis (WEE) virus, and Eastern equine encephalitis (EEE) virus. In 2013, a nationwide WNV infection outbreak in the United States resulted in 9% mortality in patients with WNV neuroinvasive disease, whereas mortality due to HSV encephalitis ranges from 30% to 60%.

Some important data to be elicited in suspected cases of encephalitis can be summarized through the use of the six Vs:

- vacation/travel (to endemic areas, foreign or domestic)
- veterinary or other animal contact (rabies)
- vectors (recent mosquito or tick bites)
- viral infections (recent or concurrent)
- vaccinations (recent for measles, varicella, rubella, rabies)
- vital statistics (contact health agencies regarding outbreaks)

Table 14.9 summarizes the distinguishing clinical features, CSF findings, MRI brain features, diagnostic studies, and treatment modalities for encephalitis.

14.8 Brain Abscess

Brain abscess is usually derived from a local infection, or hematogenous spread of a distant systemic infection. Local foci of infection include traumatic brain injury, craniotomy, mastoiditis, otitis media, dental infection, and sinusitis. Brain abscess secondary to the direct spread from a contiguous location is usually a solitary cerebral abscess. Table 14.10 lists the area of brain abscess depending on the site of local infection. Systemic sources of infection usually originate from the heart (endocarditis, cyanotic congenital heart disease with the right-to-left shunt), lung (lung abscess, empyema, or intrapulmonary arteriovenous shunts). Brain abscesses due to hematogenous dissemination are multiple lesions and are mostly distributed in the region of the middle cerebral artery. Cerebritis is defined as an early stage of brain abscess without tissue necrosis. The management of cerebritis is the same as that of brain abscess. If cerebritis is not treated, liquefactive central necrosis with brain abscess formation may occur in 2–4 weeks.

The most common clinical presenting symptoms of a brain abscess are headache, seizure, fever, and altered mental state. These symptoms may take days to weeks to present. Patients with an abscess located in the frontal and temporal lobes exhibit behavioral changes, whereas gait instability may be the presenting symptom in patients with cerebellar brain abscess.

The causal pathogens of a brain abscess depend on its etiology and the primary site of the infection (Table 14.11). Anaerobic bacteria are among the microorganisms causing a brain abscess.

In immunocompromised hosts there are other important pathogens that may contribute to brain abscesses. *Cryptococcus neoformans*, *Toxoplasma gondii*, *Nocardia* spp., or *Mycobacterium* spp. should be considered in patients with HIV infection. Primary CNS lymphoma is part of the differential diagnosis in HIV-infected patients. Invasive fungal infections, such as *Aspergillus*, *Candida*, Mucorales, *Scedosporium*, or *Nocardia* infection are important considerations of brain abscess in organ transplant recipients. Cerebral imaging with IV contrast is an important initial diagnostic tool in patients with suspected brain abscess. Cerebral MRI with gadolinium may help to differentiate brain abscess from primary, cystic, or necrotic tumors. Early consultation to neurosurgery should be obtained for stereotactic aspiration of the abscess. Treatment of brain abscesses is listed in Table 14.12.

Table 14.9 Selected causes of viral encephalitis

Etiology	Epidemiology (United States)	Clinical features	MRI brain	Diagnostic tests	Treatment
HSV-1 and HSV 2	Nationwide	Fever, headache, behavioral changes, seizures	Temporal or inferior frontal lobe hyperintensity; or bilateral temporal lobe lesions is pathognomonic	CSF PCR for HSV-1 and HSV-2	IV acyclovir 10 mg/kg every 8 hours
WNV	Nationwide Epidemic from late summer through fall Transmission reported via transfusion, transplantation, and breast-feeding	More severe in elderly persons; maculopapular rash, poliomyelitis-like flaccid paralysis, and Parkinson-like movements	Hyperintense lesions in the substantia nigra, basal ganglia, and thalami	Serum or CSF WNV-specific IgM	Supportive
St. Louis encephalitis virus	Western parts of the United States	Encephalopathy; distinctive features include urinary symptoms (dysuria, hematuria, or sterile pyuria)	Hyperintense lesions in the substantia nigra, basal ganglia, and thalami	Serum or CSF St. Louis encephalitis virus-specific IgM	Supportive
Western equine encephalitis (WEE) virus	Western parts of the United States	Headache, nausea, vomiting, neck stiffness, altered mental status, and seizures	No specific brain MRI findings are solely suggestive of WEE	Serum or CSF WEE virus-specific IgM	Supportive
Eastern equine encephalitis (EEE) virus	Atlantic and Gulf coasts of the United States Epidemic outbreak during summer	Encephalopathy, seizures; case fatality rate is 50–70% among US arboviral encephalitides	Hyperintensity in the bilateral basal ganglia	Serum or CSF EEE virus-specific IgM	Supportive

Table 14.10 Site of the primary infection with the corresponding site of brain abscess

Site of the primary local infection	Site of the brain abscess
Otitis media, mastoiditis	Inferior temporal lobe, cerebellum
Frontal or ethmoidal sinusitis	Frontal lobes
Dental infection	Frontal lobes

Table 14.11 Pathogens causing brain abscesses

The primary site of infection	Most likely microorganisms
Paranasal sinusitis	*Streptococcus* spp. (including *S. anginosus* group), *Haemophilus* spp., Enterobacteriaceae (*Escherichia coli*, *Enterobacter*, and *Klebsiella*), *Bacteroides* spp., *Fusobacterium* spp.
Otitis media or mastoiditis	*Streptococcus* spp., *Staphylococcus* spp., *Pseudomonas aeruginosa*, *Bacteroides* spp., *Prevotella* spp.
Dental infection	*Streptococcus* spp., mixed anaerobes (actinomyces, bacteroides, prevotella, and peptostreptococcus)
Neurosurgical procedures, traumatic brain injury or penetrating head trauma	*Staphylococcus aureus* (including methicillin-resistant *S. aureus*), *S. epidermidis*, *Streptococcus* spp., *Pseudomonas aeruginosa*, *Enterobacter* spp.
Hematogenous spread (from skin, lung, heart)	*Staphylococcus aureus* (including methicillin-resistant *S. aureus*), *Streptococcus* spp., *Klebsiella pneumoniae*, anaerobes

In patients with HIV infection and organ transplantation, the etiology of the brain abscess is more complicated and complex. Consultation with an infectious diseases specialist is strongly recommended for optimal therapy.

14.9 Disposition

All patients with bacterial meningitis require IV antibiotics and hospital admission. Patients with uncomplicated viral meningitis may be treated with antipyretics and supportive care and may be discharged from the ED. For patients with suspected viral meningitis who are admitted to the hospital, the decision to institute antibiotic coverage in the ED should be made by the emergency physician on the basis of the patient's clinical picture and associated risk factors.

Empiric effective antimicrobial therapy should be administered immediately in patients with suspected CNS infections. Consultation with infectious diseases, neurology, and neurosurgery should be obtained as soon as possible for optimal diagnostic and therapeutic approaches to maximize a favorable clinical outcome.

14.10 Special Considerations in Children

The presentation of infants with meningitis or CNS infections is frequently nonspecific and may be characterized by fever, increased or decreased activity, lethargy, poor tone, poor feeding, respiratory distress, or rash. While neonates are innately at greater risk due to their

Table 14.12 Treatment of brain abscesses

Primary foci of infection	Empiric treatment regimen
Sinusitis, otitis media, or mastoiditis	IV ceftriaxone 2 g every 12 hours, OR IV cefotaxime 2 g every 4–6 hours + IV metronidazole 500 mg every 8 hours
Dental infection	IV penicillin G 4 million units every 4 hours + IV metronidazole 500 mg every 8 hours
Neurosurgical procedures, traumatic brain injury, or penetrating head trauma	IV ceftazidime 2 g every 8 hours, OR IV cefepime 2 g every 8 hours, OR IV meropenem 2 g every 8 hours + IV vancomycin load with 25–35 mg/kg, then 15–20 mg/kg q 8–12 h
Hematogenous spread	IV vancomycin load with 25–35 mg/kg, then 15–20 mg/kg q 8–12 h + IV metronidazole 500 mg every 8 hours
Unknown origin	IV ceftriaxone 2 g every 12 hours, OR IV cefotaxime 2 g every 4–6 hours + IV vancomycin load with 25–35 mg/kg, then 15–20 mg/kg q8–12 h + IV metronidazole 500 mg every 8 hours

immature immune function, the risk for a misdiagnosis or a delay in treatment is greater due to the nonspecific nature of the presenting symptoms, which may go unrecognized by caregivers prior to a late presentation to the ED.

When vital signs are assessed upon presentation to the ED, pulse oximetry should be included for all patients, and for infants a head circumference as well. Findings within the assessment of cardiopulmonary status, such as increased work of breathing and poor perfusion, may be indicative of a greater severity of illness than perceived by the caregiver. An assessment of consciousness should be performed with the pediatric Glasgow Coma Scale.

14.10.1 Infants 2–24 Months of Age

After the neonatal period, aseptic meningitis overtakes bacterial meningitis as the most common CNS infection. While potentially less serious than bacterial meningitis, aseptic meningitis remains a considerable source of morbidity and mortality. Although the inflammatory reaction is less robust and the resultant cell injury is to a lesser degree, there can be associated encephalitis and increased intracranial pressure regardless of the organism.

14.10.2 Children to Pre-adolescent

Meningitis and other CNS infections occur in otherwise healthy children, and viral and bacterial forms have a very similar presentation. However, in many cases a predisposing risk factor can be discovered, such as trauma with CSF leak, surgery, recent infection or exposure, immunosuppression, asplenia, or an environmental factor such as overcrowding, participation in close group settings, or travel to an area endemic for tuberculosis, Lyme disease, or *Rickettsia*. A risk factor for *Listeria* meningitis is the consumption of *Listeria*-contaminated foods such as uncooked meats, vegetables, soft cheeses, cold cuts, and unpasteurized milk. Increasingly, under-vaccination is a risk factor for meningitis as the overall incidence of CNS infections in immunized patients has markedly declined.

14.10.3 Adolescents

Adolescents are the most likely age group to exhibit the classic meningitis findings of headache, fever, stiff neck, and may progress rapidly to altered consciousness, seizures, and focal findings. Risk factors for adolescents are group housing conditions such as dormitory, military, or overcrowding related to poverty. Vaccination status remains important because causative agents in the teenage years are frequently vaccine-preventable. Teens may not have been in an age group to have been vaccinated against *Streptococcus pneumonia*, may not have received complete vaccination against *Neisseria meningitides*, and may decline influenza vaccination due to perceived low risk.

Pearls and Pitfalls

- Consider the diagnosis of meningitis in patients with an atypical presentation.
- Consider meningitis in patients despite a negative Gram stain and/or a low CSF WBC count.
- Do not delay starting antibiotic therapy when there is a reasonable suspicion of meningitis.
- Do not delay lumbar puncture to obtain a CT scan when there are no "red flag" findings on exam.
- Hemorrhagic lesions of herpes encephalitis may lead to a false impression of a traumatic lumbar puncture.
- Nuchal rigidity is not found in children under 2 years of age.

Bibliography

Banks JT, Bharara S, Tubbs RS, et al. Polymerase chain reaction for the rapid detection of cerebrospinal fluid shunt or ventriculostomy infections. *Neurosurgery* 2005;**57**:1237–1243.

Beckham JD, Tyler KL. Encephalitis. In Bennett J, Dolin R, Blaser M (eds.) *Mandell, Douglas, and Bennett's Principles and Practice of Infectious Diseases*, 9th ed. Elsevier, 2020.

Bhimraj A. Acute community-acquired bacterial meningitis: an evidence-based review. *Cleveland Clin J Med* 2012;**79**:393–400.

Brouwer MC, Thwaites GE, Tunkel AR, Van de Beek D. Dilemmas in the diagnosis of acute community-acquired bacterial meningitis. *Lancet* 2012;**380**(9854):1684–1692.

Brouwer MC, Tunkel AR, McKhann GM 2nd, Van de Beek D. Brain abscess. *N Engl J Med* 2014;**371**(5):447–456.

Centers for Disease Control and Prevention. ACIP: Advisory Committee on Immunization Practices. Available at: www.cdc.gov/vaccines/acip.

de Gans JD, Van de Beek D, European Dexamethasone in Adulthood Bacterial Meningitis Study Investigators. Dexamethasone in adults with bacterial meningitis. *N Engl J Med* 2002;**347**:1549–1556.

Davis IRC, McNeil SA, Allen W, MacKinnon-Cameron D, et al. Performance of a Modified Two-Tiered Testing Enzyme Immunoassay Algorithm for Serologic Diagnosis of Lyme Disease in Nova Scotia. *J Clin Microbiol.* 2020;**58**(7):e01841-19.

Engorn B, Flerlage J (eds.) *The Harriet Lane Handbook: A Manual For Pediatric House Officers.* Mosby Elsevier, 2015.

Fitch MT, Van de Beek D. Emergency diagnosis and treatment of adult meningitis. *Lancet* 2007;**7**:191–200.

Halperin JJ, Shapiro ED, Logigian E, et al. Practice parameter: treatment of nervous system Lyme disease (an evidence-based review): report of the Quality Standards Subcommittee of the American Academy of Neurology. *Neurology* 2007;**69**(1):91–102.

Hasbun R, Abrahams J, Jekel J, et al. Computed tomography of the head before lumbar puncture in adults with suspected meningitis. *N Engl J Med* 2001;**345**:1727–1733.

Hasburn R, Van, de Beek D, Brouwer MC,Tunkel AR, Acute meningitis. In Bennett J, Dolin R, Blaser M (eds.) *Mandell, Douglas, and Bennett's Principles and Practice of Infectious Diseases*, 9th ed. Elsevier, 2020.

Lantos PM, Rumbaugh J ,Bockenstedt LK, et al. Clinical Practice Guidelines by the Infectious Diseases Society of America (IDSA), American Academy of Neurology (AAN), and American College of Rheumatology (ACR): 2020 Guidelines for the Prevention, Diagnosis and Treatment of Lyme Disease. *Clin Infect Dis* 2021;**72**(1);e1–e48.

Lindsey NP, Lehman JA, Staples JE, Fischer M. West Nile virus and other arboviral diseases: United States, 2013. *MMWR Morb Mortal Wkly Rep* 2013;**63**(24):521–526.

Mead P, Petersen J, Hinckley A. Updated CDC Recommendation for Serologic Diagnosis of Lyme Disease. *MMWR Morb Mortal Wkly Rep.* 2019;**68**(32):703.

MMWR, October 23, 2015, Vol 64 #41. Use of serogroup B meningococcal vaccines in adolescents and young adults: recommendations of the Advisory Committee on Immunization Practices, 2015. Available at: www.cdc.gov/mmwr/preview/mmwrhtml/mm6441a3.htm.

MMWR, March 22, 2013, Vol 62 #2. Prevention and control of meningococcal disease: recommendations of the Advisory Committee on Immunization Practices, 2013. Available at: www.cdc.govwww.cdc.gov/mmwr/preview/mmwrhtml/mm6441a3.htm.

O'Halloran JA, Franklin A, Lainhart W, et al. Pitfalls Associated With the Use of Molecular Diagnostic Panels in the Diagnosis of Cryptococcal Meningitis. *Open Forum Infect Dis.* 2017;**4**(4):ofx242.

Patel K, Clifford DB. Bacterial brain abscess. *Neurohospitalist* 2014;**4**(4):196–204.

Perfect JR, Dismukes WE, Dromer F, et al. Clinical practice guidelines for the management of cryptococcal disease: 2010 update by the infectious Diseases Society of America. *Clin Infect Dis* 2010;**50**(3):291–322.

Petersen LR, Marfin AA, Gubler DJ. West Nile virus. *JAMA* 2003;**290**:524–528.

Pickering LK, ed. *American Academy of Pediatrics Red Book: 2015 Report of the Committee on Infectious Diseases*, 30th ed. Academy of Pediatrics, 2015.

Pizon AF, Bonner MR, Wang HE, Kaplan RM. Ten years of clinical experience with adult meningitis at an urban academic center. *J Emerg Med* 2006;**30**:367–370.

Thigpen MC, Whitney CG, Messonnier NE, et al. Bacterial meningitis in the United States, 1998–2007. *N Engl J Med* 2011;**364**:2016–2025.

Thomas KE, Hasbun R, Jekel J, Quagliarello VJ. The diagnostic accuracy of Kernig's sign, Brudzinski's sign, and nuchal rigidity in adults with suspected meningitis. *Clin Infect Dis* 2002;**35**:46–52.

Tunkel AR. Approach to the patient with central nervous system infection. In Bennett J, Dolin R, Blaser M (eds.) *Mandell, Douglas, and Bennett's Principles and Practice of Infectious Diseases*, 9th ed. Elsevier, 2020.

Tunkel AR. Brain abscess. In Bennett J, Dolin R, Blaser M (eds.) *Mandell, Douglas, and Bennett's Principles and Practice of Infectious Diseases*, 9th ed. Elsevier, 2020.

Tunkel AR, Glaser CA, Bloch KC, et al. The management of encephalitis: clinical practice guidelines by the Infectious Diseases Society of America. *Clin Infect Dis* 2008;**47**(3):303–327.

Van de Beek D, de Gans J, Spanjaard L, et al. Clinical features and prognostic factors in adults with bacterial meningitis. *N Engl J Med* 2004;**351**:1849–1859.

Van de Beek D, de Gans J, Tunkel AR, et al. Community-acquired bacterial meningitis in adults. *N Engl J Med* 2006;**354**:44–53.

Van de Beek D, Drake JM, Tunkel AR. Nosocomial meningitis. *N Engl J Med* 2010;**362**(2):146–154.

Van de Beek D, Brouwer MC, Thwaites GE, Tunkel AR. Advances in treatment of bacterial meningitis. *Lancet* 2012;**380**(9854):1693–1702.

Chapter 15

Traumatic Brain Injury

Moira Davenport and James E. Wilberger

15.1 Introduction

Traumatic brain injury (TBI) is an increasingly common cause of morbidity and mortality in the United States. Rates of emergency department (ED) visits for TBI rose 70% between 2001 and 2010, with an estimated 2.5 million patients/year seeking emergency care, highlighting the increased focus on early identification and treatment of brain injuries. Hospital admission rates for TBI rose 11% in this time frame while deaths decreased 7%. Despite improvements in the management of TBI, 50,000 people die each year from this trauma (30% of all trauma-related deaths in the United States). Falls are the most common mechanism of TBI, followed by blunt trauma, motor vehicle collisions (MVCs), and assault. Men are three times more likely to sustain a TBI than their female counterparts, whereas the very young (<4 years old) and older patients (>65 years old) are more likely to sustain head trauma than those of other ages. The evaluation of these patients should follow advanced trauma life support (ATLS) guidelines. Once the primary survey has been completed, a thorough neurovascular exam should be performed to evaluate for TBI. ED imaging should be performed; a noncontrast CT scan of the head is the recommended initial imaging study. Based on this imaging, a variety of medications may be used, in conjunction with neurosurgical evaluation, to further manage the injured patient.

15.2 History

TBI is a spectrum of conditions. Overt signs of head trauma are not necessarily associated with TBI, although findings such as lacerations, contusions, abrasions, and ecchymoses should heighten physician suspicion for an underlying brain injury. Two types of brain injury should be delineated: (1) a primary brain injury results from mechanical forces disrupting the normal structure of the brain; and (2) a secondary brain injury results from the altered physiology that can occur with systemic trauma or illness. Changes in glucose metabolism, electrolyte balance, oxygenation, blood pressure, and acid–base status can all contribute to secondary brain injuries. Secondary brain injuries can significantly increase the morbidity and mortality associated with head trauma, thus highlighting the need for the emergency physician to be familiar with management of these conditions.

15.3 Differential Diagnosis

Subdural hematomas (SDH) commonly result from rapid acceleration and deceleration of the head and cervical spine, as seen in MVCs and falls from various heights. This rapid change in velocity can tear the bridging veins and result in a crescent moon-shaped density on a CT scan as blood pools between the dura mater and the actual brain parenchyma. Loss of consciousness is variable, as is patient presentation. Headache of varying intensity is the most common presenting symptom, whereas neurologic deficits can range from an essentially nonfocal examination to an obtunded state. The possibility of the patient being on chronic anticoagulation or antiplatelet agents should be considered in all cases of head trauma, even if the mechanism of injury seems relatively minor. The incidence of SDH is increasing as use of these medications increases in an aging population. Patient disposition is based on the size of the hematoma, with smaller hematomas (<3 mm) typically managed conservatively. SDH is fairly common and is estimated to be seen in 10–20% of all patients with TBI.

Epidural hematomas (EDH) are typically seen following a direct blow to the head, most commonly in the temporal area. This direct force often disrupts the middle meningeal artery resulting in a convex collection of blood on the brain parenchyma. Patients may experience a brief loss of consciousness followed by an essentially symptom-free period followed by a period of rapid clinical decline. Emergent surgical intervention is critical to limit associated morbidity and mortality.

Diffuse axonal injury (DAI) is the disruption of axons due to trauma; any mechanism can result in this condition. Any part of the brain may be affected, but the brainstem and internal capsule are the most commonly involved. This condition is difficult to diagnose on initial CT scan, as mild global cerebral edema is the most common finding. However, most patients with DAI present with profoundly altered mental status and subsequently a limited neurologic examination. Axonal regeneration is somewhat variable, particularly in severe DAI, heightening the need to limit secondary brain injury by optimizing hemodynamic parameters. Patients with DAI typically require admission to an intensive care setting.

Cerebral contusions are collections of blood within the brain parenchyma; these can result from any mechanism but are most commonly the result of direct contact between the brain and the skull. Clinical presentation is variable and depends on the location of the contusion, its size, and the amount of resulting edema and/or shift. Patient disposition is also dependent on the size of the contusion and the resultant neurologic examination.

Concussion is a change in the normal neurologic function of the brain that is rarely accompanied by acute structural changes of the brain, making this a clinical diagnosis more than an imaging-based diagnosis (Table 15.1). This condition has been the focus of considerable attention, particularly in athletes. Both direct and indirect head trauma may lead to concussion. Concussed patients typically do not lose consciousness at the time of the injury, but symptoms may persist for an extended period of time. Recovery from a concussion often follows a typical pattern, allowing for the development of return-to-play criteria for affected athletes.

15.4 ED Management

Basic trauma protocols should be followed during the initial evaluation of any patient with suspected head trauma. Airway patency, efficiency of breathing, circulatory status, initial vital signs, and the Glasgow Coma Scale (GCS; Table 15.2) should be assessed immediately. The GCS is calculated by assessing the patient's eye, verbal, and motor responses. The sum of each of these subcategories is the GCS and can then be used to assess the

Table 15.1 Symptoms and signs of concussion

Domain	Findings
Symptoms	Somatic: headache Cognitive: feeling slow Emotional: lability
Physical signs	Level of consciousness Amnesia
Behavioral changes	Irritability
Cognitive changes	Slowed reaction times
Sleep disturbance	Insomnia Increased sleep

Adapted from McCrory et al. (2013)

severity of head trauma. Minor head trauma patients have a GCS of 14 or 15, moderate head trauma victims have a GCS of 9–13, and severely head-injured patients score ≤8 on the GCS. It is imperative that the emergency physician be familiar with current diagnostic and treatment recommendations for the variety of TBI as early appropriate intervention can optimize outcomes.

Intravenous access should be obtained prior to the secondary trauma survey. A complete physical examination should be performed with particular focus on the head, neck, and the neurologic examination. Several key physical findings should raise the suspicion of a significant head injury, including depressed skull fractures, a raccoon sign, pupil abnormalities, a battle sign, otorrhea, hemotympanum, and rhinorrhea. Altered mental status may be seen in the patient with a suspected brain injury, but care should be taken to rule-out other possible causes of this change, including hypoglycemia or the use of substances of abuse. The presence of localized neurologic deficits should raise physician concern for concurrent spinal cord injury. ED management of the TBI patient should follow ATLS guidelines. Attention should be paid to the patient's hemodynamic stability to ensure that the cerebral perfusion pressure remains adequate. A systolic blood pressure <90 mm Hg has been shown to be a marker of increased morbidity and mortality. This finding may require fluid resuscitation with normal saline, lactated Ringers solution, or hypertonic saline, or blood pressure support with norepinephrine. Airway protection via rapid sequence intubation may be required and should be considered early in the evaluation process to limit hypoxia. Reversal of antiplatelet and anticoagulation agents should be considered in patients taking these medications. Recommendations for reversal of antiplatelet agents from 2016 guidelines of the Neurocritical Care Society include: (1) discontinuing antiplatelet agents when intracranial hemorrhage is suspected; (2) consideration of platelet transfusion for patients with aspirin- or adenosine diphosphate inhibitor-associated intracranial hemorrhage who will undergo a neurosurgical procedure; and (3) testing of platelet function prior to transfusion if possible. Importantly, the guidelines recommend against platelet transfusion with laboratory-documented platelet function within normal limits or documented platelet resistance.

Table 15.2 Glasgow Coma Scale

	1	2	3	4	5	6
Eye	No response	Opens to pain	Opens to verbal request	Opens spontaneously		
Verbal	No response	Random sounds	Inappropriate words	Confused	Coherent	
Motor	No response	Extends to pain	Flexes to pain	Withdraws to pain	Localizes to pain	Follows commands

Table 15.3 Reversal of low molecular weight heparins

Agent	Protamine dose
Dalteparin	1 mg protamine/100 units dalteparin in last 8 hours
Enoxaparin	1 mg protamine/1 mg enoxaparin in last 8 hours
Tinzaparin	1 mg protamine/100 units tinzaparin in last 8 hours

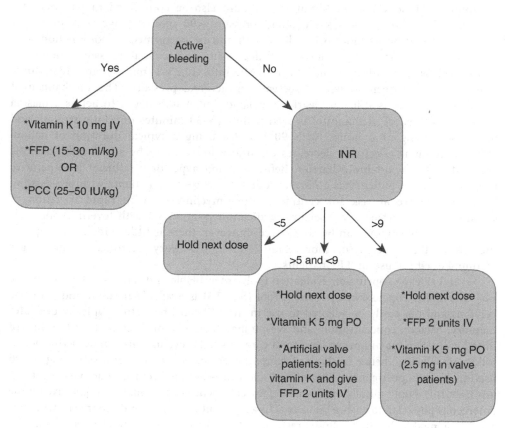

Figure 15.1 Reversal of warfarin therapy. IFFP, fresh frozen plasma; NR, international normalized ratio; PCC, platelet complex concentrates.

Several guidelines are available to facilitate the reversal of warfarin therapy (Figure 15.1).

The low molecular weight heparin (LMWH) agents can be reversed using protamine at a dose based on the amount of LMWH used in the preceding 8 hours (Table 15.3).

Use of the non-vitamin K oral anticoagulants continues to increase. Idarucizumab (5 g administered via 2.5 g/50 mL bolus with two doses within 15 minutes) has FDA approval for the reversal of dabigatran. Reversal of the other non-vitamin K oral anticoagulants (Factor Xa inhibitors) poses a clinical challenge. Four-factor platelet complex concentrate (containing factors II, VII, IX, and X, as well as protein C and protein S) and FEIBA (factors II, VII, IX, and X) have shown some ability to reverse rivaroxaban but not the other novel anticoagulant agents. If the medication history is not available and there is concern for anticoagulant use, thromboeslastography (TEG) with platelet mapping may be used to help identify the most likely agent. Cardiology and/or hematology consultation should also be considered to further risk-stratify anticoagulation reversal in patients with known valvular disease or cardiac dysrhythmia. Intracranial pressure monitoring is indicated for patients with a GCS of 3–8 and an abnormal head CT scan. Monitoring should also be considered in patients with a normal CT scan and a systolic blood pressure <90 mm Hg, age >40, or motor posturing. Insertion of monitoring devices should be performed in conjunction with neurosurgery. Pharmacologic means of decreasing intracranial pressure should be considered once monitoring has begun. Mannitol (0.25–1 mg/kg) and hypertonic saline (3%) have been shown to decrease intracranial pressure. The mechanism of action of mannitol is still not clearly elucidated, but it is believed to act as a plasma expander. The effect of mannitol is seen within 15–30 minutes of administration and may last as long as 6 hours, with 90 minutes being a typical duration of action. Hypertonic saline effectively decreases cerebral water content by altering the osmotic gradient at the blood–brain barrier. Before starting hypertonic saline it is imperative to ensure that the patient has a normal sodium level because patients with pre-existing hyponatremia are at risk for central pontine myelinolysis with rapid elevation of sodium levels. Short-term antiseizure medication prophylaxis with levetiracetam, valproic acid, or phenytoin can be considered; however, there is little evidence to support the use of these agents for more than 7 days post-injury. Steroids are no longer recommended for use in TBI patients.

Several sideline concussion evaluation tools are available and can easily be used in the ED. The sports concussion assessment tool (SCAT5) is available in adult and pediatric versions and can easily be adapted to use in the ED. Sideline testing typically evaluates memory, balance, concentration, and symptomatology. Use of these tools at the time of initial evaluation may improve long-term care as similar evaluations can be performed at follow-up, allowing better tracking of symptom resolution. Neurocognitive testing is also used to evaluate post-concussion patients and can help guide return to activity planning, however, this is not typically the domain of the emergency physician. It is imperative for the emergency physician to ensure that a concussed patient is given clear discharge instructions regarding modified activity, brain rest, use of analgesics, and referral to a concussion specialist.

15.5 Imaging

Noncontrast CT scan of the head is the imaging modality of choice for patients with suspected TBI. If there is concern for concurrent cervical spine injury based on the physical examination, a noncontrast CT scan of the cervical spine should also be performed. No widely accepted imaging guidelines exist for adult patients with suspected TBI, but patients with neurologic deficits, elderly patients, patients with alcohol intoxication and/or abuse, and patients on anticoagulants should have imaging studies performed. MRI can be considered as a second-line imaging study if more detailed evaluation of the anatomy is required, particularly if DAI is considered the primary diagnosis. The PECARN guidelines can eliminate unnecessary CT scans in the pediatric population (Figures 15.2 and 15.3).

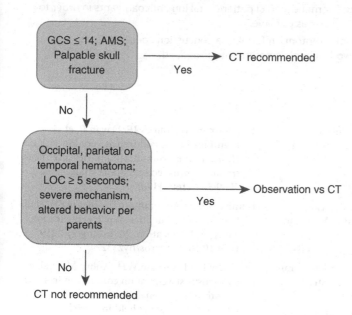

Figure 15.2 PECARN imaging guidelines for children <2 years old.

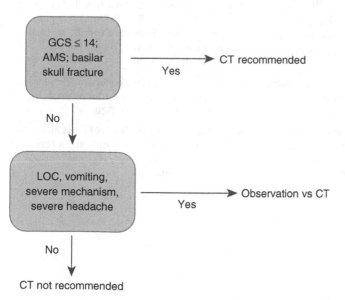

Figure 15.3 PECARN imaging guidelines for children >2 years old.

Pearls and Pitfalls

- Evaluation of the TBI patient should follow ATLS guidelines.
- Hemodynamic parameters should be closely monitored in the TBI patient.
- Efforts should be made to determine if a TBI patient is taking anticoagulants in order to start the reversal process as soon as possible.
- Concussion is a spectrum of symptoms; referral to a concussion specialist is recommended to adjust work/school commitments as needed.

Bibliography

CDC. Traumatic brain injury & concussion. Available at: www.cdc.gov/traumaticbrain injury/get_the_facts.html.

Cushman M, Lim W, Zakai NA. *Clinical Practice Guide on Anticoagulant Dosing and Management of Anticoagulant-Associated Bleeding Complications in Adults.* American Society of Hematology, 2011.

Erenberg ES, Kamphuisen PW, Sijpkens MK, et al. Reversal of rivaroxaban and dabigatran by prothrombin complex concentrate. *Circulation* 2011;**124**:1573–1579.

Faraoni D, Levy JH, Albaladejo P, et al. Updates in the perioperative and emergency management of non-vitamin K antagonist oral anticoagulants. *Critical Care* 2015;**19**:203.

Frontera JA, Lewin JJ, Rabinstein AA, et al. Guideline for reversal of antithrombotics in intracranial hemorrhage. *Neurocrit Care* 2016;**24**:6–46.

Garcia DA, Crowther MA. Reversal of warfarin: case-based practice recommendations. *Circulation* 2012;**125**:2944–2947.

Karibe H, Hayashi T, Hirano T, et al. Surgical management of traumatic acute subdural hematoma in adults: a review. *Neurol Med Chir (Tokyo)* 2014;**54**:887–894.

Kupperman N, Holmes JF, Dayan P, et al. Identification of children at very low risk of clinically-important brain injuries after head trauma: a prospective cohort study. *Lancet* 2009;**374**:1160–1170.

Lumba-Brown A, Teramoto M, Bloom OJ, et al. Concussion guidelines step 2: evidence for subtype classification. *Neurosurgery* 2019. DOI:10.1093/neuros/nyz332.

McCrory P, Meeuwisse WH, Aubry M, et al. Consensus statement on concussion in sport: the 4th International Conference on Concussion in Sport held in Zurich, November 2012. *Br J Sports Med* 2013;**47**:250–258.

Pollock CV, Reilly PA, Bernstein R et al. Design and rationale for RE-VERSE AD: a phase 3 study of idarucizumab, a specific reversal agent for dabigatran. *Thromb Haem* 2015;**114**(1):198–205.

Pollock CV, Reilly PA, Eikelboom J, et al. Idarucizumab for dabigatran reversal. *N Engl J Med* 2015;**373**(6):511–520.

Rowe AS, Goodwin H, Brophy GM et al. Seizure prophylaxis in neurocritical care: a review of evidence-based support. *Pharmacotherapy* 2014;**34**(3):396–409.

Chapter 16

Increased Intracranial Pressure and Herniation Syndromes

Diana J. Jho, Brian Rempe, James Burgess, and Alexander K. Yu

16.1 Introduction

The cranial vault in an adult is an enclosed space encased by the rigid skull. The Monro–Kellie doctrine proposed in the early nineteenth century states that the volume inside the cranium is fixed and normally filled with the brain, cerebral spinal fluid (CSF), and blood in a state of equilibrium. An increase in the volume of one of these constituents must be compensated by a decrease in another. Intracranial pressure (ICP) is the pressure inside the skull due to the volume within the cranium. Elevated ICP can be severely debilitating and even life-threatening. It is very important to quickly identify signs and symptoms of elevated ICP, diagnose the pathology, and promptly initiate treatment in the emergency setting to prevent irreparable brain damage, significant disability, or death.

16.2 Pathophysiology

In accordance with the Monro–Kellie doctrine, the intracranial space comprises three compartments. Normal brain volume is approximately 1,300–1,400 mL. CSF comprises 120–140 mL with about 40 mL within the ventricles, 30 mL in the spinal subarachnoid space, and the remainder within the intracranial cisterns and subarachnoid space. Adult cerebral blood volume is approximately 110–150 mL. The rigid, bony encasement allows an increase in any compartment or a space-occupying lesion to raise the ICP within the skull. Small amounts of changes in volume can be tolerated to a certain limit, but once the limit is reached one or more of the compartments must be displaced to compensate for the additional volume and increased pressure leading to clinically significant symptoms and potentially leading to herniation syndromes.

At rest, ICP in a supine adult is normally 5–15 mm Hg or 7.5–20 cmH$_2$O (1 mm Hg = 1.36 cmH$_2$O). ICP has been shown to be influenced by changes in intra-abdominal pressure such as coughing and the Valsalva maneuver. Abnormal pathology such as a brain tumor, subdural hematoma, epidural hematoma, cerebral edema, traumatic contusions, intracerebral hemorrhage, and hydrocephalus can lead to a life-threatening increase in ICP. The upper limit of normal ICP is 20–25 mm Hg or 27–34 cmH$_2$O and treatment should be strongly considered if ICP persists at that level. Sustained ICP values greater than 40 mm Hg indicate severe, life-threatening hypertension.

Unlike other organs, the brain is dependent on a steady arterial perfusion to meet its metabolic needs. Cerebral perfusion pressure (CPP) is an indirect measurement of cerebral blood flow (CBF). CPP is calculated by the equation:

CPP = mean arterial pressure (MAP) – ICP
MAP = 1/3 systolic blood pressure + 2/3 diastolic blood pressure.

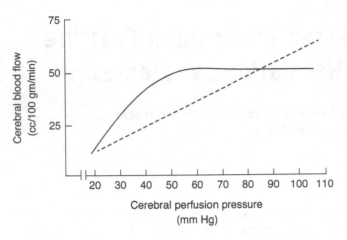

Figure 16.1 Autoregulation of CBF. Flow is plotted against CPP (MAP – ICP). The solid line describes the normal relationship. There is little change in flow over a wide range of perfusion pressures. When perfusion pressure decreases below 50–60 mm Hg, CBF begins to fall. The dashed line depicts the relation between perfusion pressures and flow when autoregulation has been lost. CBF changes passively, and in linear fashion, with the perfusion pressure. From JE McGillicuddy, Cerebral protection: pathophysiology and treatment of increased intracranial pressure. *Chest.* 1985; 87:85–93.

Cerebral autoregulation refers to the constant rate of CBF despite changes in CPP. CBF can be maintained at 50 mL/100 g of brain tissue per minute over a range of MAP from 50 mm Hg to 160 mm Hg. If MAP falls or ICP increases drastically, CPP decreases as well. As long as autoregulation is intact, CBF will remain unchanged with a decrease in CPP by the vasodilatory cascade. When the CPP falls below 50 mm Hg, the threshold for autoregulation mechanisms is surpassed, leading to a correlating decrease in CBF (Figure 16.1). Elevated ICP not only produces a physical force on the parenchyma but also decreases CPP, thereby reducing CBF and leading to ischemia. Autoregulation mechanisms include arterial dilation or constriction in response to carbon dioxide, oxygen, and neurogenic influences of the autonomic nervous system. The vasculature is more sensitive to changes in $PaCO_2$, which can cause a disproportionate change in CBF that can be manipulated to the patient's advantage for short-term treatment of increased ICP.

16.3 Types of Edema

Vasogenic edema is characterized by an increase in vascular permeability leading to plasma fluid leak into cerebral tissue. This is due to the disruption of the tight endothelial junctions that form the blood–brain barrier. Fluid accumulates predominantly in the white matter but can also build up in the gray matter. Traumatic brain injury, neoplasms, abscess, meningitis, infarction, and hemorrhage are common causes of vasogenic edema.

Cytotoxic edema occurs with dysregulation of the sodium–potassium pumps within the cellular membrane, causing cellular retention of sodium and water. The blood–brain barrier is intact, leading to an overall reduction in extracellular fluid volume as fluid collects intracellularly. Both gray and white matter are affected. Hypoxia, diabetic ketoacidosis, early ischemia, Reye's syndrome, and toxic encephalopathies are associated with cytotoxic edema.

Interstitial edema occurs from an increased amount of CSF leading to a disruption of the CSF–brain barrier. This is caused by a blockage of absorption from the arachnoid villi or from a blockage of normal CSF flow. The blood–brain barrier is intact, and generally the periventricular white matter is affected. Obstructive hydrocephalus is the main cause of interstitial edema.

Osmotic edema occurs with dilution of plasma leading to a decrease in serum osmolality in comparison to that of the CSF and extracellular fluid. Normally, the osmolality of CSF and extracellular fluid in the brain is slightly lower than that of plasma. When the serum osmolality is decreased, an abnormal pressure gradient is created, causing water to move through the intact blood–brain barrier into the brain, causing cerebral edema. This can be caused by excessive water intake, syndrome of inappropriate antidiuretic hormone (SIADH), hemodialysis, or rapid decrease in blood glucose in a hyperosmolar hyperglycemic state.

16.4 Signs and Symptoms

Patients with elevated ICP can present with a myriad of signs and symptoms including headaches, nausea, vomiting, change in vision, seizures, weakness, lethargy, coma, Parinaud syndrome, Cushing's reflex, or herniation syndromes.

Parinaud syndrome, also known as dorsal midbrain syndrome, is a vertical gaze palsy due to compression of the vertical gaze center in the rostral interstitial nucleus of the medial longitudinal fasciculus. The syndrome is a cluster of eye movement abnormalities that include paralysis of upgaze, a pseudo-Argyll Robertson pupil, convergence–retraction nystagmus, eyelid retraction (Collier's sign), and a "setting sun" sign. This syndrome is classically seen with young patients with a pineal mass, women with multiple sclerosis, or older patients following a stroke. However, any issue causing compression of the dorsal midbrain can also produce this syndrome, such as trauma, vascular lesions, metabolic lesions, infectious causes, or obstructive hydrocephalus.

Cushing's reflex – also known as the vasopressor response, Cushing's triad, Cushing's reaction, Cushing's phenomenon, and Cushing's response – is a triad of signs of elevated ICP and impending herniation. The response consists of elevated systolic and pulse pressure, bradycardia, and respiratory irregularities due to compression of the brainstem. Dr. Harvey Cushing is credited for the discovery of this response in 1901.

There are multiple types of herniation syndromes that may occur with elevated ICP (Figure 16.2). Subfalcine herniation occurs as the frontal lobe extends under the falx cerebri. Imaging characteristics include a shift of the septum pellucidum, effacement of the anterior horn of the lateral ventricle, and compression of the anterior cerebral artery against the falx. One of the risks of subfalcine herniation is compression of the anterior cerebral artery long enough to cause a stroke in that territory, typically leading to contralateral leg weakness.

Uncal herniation occurs when the medical portion of the temporal lobe (uncus) is displaced into the suprasellar and ambien cisterns, leading to pressure on the midbrain. As uncal herniation progresses, the uncus causes a mass effect on the third cranial nerve affecting the parasympathetic input to the eyes leading to pupillary dilation and decreased reactivity. Pressure is also placed on the ipsilateral cerebral peduncle, leading to contralateral hemiparesis. In some cases, the lateral translation of the midbrain is so severe that the cerebral peduncle on the opposite side is pushed against the edge of the tentorium leading to the Kernohan's notch phenomenon. A false localizing sign is produced as the contralateral

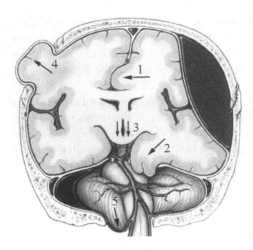

Figure 16.2 Patterns of brain herniation: (1) subfalcine (also called cingulate) herniation; (2) uncal herniation through the tentorial incisura; (3) central transtentorial herniation; (4) transcalvarial herniation; and (5) cerebellar tonsillar herniation through the foramen magnum. Adapted from CEN Brain Herniation Overview (2020) Elite Review, elitereview.net.

cerebral peduncle is affected, leading to ipsilateral hemiparesis. Another key feature to uncal herniation is a decreasing level of consciousness as the ascending arousal system is compressed.

Central herniation produces symptoms similar to those of uncal herniation as the diencephalon (i.e., thalamus and hypothalamus) is forced through the tentorial opening, leading to compression of the midbrain. The early diencephalic stage is reversible and is characterized by a decreasing level of consciousness, with difficulty concentrating, agitation, and drowsiness, small but reactive pupils, intact ciliospinal reflex (pupils dilate in response to a pinch of the skin on the neck), intact oculocephalic reflex (doll's eyes), flexor plantar responses, and deep sighs and yawns with respirations. In the late diencephalic stage the patient becomes more difficult to arouse, localizing motor response to pain disappears, and decorticate posturing appears with eventual progression to decerebrate posturing. Progressive diencephalic impairment is thought to be due to the stretching of small penetrating vessels of the posterior cerebral and associated perforating arteries that supply the hypothalamus and thalamus. As herniation progresses to the midbrain stage, signs of oculomotor failure appear, with pupils becoming irregular then fixed at midposition, oculocephalic reflexes become more difficult to elicit, and motor tone is increased and plantar responses are extensor.

Cerebellar tonsillar herniation occurs when the cerebellar tonsils herniate through the foramen magnum, causing compression of the medulla oblongata and upper cervical spinal cord. It is typically observed in the setting of a posterior fossa mass lesion, but can also occur with supratentorial lesions. Areas controlling respiration and hemodynamic stability are located in the medulla and may become compromised with severe compression. In the general population, the position of the cerebellar tonsils may extend up to 3 mm below the foramen magnum. In patients with a Chiari malformation, the tonsils typically extend 5 mm or greater below the foramen magnum but must be considered within the clinicopathological context because there are patients with Chiari malformation symptoms with less than 5 mm tonsillar herniation and vice versa.

16.5 Differential Diagnosis

16.5.1 Trauma

Traumatic injury to the skull or brain can lead to elevated ICPs in accordance with the Monro–Kellie doctrine. A depressed skull fracture may lead to diminished intracranial volume within the skull as well as injury to the underlying brain tissue. A subdural hemorrhage (SDH) or epidural hematoma (EDH) leads to an additional mass within the cranial vault. Intracerebral contusions as well as cerebral edema expand the cerebral volume. Traumatic brain injury (TBI) is the most common cause for elevated ICP.

16.5.2 Mass Lesions

Mass lesions such as tumors, aneurysms, or vascular malformations can cause a myriad of symptoms, depending on their location as well as the rate of growth and amount of related brain edema. Intracerebral hemorrhage increases the volume of blood within the cranium. Infarction or ischemic stroke leads to cerebral edema and expansion of the brain volume.

16.5.3 Idiopathic Intracranial Hypertension

Idiopathic intracranial hypertension, also known as pseudotumor cerebri, is a condition with elevated ICP without an obvious pathology or disease. It is theorized that venous outflow obstruction and/or dural venous stenosis is a possible causative phenomenon leading to this condition. Patients are most commonly young, overweight females with an incidence of 20 per 100,000 persons. Typically, they present with throbbing headaches that are worse with activities that increase ICP such as coughing, Valsalva maneuvers, or bending over. Nausea and vomiting may accompany the headaches. The most concerning symptom is change in vision and will lead to blindness secondary to papilledema if ICP is not controlled quickly. With chronic persistent elevated ICP, papilledema leads to damage of the optic nerve. Imaging studies such as CT or MRI likely will be normal, although they may show an empty sella turcica, distention of the optic nerve sheath, and posterior globe flattening. It is important to obtain an ophthalmology consult to formally document visual fields and assess the degree of papilledema.

16.5.4 Chiari Malformations

There are four traditional types of Chiari malformations with varying degrees of cerebellum and/or brainstem herniation through the foramen magnum leading to a disruption of the normal flow of CSF through the ventricles. This disruption of CSF flow may lead to the development of hydrocephalus or the formation of syringomyelia or syrinx (a CSF-filled tubular cyst within the central canal) in any region of the spinal cord. Patients may present with a myriad of symptoms such as headaches made worse with coughing or straining, neck pain, balance problems, numbness or paresthesia in arms or legs, difficulty swallowing, dizziness, nausea, vomiting, visual problems, hearing loss, insomnia, or depression.

16.5.5 CNS Infections

Meningitis, especially bacterial meningitis, can cause elevated ICP and is believed to be a major contributor to morbidity and mortality. It has been reported that up to 85–95% of patients with acute bacterial meningitis have elevated ICP. In patients with acute bacterial meningitis who present with severe impaired mental status, early neuro-intensive care using ICP-targeted therapy has shown improved functional recovery and decreased mortality when compared to standard intensive care therapy.

Intracranial abscesses are mass lesions associated with a subacute or chronic rise in ICP, tissue destruction, and vasogenic edema. Patients may present with fever, headache, focal neurologic symptoms depending on the location, or seizures, but can also have relatively mild symptoms.

16.5.6 Oral Contraceptives and Intrauterine Levonorgestrel

Oral contraceptives have been associated with benign intracranial hypertension, with the first case reported as far back as 1978. Patients have been reported to develop severe headaches and papilledema, with resolution of symptoms after discontinuing the medication. Obese middle-aged women appear to be most at risk for developing this disease. This association has also been found with the intrauterine form of levonorgestrel (Mirena®) and can develop even after long-term use. Females on oral contraceptives or with intrauterine levonorgestrel who develop headaches and visual disturbance should have a funduscopic examination to assess for papilledema, and discontinuation of hormone therapy should be considered.

16.6 Management

The initial management, especially in a lethargic or comatose patient, should focus on airway, breathing, and circulation. Endotracheal intubation may be necessary to perform controlled ventilation. Once the patient is hemodynamically stable, a focused neurologic examination should be performed. In a trauma patient, these steps are a part of the primary survey, with the addition of a cervical collar to stabilize the spine. If elevated ICP is suspected in a patient, initial management steps are geared toward avoiding factors that may aggravate or precipitate elevated ICP. Specific factors include obstruction of cerebral venous outflow (head position, agitation, elevated intrathoracic or intra-abdominal pressures), respiratory problems (airway obstruction, hypoxia, hypercapnia), fever, severe hypertension, hyponatremia, anemia, and seizures.

To minimize venous outflow obstruction, elevating the head of the bed to 30 degrees is a quick and simple step that can be performed in the pre-hospital setting and can reduce ICP. Trauma patients are given various types of cervical collars as part of the spine stabilization step. If the brace is too tight it can cause physical compression of the jugular veins, leading to venous obstruction and exacerbation of intracranial hypertension. Although it is important to maintain spinal precautions, the cervical collar must be adequately placed to prevent spinal injury but not so tightly as to cause elevated ICP. Agitation and pain increases blood pressure while it obstructs venous outflow, leading to increased ICP. An adequate level of sedation with various medications may be needed to decrease ICP. Increased intrathoracic or intra-abdominal pressure, such as with a hemo- or pneumothorax or abdominal compartment syndrome, can also lead to elevated ICP, presumably by obstructing cerebral venous outflow. Several case reports have indicated immediate reduction in ICP with decompressive laparotomy for an abdominal compartment syndrome that is refractory to medical treatment following TBI.

16.6.1 Hyperventilation

Hyperventilation decreases $PaCO_2$, which can lead to constriction of cerebral arteries by alkalinizing the CSF. The resulting reduction in cerebral blood volume decreases ICP.

The vasoconstrictive effect on cerebral arterioles lasts only 11–20 hours due to the rapid equilibration of the pH of the CSF. As the pH equilibrates, the cerebral arterioles redilate, possibly to a larger caliber than at baseline. This may lead to a rebound phase of increased ICP. Routine chronic hyperventilation (to a $PaCO_2$ of 20–25 mm Hg) should be avoided especially during the first 5 days due to evidence showing detrimental effect on outcome. Hyperventilation (to $PaCO_2$ of 25–30 mm Hg) should only be used acutely to allow time for more definitive treatments and should not be used routinely in all head injury patients.

16.6.2 Hyperosmolar Therapy

Mannitol is the most commonly used hyperosmolar agent for the acute treatment of intracranial hypertension. Common dosage is 0.25–1 mg/kg as an initial loading dose, then 0.25–0.5 mg/kg every 2–6 hours. An intravenous mannitol bolus lowers the ICP in 1–5 minutes, with a peak effect at 20–60 minutes. The effect of mannitol lasts from 1.5 to 6 hours, depending on the clinical condition. Contraindications to mannitol therapy include hypotension, hypovolemia, and renal failure. In addition to the osmotic properties, mannitol also has rheologic effects with an expansion of plasma volume and a reduction in hematocrit and blood viscosity, which may increase CBF in patients with intact cerebral autoregulation. Mannitol opens up the blood–brain barrier and may cross into the brain parenchyma, leading to a rebound exacerbation of vasogenic and osmotic edema.

Hypertonic saline is given in concentrations from 3% to 23.4%. Both mannitol and hypertonic saline create an osmotic force to draw water from the interstitial space of the brain parenchyma into the intravascular space. Hypertonic saline may be administered as a bolus for an acute decrease in ICP or as a continuous infusion for long-term management of ICP. Sodium levels and osmolality should be measured regularly while on hypertonic saline. There is a clear advantage with hypertonic saline use compared with mannitol in hypovolemic and hypotensive patients. Mannitol acts as a diuretic and can decrease blood pressure and volume status, whereas hypertonic saline augments intravascular volume and may increase blood pressure in addition to decreasing ICP. Hypertonic saline has not been associated with the rebound edema that is associated with mannitol, as the reflection coefficient for hypersonic saline is 1.0, whereas mannitol has a reflection coefficient of 0.9. The reflection coefficient is a measure of the relative impermeability of solutes. Mannitol can cross from intravascular spaces, causing the rebound edema effect.

16.6.3 Hypothermia

The NABIS trial, a multicenter randomized clinical trial of very early hypothermia induction in severe TBI, did not show a beneficial effect on neurological outcome, but it was noted that fewer patients randomized to moderate hypothermia had intracranial hypertension. A pilot randomized clinical trial of moderate hypothermia in children with TBI found similar findings, with a reduction of ICP during hypothermia treatment but no improvement in neurological outcome. Routine induction of hypothermia is not indicated at present, but it may be an effective adjunctive treatment for elevated ICP refractory to other medical management.

16.6.4 Steroids

Steroids are not recommended for patients with elevated ICP due to TBI, but are commonly used for primary or metastatic brain tumors to decrease the amount of vasogenic edema. Dexamethasone given at 4 mg every 6 hours is the typical dose used for tumors, and improvement in focal neurological signs and improved mental status owing to surrounding edema typically can be seen within hours. For TBI or spontaneous intracerebral hemorrhage, steroids have not shown any benefit and in some studies have been found to have detrimental effects. The CRASH trial, a large placebo-controlled randomized clinical trial of methylprednisolone for 48 hours in patients with TBI, showed a significant increase in the risk of death from 22.3% to 25.7% (relative risk 1.15, 95% confidence interval 1.07–1.24). This trial confirmed previous studies and guidelines that routine administration of steroids is not indicated for patients with TBI.

16.6.5 Barbiturate Coma

Barbiturate coma should only be considered for patients with refractory intracranial hypertension due to the serious complications associated with the use of high-dose barbiturates and the compromised neurological examination for several days as pentobarbital's half-life is 15–50 hours in adults. Pentobarbital is administered in a loading dose of 10 mg/kg followed by 5 mg/kg each hour for three doses. Maintenance dose is 1–2 mg/kg/h, titrated to a serum level of 30–50 µg/mL or until the electroencephalogram (EEG) shows a burst suppression pattern. Continuous EEG is utilized to monitor an effective burst suppression pattern. A randomized multicenter trial showed that instituting barbiturate coma in patients with refractory intracranial hypertension resulted in a twofold greater chance of controlling ICP. Complications occurring during treatment with barbiturate coma include hypotension, hypokalemia, respiratory problems, infections, hepatic dysfunction, and renal dysfunction.

16.6.6 Surgical Management

Decompressive craniectomy should be considered when elevated ICP is refractory to medical management. The surgical removal of part of the calvarium negates the Monro–Kellie doctrine by eliminating the rigid enclosure allowing for the swollen brain to herniate out of the bone window. This surgical treatment has been used to treat uncontrolled intracranial hypertension of various origins, including infarction, trauma, subarachnoid hemorrhage, and spontaneous hemorrhage.

Hydrocephalus and elevated ICP associated with intraventricular hemorrhage may be managed with external ventricular drainage. Obstructive hydrocephalus may occur when intraventricular blood obstructs normal CSF pathways. External ventricular drainage may assist in resolution of the intraventricular hemorrhage. Open surgical craniotomy is typically not performed to evacuate intraventricular hemorrhage; minimally invasive techniques are currently being studied. The Clot Lysis: Evaluating Accelerated Resolution of Intraventricular Hemorrhage Phase III (CLEAR-III) trial showed that patients with an intraventricular hemorrhage and an external ventricular drain irrigated with alteplase did not substantially improve outcome compared with irrigation with saline. Newer devices utilizing minimally invasive clot evacuation of intraventricular hemorrhage are available and under evaluation.

Craniotomy for evacuation of mass lesions, including intracranial hemorrhage, are options in select cases. Patient age, comorbidities, neurological status, and patient expectations should be considerations when deciding who would benefit from surgical treatment.

16.7 Methods for Measuring Intracranial Pressures

Lumbar puncture (LP) is the most common way of measuring ICP in the emergency setting. It is important to obtain a noncontrast CT scan of the brain to ensure that there is no mass lesion or obstructive cause for elevated ICP as performing a LP can cause herniation syndromes and even death. LPs can be performed with the patient lying on their side or sitting up. However, to obtain an accurate opening pressure that truly reflects the ICP it is necessary to have the patient positioned lying on their side with the head at the same horizontal level as the lumbar spine and their legs fully extended. Opening pressure should be measured prior to draining off any CSF to obtain an accurate measurement. Please see Chapter 4 for more specific instructions on the procedure.

The gold standard method for monitoring ICP is with an intraventricular catheter. The catheter is inserted through a burr hole over the convexity anterior to the coronal suture and directed to a point in line with the medial ipsilateral canthus and just anterior to the tragus. This projection typically lands the tip of the catheter in the lateral ventricle pointed toward the foramen of Monro. The catheter allows for the transduction of ICP as well as drainage of CSF for refractory elevated ICP. Other methods for monitoring ICP include a parenchymal pressure bolt, subdural pressure bolt, and epidural sensor.

Pearls and Pitfalls
• CPP = MAP − ICP.
• MAP = 1/3 systolic blood pressure + 2/3 diastolic blood pressure.
• Parinaud syndrome is a cluster of eye movement abnormalities that include paralysis of upgaze, a pseudo-Argyll Robertson pupil, convergence–retraction nystagmus, eyelid retraction (Collier's sign), and a "setting sun" sign.
• Cushing's response of impending herniation: elevated systolic and pulse pressure, bradycardia, and respiratory irregularities due to compression of the brainstem.
• Females on oral contraceptives or with intrauterine levonorgestrel who develop headaches and visual disturbance should have a funduscopic examination to assess for papilledema along with other signs of elevated ICP.
• To minimize venous outflow obstruction, elevating the head of the bed to 30 degrees is a quick simple step that can be performed in the pre-hospital setting to reduce ICP.
• Hyperventilation (to PaCO$_2$ of 25–30 mm Hg) for increased ICP should only be used acutely to allow time for more definitive treatments.
• Hypertonic saline has not been associated with the rebound edema that is associated with mannitol, and is the osmotic agent of choice when the patient is hypotensive.
• Steroids are not recommended for patients with elevated ICP caused by TBI, but are commonly used for primary or metastatic brain tumors.

Bibliography

Adelson PD, Ragheb J, Kanev P, et al. Phase II clinical trial of moderate hypothermia after severe traumatic brain injury in children. *Neurosurgery* 2005;56(4):740–754.

Ashwal S. Neurologic evaluation of the patient with acute bacterial meningitis. *Neurol Clin* 1995;13(3):549–577.

Bader MK, Arbour R, Palmer S. Refractory increased intracranial pressure in severe traumatic brain injury: barbiturate coma and bispectral index monitoring. *AACN Clin Issues* 2005;16(4):526–541.

Brain Trauma Foundation, American Association of Neurological Surgeons, Joint Section on Neurotrauma and Critical Care. Hyperventilation. *J Neurotrauma* 2000;17 (6–7):513–520.

Clifton GL, Miller ER, Choi SC, et al. Lack of effect of induction of hypothermia after acute brain injury. *N Engl J Med* 2001;344 (8):556–563.

Clifton GL, Valadka A, Zygun D, et al. Very early hypothermia induction in patients with severe brain injury (the National Acute Brain Injury Study: Hypothermia II): a randomised trial. *Lancet Neurol* 2011; 10(2):131–139.

Cushing H. Concerning a definite regulatory mechanism of the vaso-motor centre which controls blood pressure during cerebral compression. *John Hopkins Hosp Bull* 1901;12:290–292.

De Simone R, Ranieri A, Montella S, Bilo L, Cautiero F. The role of dural sinus stenosis in idiopathic intracranial hypertension pathogenesis: the self-limiting venous collapse feedback-loop model. *Panminerva Med* 2014;56(3):201–209.

Diringer MN, Videen TO, Yundt K, et al. Regional cerebrovascular and metabolic effects of hyperventilation after severe traumatic brain injury. *J Neurosurg* 2002;96(1):103–108.

Doczi T. Volume regulation of the brain tissue: a survey. *Acta Neurochir (Wien)* 1993;121:1–8.

Dorfman JD, Burns JD, Green DM, DeFusco C, Agarwal S. Decompressive laparotomy for refractory intracranial hypertension after traumatic brain injury. *Neurocrit Care* 2011;15(3):516–518.

Edwards P, Arango M, Balica L, et al. Final results of MRC CRASH, a randomised placebo-controlled trial of intravenous corticosteroid in adults with head injury: outcomes at 6 months. *Lancet* 2005;365 (9475):1957–1959.

Eisenberg HM, Frankowski RF, Contant CF, Marshall LF, Walker MD. High-dose barbiturate control of elevated intracranial pressure in patients with severe head injury. *J Neurosurg* 1988;69(1):15–23.

Etminan M, Luo H, Gustafson P. Risk of intracranial hypertension with intrauterine levonorgestrel. *Ther Adv Drug Saf* 2015; 6(3):110–113.

Feigin VL, Anderson N, Rinkel GJ, et al. Corticosteroids for aneurysmal subarachnoid haemorrhage and primary intracerebral haemorrhage. *Cochrane Database Syst Rev* 2005;20(3):CD004583.

Feldman Z, Kanter MJ, Robertson CS, et al. Effect of head elevation on intracranial pressure, cerebral perfusion pressure, and cerebral blood flow in head-injured patients. *J Neurosurg* 1992;76(2):207–211.

Fodstad H, Kelly PJ, Buchfelder M. History of the Cushing reflex. *Neurosurgery* 2006; 59(5):1132–1137.

Gean AD. *Imaging of Head Trauma*. Lippincott Williams & Wilkins, 1994.

Glimåker M, Johansson B, Halldorsdottir H, et al. Neuro-intensive treatment targeting intracranial hypertension improves outcome in severe bacterial meningitis: an intervention–control study. *PLoS One* 2014; 9(3):e91976.

Gobiet W, Grote W, Bock WJ. The relation between intracranial pressure, mean arterial pressure and cerebral blood flow in patients with severe head injury. *Acta Neurochir (Wien)* 1975;32:13–24.

Gudeman SK, Miller JD, Becker DP. Failure of high-dose steroid therapy to influence intracranial pressure in patients with severe head injury. *J Neurosurg* 1979;51(3):301–306.

Hlatky R, Valadka A, Robertson CS. Prediction of a response in ICP to induced hypertension using dynamic testing of cerebral pressure autoregulation. *J Neurotrauma* 2004;21:1152.

Jandolo B, Casaglia P, Morace E. Cerebral pseudotumor and oral contraceptives (cerebral case). *Riv Neurobiol* 1978;24 (1–2):106–108.

Joseph DK, Dutton RP, Aarabi B, Scalea TM. Decompressive laparotomy to treat intractable intracranial hypertension after traumatic brain injury. *J Trauma* 2004;57(4):687–693.

Kaal EC, Vecht CJ. The management of brain edema in brain tumors. *Curr Opin Oncol* 2004;16(6):593–600.

Kellie G. An account of the appearances observed in the dissection of two of the three individuals presumed to have perished in the storm of the 3rd, and whose bodies were discovered in the vicinity of Leith on the morning of the 4th November 1821 with some reflections on the pathology of the brain. *Trans Med Chir Sci Edinburgh* 1824;1:84–169.

Knapp JM. Hyperosmolar therapy in the treatment of severe head injury in children: mannitol and hypertonic saline. *AACN Clin Issues* 2005;16(2):199–211.

Martinez H, Arana H, Gancedo B, Larel M, De Virgillis M. A typical pseudotumor cerebri. *Neuroophthalmology* 2010;34:131–288.

McGillicuddy JE. Cerebral protection: pathophysiology and treatment of increased cranial pressure. *Chest* 1985;87:85–93.

Mokri B. The Monro–Kellie hypothesis: applications in CSF volume depletion. *Neurology* 2001;56(12):1746–1748.

Monro A. *Observations on the Structure and Function of the Nervous System.* Creech & Johnson, 1783.

Ng I, Lim J, Wong HB. Effects of head posture on cerebral hemodynamics: its influences on intracranial pressure, cerebral perfusion pressure, and cerebral oxygenation. *Neurosurgery* 2004;54 (3):593–597.

Pickard JD, Czosnyka M. Management of raised intracranial pressure. *J Neurol Neurosurg Psychiatry* 1993;56:845–858.

Pickard JD, Czosnyka M. Raised intracranial pressure. In Hughes RAC (ed.) *Neurological Emergencies.* BMG, 1994.

Rangel-Castillo L, Gopinath S, Robertson CS. Management of intracranial hypertension. *Neurol Clin* 2008;26(2):521–541.

Rosner MJ, Coley IB. Cerebral perfusion pressure, intracranial pressure, and head elevation. *J Neurosurg* 1986;65:636–641.

Saul TG, Ducker TB, Salcman M, Carro E. Steroids in severe head injury: a prospective randomized clinical trial. *J Neurosurg* 1981; 54(5):596–600.

Schalén W, Sonesson B, Messeter K, Nordström G, Nordström CH. Clinical outcome and cognitive impairment in patients with severe head injuries treated with barbiturate coma. *Acta Neurochir (Wien)* 1992;117 (3–4):153–159.

Sheehan JP. Hormone replacement treatment and benign intracranial hypertension. *Br Med J (Clin Res Ed)* 1982;284(6330):1675–1676.

Stocchetti N, Maas AI, Chieregato A, van der Plas AA. Hyperventilation in head injury: a review. *Chest* 2005;127(5): 1812–1827.

Traumatic and Nontraumatic Spinal Cord Disorders

Thomas F. Scott, Nestor Tomycz, and David Jho

17.1 Introduction

Traumatic spinal cord injury requires urgent imaging and decision-making involving a team approach. Causes of nontraumatic spinal cord injury are protean and can be roughly divided into compressive and non-compressive disease states. In general, it is the scenario of compressive spinal injury that needs to be identified quickly for possible urgent surgical decompression, whereas non-compressive injury requires a systematic work-up, which is somewhat less urgent. MRI is the imaging modality of choice for essentially all acute spinal cord disorders presenting to the ED, and the physician is charged with expeditious performance of this testing whenever spinal cord compression is deemed a likely possibility.

17.2 Presentation

Key history: The history of the patient provides invaluable information when considering which direction to take in the ED setting. When historical information is not available, especially in the setting of trauma, evidence of spinal injury should be sought, and spinal instability may be assumed until proven otherwise. This is true for all comatose patients and patients with altered mentation who are not able to cooperate with an exam on arrival.

The temporal evolution of spinal or myelopathic symptoms is often the most important element of the formulation. Apoplectic nontraumatic onset of myelopathy is rare and suggests vascular insult (infarct or hemorrhagic rupture into tumor or an arteriovenous malformation). Acute idiopathic transverse myelitis evolves over hours or days, although milder forms of idiopathic or demyelinating myelopathies (partial transverse myelitis) can evolve over weeks or months. Extradural compression from neoplasm or infection may evolve rapidly in terms of motor and sensory loss, but this generally occurs after a prodrome of many days of neck or back pain.

Past medical history and review of systems (generally for nontraumatic myelopathy) that includes a history of neoplasia, autoimmunity, or any systemic disorder often provides the key clue to a diagnosis. The review of systems parallels this search, which encompasses a long list of possibilities for acute and subacute myelopathies. Constitutional symptoms (e.g., weight loss, fatigue) and nonspecific complaints (e.g., arthralgias, rash, night sweats) tend to support either neoplasia or autoimmunity. Other useful review questions search for sicca syndrome (suggesting Sjögren's myelitis), hypercoagulable syndromes (lupus myelitis), and dry cough (sarcoid myelitis). A history of fevers is sought (infection, vasculitis). A pitfall is to dismiss infection when fevers are absent (epidural abscess).

Once a myelopathy is considered, based usually on sensory and motor complaints, specific queries regarding sensation are often useful. Is Lhermitte's phenomenon present?

Is there a sensation of a hug, or squeezing band sensation present (suggesting a sensory level). Queries regarding bowel and bladder function are mandatory. Patients may be embarrassed concerning the specific area of the saddle and genitalia, but the physician should specifically inquire about subjective experience in these areas.

17.3 Key Findings on Exam

The examination of a patient with suspected spinal cord pathology should be complete in terms of both general examination and also detailed in terms of signs relating to the spinal cord. Findings suggestive of systemic disorders covered in the review of systems include fever, rash, joint tenderness, and general appearance. A complete neurological exam is undertaken to search for the possibility of multifocal lesions. Myelopathy in this setting of multifocal lesions suggests autoimmunity, primarily multiple sclerosis (MS), but other possibilities are also considered (e.g., multiple neoplastic lesions or neurosarcoidosis). Specific findings relating to a focal lesion of the spinal cord are more often a mixture of motor and sensory abnormalities than pure sensory and rarely pure motor. A spinal shock picture with paraplegia, a sensory level, a flaccid bladder and areflexia is generally only seen in hyperacute spinal injury such as trauma or cord infarct. For all cases a sensory level is sought using light touch, pin prick, and temperature testing (an exam glove filled with ice water is often used), and may identify the uppermost level of the lesion, though findings are often at a level below lesions seen on MRI. Once an upper motor neuron lesion has been present for more than a hyperacute phase, hyperactive deep tendon reflexes predominate.

Typical patterns of sensory and motor loss: The Brown–Sequard syndrome of hemi-cord dysfunction (ipsilateral motor and contralateral sensory loss) may be seen with both intramedullary and extramedullary lesions, sometimes with an additional finding of a sensory dermatome ipsilateral to the spinal lesion. The cauda equina syndrome combines "saddle numbness" with bowel and bladder dysfunction and varying degrees of polyradiculopathy of lumbosacral nerve roots. The "anterior spinal artery syndrome" refers to sparing of the posterior columns (vibratory sensation) generally seen in spinal ischemic conditions. Mild "partial transverse myelitis" often presents with asymmetrical patchy sensory loss, and may mimic acute peripheral neuropathy with only mild bilateral distal paresthesias.

17.4 Neuroimaging

The delineation of traumatic injury and differential diagnosis of nontraumatic lesions are largely CT/MRI-dependent. MRI allows compartmentalization of lesions into intramedullary, extramedullary intradural, and extradural, with both specific and nonspecific MRI patterns characterizing the various disorders considered (Table 17.1).

17.5 Specific Disorders

17.5.1 Spinal Cord Infarct

Spinal cord infarct is rare and predominantly affects the elderly. The presentation is generally hyperacute, but can be stuttering. Arteriosclerotic thrombosis of key segmental arteries is seen in those with typical risk factors, but spinal infarction is rare vs cerebral thrombosis due to the rich network of anastomotic vessels enveloping the spinal cord. Due

Table 17.1 Common and rare nontraumatic spinal lesions by compartment and typical MRI characteristics

Intramedullary	Extramedullary intradural	Extradural
Myelitis (enhancing as ring, diffusely, or speckled, within a T2 lesion that may be small or extend over many levels, mild expansion of the cord if any, enhancement resolves within days if inflammation is mild); see Figure 17.1.	Meningioma (diffusely enhancing, sarcoid may mimic) abscess (inflamed cord surface may enhance adjacent to abscess).	Herniated disc (nonenhancing, cord is indented by disc with a small area of reactive edema; increased T2 within cord).
Neoplasm (nonenhancing if low-grade glioma, enhancing if metastasis, oligodendroglioma, or lymphoma, with cord enlargement, sarcoid may mimic).	Hematoma (MRI pattern of blood is age-dependent, complex).	Neoplasia (enhancing, destructive lesion of vertebral body).
Infections (ring enhancement, surrounding edema).	Sarcoidosis (enhancing).	

to the rarity of spinal infarction, hypercoagulable and embolic states should be considered. Young patients with spinal infarction may suffer from cartilaginous emboli (disc material), perhaps triggered by heavy lifting, and this type of spinal infarction has also been reported in cows and dogs. One special scenario for spinal infarction is the syndrome of dissection of the abdominal aorta with accompanying acute renal failure.

17.5.2 Spinal Cord Hemorrhage

Conditions causing spinal cord hemorrhage are exceedingly rare. Arteriovenous malformations rarely bleed into the spinal cord parenchyma or subarachnoid space. Although spinal gliomas are also rare, a notable proportion of oligodendrogliomas may bleed and cause sudden-onset myelopathy. These conditions are first identified by MRI, and urgent neurosurgical consultation is warranted for consideration of clot evacuation.

17.5.3 Spinal Infections

Spinal and paraspinal tissues can be infected by hematogenous spread of bacteria, and presentations are generally nonspecific in nature. Epidural abscess at first evaluation may present with localized pain without any neurological deficits, or severe spinal level deficits of motor and sensory function. A clue to infection is local tenderness, but an elevated sedimentation rate (ESR) can more reliably distinguish infection from benign back pain. Fever and leukocytosis may be absent, therefore an ESR should be considered in the ED setting. Discitis is exquisitely painful, and may occur with or without epidural abscess. The finding of a compressive epidural abscess is generally a surprise in the ED setting, considering the multitude of benign back pain issues physicians encounter. The early identification of an epidural abscess may prevent disastrous progression to severe paraparesis. Frequently the diagnosis is delayed until after the progression of deficits beyond those seen at presentation. A source of infection is generally not found. Even more rare and mysterious, an intramedullary abscess of the spinal cord may also be due to seeding from an unknown source (often streptococcal species). Tuberculosis is a consideration in at-risk populations.

Nonbacterial infections of the spinal cord are very rare. The most common is perhaps extension of typical herpes zoster from the nerve root into the spinal cord, with herpetic infections limited to the spinal cord being much more rare, and generally "proven" by CSF PCR for virus. Lyme disease of the spinal cord is also classically a myeloradiculopathy rather than a pure myelopathy. In endemic areas, schistosomiasis is considered.

17.5.4 Spinal Neoplasia

Spinal tumors generally present with a story of weeks of pain or minor neurological complaints, with some type of more acute superimposed complaint. Neoplastic myelopathy most often results from metastatic lesions of the vertebral bodies, and both primary tumors and metastases rarely involve the intramedullary compartment. The most common of these rare tumors is perhaps a low-grade oligodendroglioma, which may present with apoplectic bleeding. Lymphoma is a consideration for enhancing mass lesions, and sarcoidosis mimics all forms of spinal neoplastic tumors (intramedullary and extramedullary).

17.5.5 Transverse Myelitis

Severe acute transverse myelitis (ATM) is usually an idiopathic process and is seen in pediatric and adult populations (Figure 17.1). A postinfectious immune process has been proposed, and post-vaccinal cases are also reported. Patients present with moderate to severe sensory and motor dysfunction evolving over several hours to days. Bladder dysfunction ensues in almost all patients within several days of onset of weakness, as does a sensory level on exam. Mild acute partial transverse myelitis (APTM) may lack some or all of these cardinal features, presenting in a subtle fashion (usually first evaluated in an outpatient setting). The differential diagnosis for both ATM and APTM includes MS, systemic lupus erythematosus, sarcoidosis, and rarer dysimmune disorders. Both are usually idiopathic, with ATM having a higher likelihood of neuromyelitis optica (up to 40% in the setting of a longitudinally extensive lesion on MRI), and APTM having a higher likelihood of MS (about 20% for the next decade of life in the setting of a normal cerebral MRI). A cerebral MRI consistent with MS in the setting of APTM is virtually diagnostic of MS if the review of systems is negative for other more rare types of autoimmunity.

The nadir of weakness in ATM is often unclear when patients present to the ED, and patients are generally admitted for treatment with high-dose steroids (no class 1 or class 2 evidence), and for plasma exchange in the most severe cases (class 2 evidence). Cases involving cervical myelitis are especially worrisome, as progression into the high cervical levels or brainstem has been associated with respiratory failure.

17.6 Chronic Myelopathies

The differential diagnosis for chronic myelopathies is essentially distinct from acute disorders, and will most often be noted in the ED setting as an incidental finding or as a complicating issue separate from the primary complaint. In elderly patients cervical spine stenosis is often undetected until an examining physician makes note of spastic legs (hyperreflexia, plantar extensor responses). Thus, it is sometimes a challenge to untangle

(a)

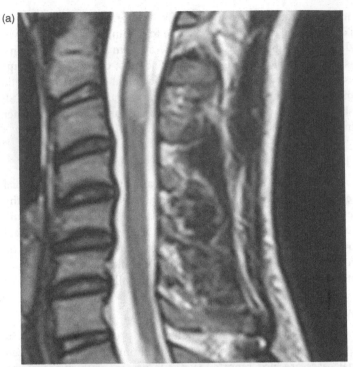

Figure 17.1 (a) Idiopathic acute transverse myelitis. (b) Mild partial myelitis as a presentation for MS.

(b)

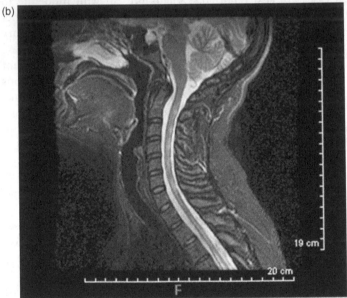

chronic incidental findings from more acute neurological issues. Consideration should be given toward work-up of possible chronic myelopathies (e.g., B12 level might be drawn, nonurgent imaging can be considered), but this should not detract from more acute issues.

In a middle-aged patient, primary progressive MS should be considered. Other considerations for chronic myelopathies include genetic disorders (e.g., familial spastic paraparesis and olivopontocerebellar atrophies) and rare deficiency states such as copper deficiency.

When MRI imaging or the elements of the case have established an intramedullary process, a decision is made concerning the extent of further work-up in the ED and disposition. Some myelopathies can be appropriately worked-up in an outpatient setting (e.g., mild APTM). Primary concerns are autoimmune disorders, infections, and neoplasia. Some considerations can be ruled out in the ED setting, whereas other considerations may require a stepwise extensive approach evolving over days or weeks. For example, deficiency of vitamin B12 rarely has a subacute myelopathic picture (usually weeks of stocking glove neuropathy symptoms at presentation), but is easily ruled out by a serum B12 level. By comparison, although an autoimmunity work-up can be initiated in the ED (e.g., ESR, antinuclear antibodies, SS-A antibodies, coagulation studies, selective imaging such as chest x-ray), other elements such as evoked potentials, spinal fluid analysis for IgG abnormalities, and highly specialized auto-antibody testing for neuromyelitis optica may be better left for an outpatient clinic. A neurologist will assist the ED physician in planning important disposition issues.

17.7 Evaluation of Cervical Spine Trauma

Cervical spine injury is common in the polytrauma patient and even patients with isolated cervical spine injury are often transferred to level I trauma centers for emergency evaluation and treatment. Approximately 40% of cervical spine injuries are associated with neurological damage and there are several unique cervical spinal cord syndromes that may occur in the setting of trauma. Elderly patients with advanced spine degenerative disease or other disorders such as ankylosing spondylitis are especially prone to cervical spine injuries and spinal cord injury after even minor trauma. In addition, elderly patients may be more prone to acute spinal hematomas in the setting of trauma due to frequent use of anticoagulant medications. The cervical spinal canal in the subaxial spine significantly narrows during extension, which explains why mild hyperextension injuries of the cervical spine may be associated with severe neurological complications. Cervical spinal cord injury may be life-threatening by its ability to engender hemodynamic instability and respiratory failure. Moreover, cervical spine trauma carries a risk of vascular injury to the carotid arteries but more commonly the vertebral arteries, which can cause immediate or delayed ischemic strokes. Survival and neurologic outcomes are optimized with rapid diagnosis and treatment.

17.8 Neurogenic Shock and Spinal Shock

Neurogenic shock describes the sudden bradycardia and hypotension that may result from a loss of autonomic tone after spinal cord injury. Neurogenic shock occurs with injuries above T6 and may require urgent treatment with vasoconstrictors, ionotropes, and chronotropes. In addition to hypotension and bradycardia, patients may exhibit warm, flushed skin and male patients may exhibit priapism. Hypothermia is a consequence of neurogenic shock that may also require treatment. Aggressive fluid resuscitation is necessary to treat a commonly depressed central venous pressure. Rapid atropine administration or even cardiac pacing may be necessary in patients with higher (C1–C5) spinal cord injuries. Neurogenic shock should only be considered the diagnosis for cardiovascular instability in a trauma patient once hemorrhagic shock has been ruled out. Aggressive treatment is necessary for hypotension since this is a well-established risk factor for secondary injury in traumatic brain injury and spinal cord injury. Phenylephrine, norepinephrine, and vasopressin may be helpful to support blood pressure in such patients; however, there is only low-quality evidence that there is a benefit of elevating the mean arterial pressure in patients with spinal cord injury. Neurogenic shock may persistent for weeks and evolve into a chronic state of dysautonomia in which patients experience low resting blood pressure, orthostatic hypotension, and autonomic dysreflexia with dangerous episodic hypertension and tachycardia.

Spinal shock refers to the sudden and often reversible loss of motor, sensory, and reflex function below the level of a spinal cord injury. Spinal shock is characterized by flaccidity, loss of bowel/bladder control, loss of plantar responses, and loss of spinal reflexes such as the anal wink and bulbocavernosus reflex. This form of shock may last days but eventually many spinal reflexes may recover. Some consider return of the bulbocavernosus reflex as a sign of recovery from spinal shock. The presence or absence of spinal shock does not have much prognostic significance in comparison to the ASIA (American Spinal Injury Association) motor examination. Digital rectal exam has poor sensitivity but high specificity in the diagnosis of a spinal cord injury and becomes quite important in the subacute setting to differentiate different ASIA spinal cord injury scores.

17.9 Classification of Spinal Cord Injury (ASIA Scale)

Spinal cord injuries are grossly classified as complete (no motor or sensory function below the lesion) or incomplete. Patients with no voluntary anal contraction or sensation in the S4, S5 dermatomes and no sensation with deep anal pressure are considered to have a complete injury. Although multiple scales are available to classify spinal cord injury, the ASIA scale is currently the most commonly used (Figure 17.2). This classification system has good inter-rater validity and reliability and has been shown to be a strong prognostic tool for recovery in spinal cord injury patients. Because of spinal shock, the ASIA score first begins to be prognostic 48 hours after the injury.

17.10 Imaging and Clearing the Traumatic Cervical Spine

In the alert and cooperative patient, the National Emergency X-ray Utilization Study (NEXUS) criteria and the Canadian C-spine rule have been designed to determine the need for radiographic imaging. The NEXUS criteria state that a patient can be cleared without further imaging if the following five rules are met:

- absence of midline tenderness
- normal level of alertness
- no evidence of intoxication
- no neurological findings
- no painful distracting injuries

Both the NEXUS and Canadian C-spine rule criteria are supported as safe and effective criteria for cervical collar clearance of a subgroup of patients without the need for radiographs. For patients that require radiographic imaging due to a high-risk mechanism,

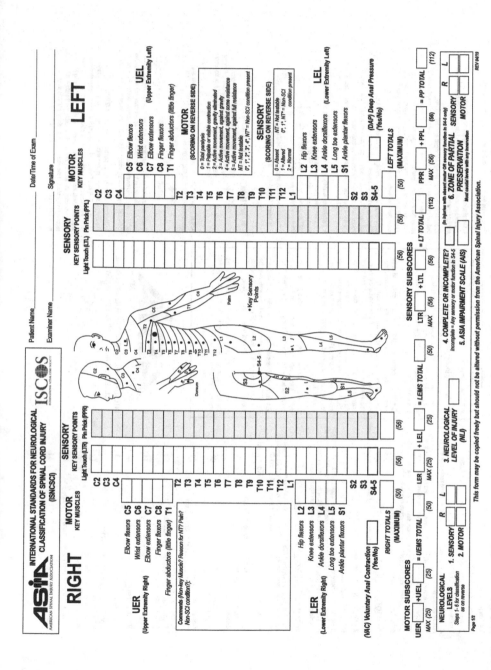

Figure 17.2 The ASIA scale.

Muscle Function Grading

0 = Total paralysis

1 = Palpable or visible contraction

2 = Active movement, full range of motion (ROM) with gravity eliminated

3 = Active movement, full ROM against gravity

4 = Active movement, full ROM against gravity and moderate resistance in a muscle specific position

5 = (Normal) active movement, full ROM against gravity and full resistance in a functional muscle position expected from an otherwise unimpaired person

NT = Not testable (i.e. due to immobilization, severe pain such that the patient cannot be graded, amputation of limb, or contracture of > 50% of the normal ROM)

0*, 1*, 2*, 3*, 4*, NT* = Non-SCI condition present *

Sensory Grading

0 = Absent   1 = Altered, either decreased/impaired sensation or hypersensitivity

2 = Normal   NT = Not testable

0*, 1*, NT* = Non-SCI condition present *

Note: Abnormal motor and sensory scores should be tagged with a "" to indicate an impairment due to a non-SCI condition. The non-SCI condition should be explained in the comments box together with information about how the score is rated for classification purposes (at least normal / not normal for classification).

When to Test Non-Key Muscles:

In a patient with an apparent AIS B classification, non-key muscle functions more than 3 levels below the motor level on each side should be tested to most accurately classify the injury (differentiate between AIS B and C).

Movement	Root level
Shoulder: Flexion, extension, abduction, adduction, internal and external rotation Elbow: Supination	C5
Elbow: Pronation Wrist: Flexion	C6
Finger: Flexion at proximal joint, extension Thumb: Flexion, extension and abduction in plane of thumb	C7
Finger: Flexion at MCP joint Thumb: Opposition, adduction and abduction perpendicular to palm	C8
Finger: Abduction of the index finger	T1
Hip: Adduction	L2
Hip: External rotation	L3
Hip: Extension, abduction, internal rotation Knee: Flexion Ankle: Inversion and eversion Toe: MP and IP extension	L4
Hallux and Toe: DIP and PIP flexion and abduction	L5
Hallux: Adduction	S1

ASIA Impairment Scale (AIS)

A = Complete. No sensory or motor function is preserved in the sacral segments S4-5.

B = Sensory Incomplete. Sensory but not motor function is preserved below the neurological level and includes the sacral segments S4-5 (light touch or pin prick at S4-5 or deep anal pressure) AND no motor function is preserved more than three levels below the motor level on either side of the body.

C = Motor Incomplete. Motor function is preserved at the most caudal sacral segments for voluntary anal contraction (VAC) OR the patient meets the criteria for sensory incomplete status (sensory function preserved at the most caudal sacral segments S4-5 by LT, PP or DAP), and has some sparing of motor function more than three levels below the ipsilateral motor level on either side of the body.
(This includes key or non-key muscle functions to determine motor incomplete status.) For AIS C – less than half of key muscle functions below the single NLI have a muscle grade ≥ 3.

D = Motor Incomplete. Motor incomplete status as defined above, with at least half (half or more) of key muscle functions below the single NLI having a muscle grade ≥ 3.

E = Normal. If sensation and motor function as tested with the ISNCSCI are graded as normal in all segments, and the patient had prior deficits, then the AIS grade is E. Someone without an initial SCI does not receive an AIS grade.

Using ND: To document the sensory, motor and NLI levels, the ASIA Impairment Scale grade, and/or the zone of partial preservation (ZPP) when they are unable to be determined based on the examination results.

Steps in Classification

The following order is recommended for determining the classification of individuals with SCI.

1. Determine sensory levels for right and left sides.
The sensory level is the most caudal, intact dermatome for both pin prick and light touch sensation.

2. Determine motor levels for right and left sides.
Defined by the lowest key muscle function that has a grade of at least 3 (on supine testing), providing the key muscle functions represented by segments above that level are judged to be intact (graded as a 5).
Note: In regions where there is no myotome to test, the motor level is presumed to be the same as the sensory level, if testable motor function above that level is also normal.

3. Determine the neurological level of injury (NLI).
This refers to the most caudal segment of the cord with intact sensation and antigravity (3 or more) muscle function strength, provided that there is normal (intact) sensory and motor function rostrally respectively.
The NLI is the most cephalad of the sensory and motor levels determined in steps 1 and 2.

4. Determine whether the injury is Complete or Incomplete.
(i.e. absence or presence of sacral sparing)
If voluntary anal contraction = No AND all S4-5 sensory scores = 0
AND deep anal pressure = No, then injury is Complete.
Otherwise, injury is Incomplete.

5. Determine ASIA Impairment Scale (AIS) Grade.
Is injury **Complete?** If YES, AIS=A

NO ↓   YES ↓

Is injury **Motor Complete?** If YES, AIS=B

NO ↓   (No=voluntary anal contraction OR motor function more than three levels below the motor level on a given side, if the patient has sensory incomplete classification)

Are at least half (half or more) of the key muscles below the neurological level of injury graded 3 or better?

NO ↓   YES ↓

AIS=C   AIS=D

If sensation and motor function is normal in all segments, AIS=E
Note: AIS E is used in follow-up testing when an individual with a documented SCI has recovered normal function. If at initial testing no deficits are found, the individual is neurologically intact and the ASIA Impairment Scale does not apply.

6. Determine the zone of partial preservation (ZPP).
The ZPP is used only in injuries with absent motor (no VAC) OR sensory function (no DAP, no LT and no PP sensation) in the lowest sacral segments S4-5, and refers to those dermatomes and myotomes caudal to the sensory and motor levels that remain partially innervated. With sacral sparing of sensory function, the sensory ZPP is not applicable and therefore "NA" is recorded in the block of the worksheet. Accordingly, if VAC is present, the motor ZPP is not applicable and is noted as "NA".

AMERICAN SPINAL INJURY ASSOCIATION

INTERNATIONAL STANDARDS FOR NEUROLOGICAL CLASSIFICATION OF SPINAL CORD INJURY

ISCOS
INTERNATIONAL SPINAL CORD SOCIETY

Figure 17.2 (cont.)

helical CT has become the primary screening tool. Multiple studies have revealed that the sensitivity of helical CT is much greater than that of plain x-rays and helical CT has therefore eliminated the need for screening plain radiographs in the polytrauma patient. In the setting of neurologic weakness or sensory deficits, MRI is strongly recommended in addition to CT.

Cervical spine clearance in the obtunded patient is more controversial because the neurologic examination is not reliable and MRI has often been utilized as an adjunct to CT. The concern is that an unstable ligamentous injury might be missed by bony imaging such as CT, and MRI is often ordered even if a helical cervical CT is negative. However, the evidence that helical CT alone can be utilized safely to clear the cervical spine in obtunded trauma patients has been steadily increasing and many countries have safely adopted CT alone clearance protocols for obtunded or intubated trauma patients. A meta-analysis with 17 studies and 14,327 patients concluded that modern CT alone was sufficient to detect unstable injuries in obtunded or intubated trauma patients. MRI has greater soft tissue resolution and clearly elucidates more degenerative and ligamentous pathology than CT, yet there is scant evidence that MRI will reveal an unstable injury requiring immobilization or surgery in a patient with a negative-read modern helical CT.

17.11 Spinal Cord Syndromes

There are several unique spinal cord injury syndromes and recognition of these syndromes can facilitate rapid diagnosis and treatment of different spinal cord injuries.

- Central cord syndrome is the most common spinal cord syndrome and is characterized by disproportionately greater upper extremity weakness compared with lower extremity weakness. Patients also manifest upper extremity hypesthesia, dysesthesia, or hyperesthesia. The mechanism is usually cervical hyperextension in patients with pre-existing cervical stenosis, typically elderly patients. The narrowing of the subaxial cervical spine canal that occurs with extension explains why even mild hyperextension in the setting of degenerative stenosis can lead to significant neurologic complications. Most patients show neurologic recovery with collar immobilization alone; however, surgery may be recommended if imaging reveals high-grade cord compression.
- Anterior cord syndrome results from injury to the anterior half of the spinal cord and has a worse prognosis than central cord syndrome. The mechanism of injury is typically axial loading or hyperflexion and patients manifest with complete motor deficit at the level of injury with loss of pain and temperature sensation beginning a few levels below that of motor loss.
- Posterior cord syndrome is rare and results from selective injury to the posterior spinal dorsal columns. Patients may exhibit preserved strength but loss of vibration sense and proprioception (Figure 17.3).

17.12 Cervical Spine Fracture Patterns

There are numerous cervical fracture patterns that are commonly seen after trauma, and various classification schemes have been assigned to different subtypes. The most common subtypes are briefly summarized below. Cervical injuries can be classified into upper cervical injuries (craniocervical junction, C1, and C2) and subaxial (below C2) cervical spine injuries.

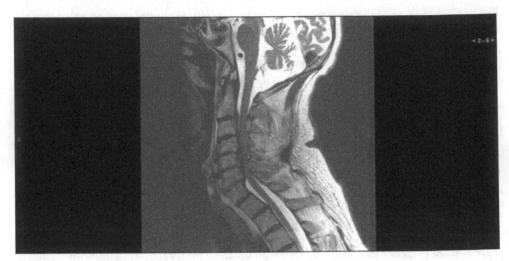

Figure 17.3 Central cord syndrome. A 71-year-old man with severe upper extremity weakness after a motor vehicle accident which caused neck hyperextension. MRI cervical spine reveals severe multilevel cervical stenosis.

17.12.1 Upper Cervical Injuries

Craniocervical disruption (CCD) refers to distractive injuries between the skull and C2. The most common types are atlanto-occipital dislocation (AOD), a disruptive injury between the skull base and the C1 vertebrae, and atlanto-axial dislocation (AAD), a distractive injury to the C1–C2 motion segment. AOD results from ligamentous damage at the atlanto-occipital joint and is often fatal before the patient reaches the hospital. According to the classification by Traynelis, the skull in an AOD either dislocates from the rest of the spine anteriorly (type I), longitudinally (type II), or posteriorly (type III). There are several measurement parameters that can help to confirm an AOD, including a Powers ratio >1:

Powers ratio = distance from the basion to the posterior arch of C1 / distance from the opisthion to the anterior arch of the atlas.

17.12.2 Atlas (C1) and Axis (C2) Fractures

Isolated atlas fractures rarely cause neurologic deficits and most are managed with collar immobilization alone. The most common subtype of atlas fracture is the Jefferson fracture, which is a burst-type fracture that classically involves four fractures (two anterior and two posterior) in the ring of C1. The Jefferson fracture does carry a risk of instability when there is concomitant injury to the transverse atlantal ligament. The magnitude of displacement of the lateral masses of C1 on C2 when viewed on an open mouth odontoid view radiograph or coronal CT reconstruction may be used to predict disruption of the transverse atlantal ligament (Figure 17.4).

C2 fractures, particularly odontoid process fractures, are quite common and may account for as much as 20% of cervical spine injuries. The three-part classification of odontoid or "dens" fractures by Anderson and D'Alonzo remains in widespread use and helps to guide treatment. Type I odontoid fractures (fracture through the odontoid tip) are considered stable and nonoperative management with collar immobilization yields

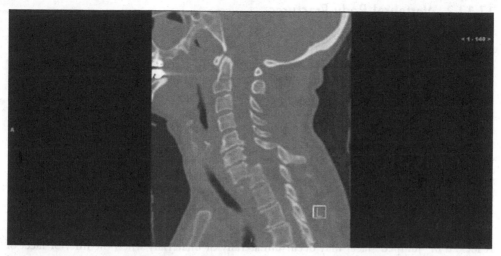

Figure 17.4 Cervical fracture-dislocation. A 52-year-old woman hit on the head by a falling tree branch. CT scan sagittal reconstructions revealed a fracture-dislocation of C7–T1 with marked C7–T1 anterolisthesis.

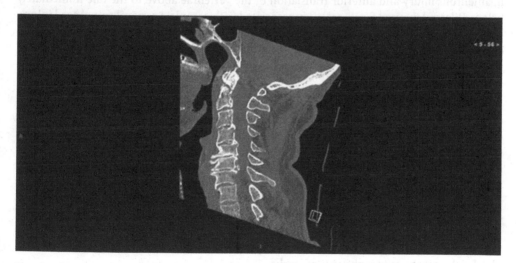

Figure 17.5 Odontoid fracture. A 71-year-old man with a fall from a motorcycle. CT cervical spine sagittal reconstructions reveals type II odontoid fracture.

excellent results. Management of type II (fracture through the base of the odontoid) and type III (fracture involving the body of C2) odontoid fractures remain more controversial and are age-dependent. Many type II and III fractures are considered unstable and may require halo immobilization or surgery. Traumatic spondylolisthesis or "hangman's fracture" is a special type of C2 fracture that involves fractures bilaterally through the pedicles or par interarticularies with varying degrees of ligamentous and C2–C3 disc space and facet disruption. Hangman's fractures with unilateral or bilateral C2–C3 facet dislocation should be treated surgically (Figure 17.5).

17.12.3 Vertebral Body Fractures

Vertebral body fractures of the subaxial cervical spine include *compression fractures*, *burst fractures*, and *teardrop fractures*. *Compression fractures* involve structural failure of the anterior half of the vertebral body and are generally considered stable. *Burst fractures* involve injury to the entire vertebral body and are commonly associated with retropulsion of bony fragments into the spinal canal. Anterior cord syndrome or complete spinal cord injury is common and these fractures are therefore highly unstable. Surgery is commonly required and may involve anterior corpectomy (complete resection of the fractured vertebral body) with a second stage posterior fixation approach. *Teardrop fractures* are highly unstable fractures that result from hyperflexion or hyperextension and involve severe disruption of the ligaments, intervertebral disc, and bilateral facets. Imaging may reveal a small triangular fracture from the anteroinferior aspect of the vertebral body.

17.13 Facet Fracture/Dislocation

A locked or "jumped" facet may occur unilaterally or bilaterally when the inferior facet of the upper vertebrae dislocates anterior to the superior facet of the lower vertebrae. Perched facet represents a milder degree of facet dislocation when the upper inferior facet is suspended over the lower superior facet. Jumped facets are usually associated with severe ligamentous injury and anterior translation of the vertebrae above to the one immediately below. Bilateral jumped facets are often associated with complete cervical spinal cord injury. Unilateral injuries may have a much milder neurologic deficit, such as a single nerve root compression syndrome. Most facet injuries are unstable and require surgical management with or without preoperative closed reduction with Gardner–Wells tongs (Figure 17.6).

17.14 Vascular Imaging

Cervical injury may be associated with injury to the vertebral arteries and less likely the carotid arteries. Digital subtraction angiography (DSA) has been considered the gold standard, but has been increasingly replaced with CT angiography, which is more rapid and noninvasive. Penetrating cervical trauma has a much higher risk for vascular injury than blunt cervical trauma. However, patients sustaining high (C1–C3) cervical spine fractures, cervical fractures with subluxation-dislocation, or those with fractures that come near or involve the foramen transversarium should undergo CT angiography to rule-out vertebral artery injury. Vertebral artery dissection or other injury may change the timing of operative intervention and require treatment with anticoagulation or anti-platelet therapy to reduce the risk of stroke.

17.15 Traumatic Disorders of the Thoracic and Lumbar Spine

Traumatic injuries of the thoracic and lumbar spine (T/L-spine) may be grouped into minor and major injuries. Minor injuries may comprise mechanisms such as a short-distance fall, being struck by a blunt object, or moderate-speed motor vehicle collision (MVC). Minor injuries may involve direct impact with transverse process and/or spinous process fractures, which are components of the T/L-spine that do not provide any significant biomechanical support. Minor injuries may also include traumatic disc herniations and lumbar sprains. Major injuries involve structural components of the spinal column and can compromise the stability of the T/L-spine. Major injuries often involve a

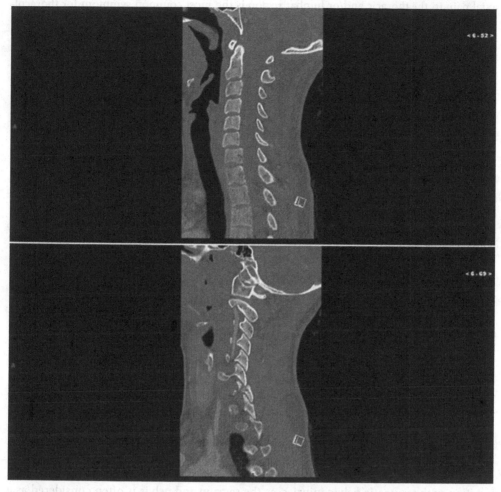

Figure 17.6 Cervical facet fracture-dislocation. A 25-year-old woman with fall from a horse. Examination revealed left arm radicular pain and left triceps weakness. CT cervical spine sagittal reconstructions reveal left C7 superior articular facet fracture and anterior displacement of C6 inferior articular facet.

long-distance fall, high-speed MVC, or penetrating trauma with gunshot as a separate category than the more common blunt injury. In terms of basic patterns of major blunt injury of the T/L-spine, there are four general types: (1) compression fractures, (2) burst fractures, (3) Chance fractures, and (4) fracture-dislocations.

For minor traumatic injuries of the T/L-spine with an intact primary survey, much of the initial evaluation consists of symptoms described by the patient along with the neurologic exam. There are guidelines such as the Canadian C-Spine Rule and NEXUS Criteria for determining which patients with traumatic injuries should undergo CT cervical spine (C-spine) imaging for further evaluation, and the evaluation of the T/L-spine for CT imaging selection is similar. For the patient to be cleared for thoracolumbar injuries without imaging, the patient should be awake/alert and not intoxicated, neurologically intact, and without midline tenderness on palpation of the T/L-spine. Acute focal axial pain in the thoracic and/or lumbar region is the most common symptom for thoracolumbar fractures, and spine pain may often be the only associated symptom. Clinical suspicion for fractures should be followed-up by noncontrast CT T/L-spine imaging for further evaluation, with MRI typically reserved for significant neurological deficits or preoperative planning evaluation. Plain spine x-rays can miss significant spine injuries and would be inadequate for determining management in many fractures, and relying on plain x-rays of the spine in trauma assessment is not recommended when CT is available.

For major traumatic injuries it may even be apparent initially in the field whether a patient has complete or incomplete spinal cord injury, but all patients with major traumatic injuries are treated with spine precautions from the start. The C-spine remains immobilized initially, and logroll precautions are maintained for the T/L-spine. Following the primary survey, the secondary survey is useful in identifying regions on which to focus further imaging studies, and the tertiary survey after CT imaging may involve spine specialist consultants (typically neurosurgery or orthopedic surgery) for assistance with management. Many patients with major traumatic injuries undergo CT of the chest/abdomen/pelvis, which can be reconstructed as CT T/L-spine studies.

17.16 T/L-Spine Fracture Patterns

The T1–T10 region is protected by the unified rib cage and associated muscles, such that injuries typically involve high-velocity mechanisms in the young vs an osteoporotic bony substrate with low-velocity mechanisms in the elderly. Fractures in the T1–T10 region comprise approximately 16% of traumatic spine fractures, with the most common subtype being compression fractures, with only a small minority(<15%) having associated spinal cord injury. The T11–L5 region includes the lower thoracic spine with floating ribs at the thoracolumbar junction and the lumbar spine, which is a more highly mobile segment of the spine and is more prone to fracture mechanisms, with three times more fractures in the T11–L5 region than the T1–T10 region. Approximately 60% of all thoracolumbar fractures are focused at the T12–L2 levels of the thoracolumbar junction, where the inflexible thoracic spine transitions to the flexible lumbar spine.

Sacral fractures will not be included in this discussion, which are assessed in conjunction with traumatic pelvic injuries, as the sacrum and pelvis is often considered as a single unit for stability consideration. We will also focus on blunt trauma of the T/L-spine, which is much more prevalent than penetrating trauma and produces reproducible patterns of injury, whereas penetrating trauma creates individual patterns based on bullet trajectory. Penetrating trauma to the T/L-spine is often managed nonsurgically, with orthosis if needed. Surgical indications for penetrating trauma with gunshot wound (GSW) to the spine would include: progressive neurological deficits with compression of neural elements, intractable CSF leak that may include external leakage component, or progressive spinal instability, with other indications being rare. Most penetrating injury to the spine is not significantly unstable and many advocate conservative treatment regardless of the extent of neurologic injury because most fail to show recovery after surgery with potential increase in CSF leak, infection, and even instability after surgery. Mechanisms of blunt T/L-spine injury can involve a combination of six basic forces, with four paired as opposing forces with compression vs distraction, flexion vs extension, and the remaining two being rotation and shear. The most common mechanisms are axial compression and flexion, which are involved in compression fractures and burst fractures, along with flexion or flexion-distraction playing a major role in Chance fractures.

Clinical spine instability is defined as the loss of ability for the spine to support physiologic loads such that the result may be progressive major deformity, progressive neurological deficits, and/or incapacitating mechanical pains with spinal loading. Spinal instability is a spectrum rather than an all-or-nothing phenomenon, given that there are varying degrees of instability. The most common stability model for clinical use is the Denis three-column model, with division of the structural T/L-spine vertebral column into three vertical segments based on sagittal CT sequences, with the anterior column including the anterior longitudinal ligament and anterior portion (half to two-thirds) of the vertebral body plus discs, middle column including the posterior portion (half to one-third) of the vertebral body plus discs and posterior longitudinal ligament, and posterior column including the pedicles plus facets and pars interarticularis bordering the lamina with associated ligaments of the posterior ligamentous complex. Fractures or injuries that involve two or three columns at the same level are considered unstable. In addition, fractures that involve the same column (such as the anterior column) in two adjacent levels are considered to be unstable, and bilateral articular injuries involving the facets and/or pars interarticularis are more unstable than unilateral facet or pars injuries. There are four general types of T/L-spine major injury patterns: (1) compression fractures, (2) burst fractures, (3) Chance fractures, and (4) fracture-dislocations.

As with cervical-level injuries, the degree of neurological deficit may be classified as complete or incomplete spinal cord injury, with outcomes for incomplete spinal cord injury being better for potential functional improvements. Autonomic dysreflexia with swings in blood pressure and disinhibited sympathetic stimulation can occur for spinal cord injury above the T6 level, and sacral parasympathetic deficits can also occur with spinal cord injury. It is more common for lumbar spine fractures to compress lumbosacral nerve roots of the cauda equina rather than the spinal cord, since the conus medullaris typically ends at T11–L2 (most commonly at T12 or L1). Toward the severe end of the spectrum for nerve root compression, cauda equina syndrome (CES) can be caused by fracture fragments or very large disc herniations, and consists of weakness in the lower extremities along with saddle anesthesia or loss of perineal sensation, plus bladder/bowel retention. CES may be complete-CES, with the classic triad of symptomatology, or incomplete-CES (also termed "cauda-in-evolution") in which the symptoms may be partial and involve a progressive process.

17.17 Compression Fracture (T/L-Spine)

Anterior wedge compression fractures involve compression and flexion mechanisms, which predominantly has anterior column injury. The radiographic components to be assessed include level(s) involved, percentage loss of height (LOH) of the vertebral body, any retropulsion into the spinal canal (typically none for true compression fractures), and angulation. Most compression fractures are relatively stable or mildly unstable along the stability spectrum, such that these can often be treated with orthosis for several weeks to a few months. Compression fractures may be more unstable if there is >1 contiguous segment involved, >50% LOH, and/or >25–30° kyphosis. These are not usually associated with spinal cord injury unless there is marked severity such as multiple contiguous levels or >30° kyphosis or progressive kyphotic deformity, which may then need to be considered for surgical fusion (Figure 17.7).

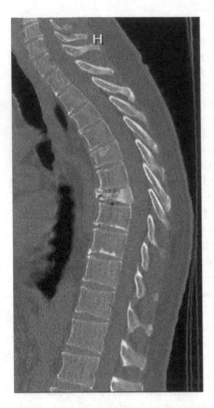

Figure 17.7 Compression fracture (T/L-spine). A 49-year-old male fell from a ladder with local evaluation that initially included only x-rays, which missed the T5 superior end-plate compression fracture and severe T7 compression fracture, with initial diagnosis of rib fractures only. He had maintained full strength and sensation. His thoracic back pains and kyphotic deformity progressed over months as he continued to do construction work, until his primary care physician ordered a CT thoracic spine without contrast (sagittal sequence shown) 6 months after his initial injury, which showed his previously missed fractures with marked LOH of the T7 compression fracture, and he was referred to neurosurgery at that time.

17.18 Burst Fracture (T/L-Spine)

Burst fractures also involve compression and flexion mechanisms, with injury to the anterior and middle columns with comminuted vertebral body fragments, and can sometimes involve the posterior column as well. The key descriptors include the level(s) involved, percentage LOH of the vertebral body, retropulsion into the spinal canal (in millimeters or percent of canal compromise), and angulation. There can be increased interpedicular distance with burst fracture and possible posterior column injuries to the pedicles, facets, lamina, and posterior ligamentous complex. There is a spectrum of stability in burst fractures with variable severity, ranging from relatively stable burst fractures (mildly to moderately unstable, similar to the configuration of compression fractures) to unstable burst fractures. Severe unstable burst fractures are often associated with spinal cord injury or injury to lumbosacral nerve roots of the cauda equina (Figure 17.8). Treatment can range from orthosis to various surgical fusion and decompression options.

17.19 Chance Fracture (T/L-Spine)

Chance fractures involve flexion-distraction at the thoracolumbar junction, considered a seatbelt (lapbelt) type of injury, although various situations may be involved. Chance fractures occur at the T11–L1 region and can be subdivided into bony Chance fractures, nonbony Chance injury (through ligaments and disc), and combination injuries. Most Chance fractures involve a combination of bony Chance fracture through the vertebral

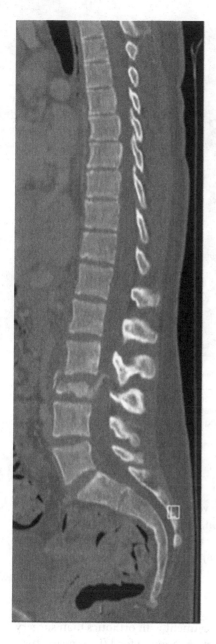

Figure 17.8 Burst fracture (T/L-spine). A 20-year-old female illicit drug dealer jumped from a second story window onto concrete to escape law enforcement, sustaining a right wrist fracture, left ankle fracture, and severe L3 burst fracture with marked LOH and retropulsion with spinal canal compromise and compression of lumbosacral nerve roots with CT thoracic and lumbar spine reconstructions (sagittal sequence shown).

body and posterior ligamentous injury. When there is not much displacement or kyphotic angulation, with significant bony component that has the opportunity to result in bony healing, these may sometimes be treated with a thoracic-lumbar-sacral orthosis (TLSO) brace over months. However, if there is involvement of bilateral pedicles or facets (or pars interarticularis), marked displacement or kyphotic angulation, and soft tissue injury components (ligaments and/or disc), these may require posterior instrumented fusion (Figure 17.9).

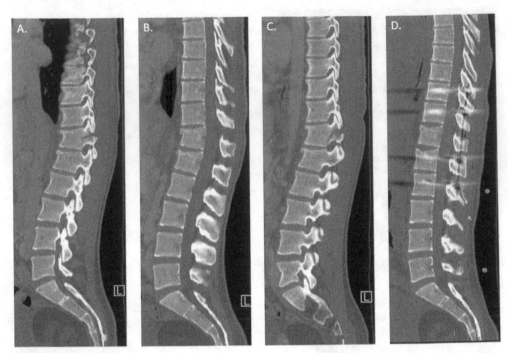

Figure 17.9 Chance fracture (T/L-spine). A 22-year-old female restrained backseat van passenger in an MVC, with back pain and without spinal cord injury, sustaining a severe T12 Chance fracture and a mild L1 superior end-plate compression fracture. CT T/L-spine without contrast (sagittal sequences) show (a) right pedicle fracture involvement at T12, (b) Chance fracture at T12 with kyphotic angulation, (c) left pedicle fracture involvement at T12, and (d) reduction of kyphotic deformity with restoration of sagittal alignment with posterior instrumented fusion from T10 to L2.

17.20 Fracture-Dislocation (T/L-Spine)

Fracture-dislocations are a miscellaneous group of severe injuries with a combination of mechanisms that can range from flexion or extension, compression or distraction, combined with shear and/or rotation. All three columns are involved, and these are highly unstable fractures often associated with spinal cord injury. Fracture-dislocations typically require surgical fusion for stabilization.

17.21 Management

It is more common for T/L-spine injuries to require treatment with orthotics than surgery. There are multiple different types of orthotics, but the most common for T/L-spine fractures is the TLSO brace in the clamshell or body jacket format, which is customized to fit the patient and stabilizes to the ribcage and torso as a total-contact brace. The selected orthotic should be considered akin to a cast, in that the fracture should be stabilized above and below along the spinal column. Using an inappropriate brace, such as a lumbar-sacral orthosis (LSO) brace for fractures at the thoracolumbar junction can result in worsening of spinal deformity by focusing the biomechanical stresses at the unsupported end (Figure 17.10).

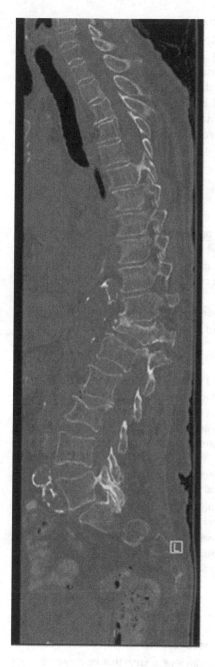

Figure 17.10 Fracture-dislocation (T/L-spine) T12 and L1 compression fractures. An 87-year-old female with osteoporosis and rheumatoid arthritis had acute-onset severe thoracolumbar back pain after picking up bags of cat food, sustaining T12 and L1 compression fractures that were treated at an outside hospital facility with inappropriate LSO that stopped superiorly at the thoracolumbar junction. She had worsening back pain and weakness in her bilateral lower extremities over months, having developed progressive severe kyphotic deformity at the thoracolumbar junction on follow-up noncontrast CT of the T/L-spine (sagittal sequence shown).

Surgical fusion for stabilization of the spinal column and surgical decompression for neural elements should be customized for the individual patient's fracture configuration and spinal anatomy, which should be determined by a spine surgical specialist.

With regard to the controversial topic of corticosteroids for spinal cord injury, the American Association of Neurological Surgeons (AANS) and Congress of Neurological Surgeons Joint Section for Spine Trauma 2002 discussed and officially commented that the methylprednisolone protocols from the NASCIS studies were reviewed, and overall studies to date have shown that the option of methylprednisolone for spinal cord injury may be considered only with the knowledge that the evidence suggesting possible harmful side effects is more consistent than any suggestion of clinical benefit, such that many institutions have established policies to decline the routine use of corticosteroids in spinal cord injury to minimize potential harmful side effects. Although the methylprednisolone protocol for SCI has fallen increasingly out of favor at many institutions, surgeons may choose to use corticosteroids in a perioperative fashion on an individual patient basis.

Pearls and Pitfalls

Patients with nontraumatic myelopathy:

- Consider epidural abscess in all patients with back or neck pain, even in the absence of neurological deficits, and consider obtaining an ESR.
- Patients with acute transverse myelitis can decline rapidly, with complete loss of bladder function (requiring catheterization), and ascending cervical lesions (requiring ventilator support).
- Consider occult spinal instability and injury in all patients with severe altered mentation.
- Consider intensive monitoring of acute cervical cord myelitis (may ascend to brainstem level with ensuing respiratory failure).

Patients in the setting of trauma:

- Modern multidetector helical CT is the gold standard for diagnosing cervical spine injuries and should be used instead of radiographs. MRI should be ordered after CT for patients with neurologic deficits such as suspected spinal cord injury.
- Spinal cord injury above T6 level may be accompanied by neurogenic shock that may require urgent supportive treatment with vasoconstrictors, ionotropes, and chronotropes.
- Spinal cord injuries are classified as complete or incomplete based on the presence or absence of voluntary anal sphincter contraction and sensation.
- Elderly patients with cervical spinal stenosis may suffer significant neurologic deficits from spinal cord injury from cervical hyperextension during trauma.
- CT angiography of the cervical spine should be considered to rule-out vascular injury, most commonly vertebral artery injury, in blunt trauma patients with high cervical fractures (C1–C3), fractures involving the foramen transversarium, and cervical fractures associated with subluxation-dislocation.
- NEXUS criteria and Canadian C-spine rule are safe and effective means for clearing a cervical collar in awake patients. It remains controversial but there is increasing evidence that even obtunded or comatose patients can be cleared of unstable cervical spine injuries with modern helical CT alone, without the need for MRI.
- Many significant T/L-spine fractures are missed by plain x-rays, such that history and examination should be used in conjunction with CT imaging if needed. If there is very low suspicion for spine fractures, then an accurate history and examination can suffice. If there is any significant suspicion for spine fractures, then CT imaging should be used.
- There are four basic types of major T/L-spine injury patterns: (1) compression fracture, (2) burst fracture, (3) Chance fracture, and (4) fracture-dislocation.

Bibliography

Biello JF, Davis JW, Cunningham MA, et al. Cervical spinal cord injury and the need for cardiovascular intervention. *Arch Surg* 2003;**138**:1127–1129.

Casha S, Christie S. A systematic review of intensive cardiopulmonary management after spinal cord injury. *J Neurotrauma* 2010;**27**:1–17.

Denis F. The three column spine and its significance in the classification of acute thoracolumbar spinal injuries. *Spine* 1983; **8**(8):817–831.

Denis F. Spinal instability as defined by the three-column spine concept in acute spinal trauma. *Clin Orthop Relat Res* 1984;**189**:65–76.

Hagedorn JC 2nd, Emery SE, France JC, et al. Does CT angiography matter for patients with cervical spine injuries. *J Bone Joint Surg Am* 2014;**4**(96):951–955.

Hoffman JR, Schriger DL, Mower W, Luo JS, Zucker M. Low-risk criteria for cervical-spine radiography in blunt trauma: a prospective study. *Ann Emerg Med* 1992;**21** (12):1454–1460.

Hurlbert RJ. The role of steroids in acute spinal cord injury: an evidence-based analysis. *Spine* 2001;**26**(24 Suppl.):S39–S46.

Krassioukov A, Karlsson A, Wecht JM, et al. Assessment of autonomic dysfunction following spinal cord injury: rationale for additions to international standards for neurological assessment. *J Rehab Res Dev* 2007;**44**(1):103–112.

Mack EH. Neurogenic shock. *Open Pediatr Med J* 2013;**7**(1):16–18.

Madsen III PW, Eismont FJ, Green BA. Diagnosis and management of thoracic spine fractures. In Winn HR, Sonntag VKH, Vollmer DG (eds.) *Youmans Neurological Surgery*, 5th ed. Elsevier, 2003.

Mathen R, Inaba K, Munera F, et al. Prospective evaluation of multislice computed tomography versus plain radiographic cervical spine clearance in trauma patients. *J Trauma* 2006;**61**:1427–1431.

Mirza SK, Mirza AJ, Chapman JR, Anderson PA. Classifications of thoracic and lumbar spine fractures: rationale and supporting data. *J Am Acad Orthop Surg* 2002;**10**(5):364–377.

Molligaj G, Payer M, Schaller K, et al. Acute traumatic central cord syndrome: a comprehensive review. *Neurochirurgie* 2014;**60**(1–2):5–11.

Nockels RP, York J. Diagnosis and management of thoracolumbar and lumbar spine injuries. In Winn HR, Sonntag VKH, Vollmer DG (eds.) *Youmans Neurological Surgery*, 5th ed. Elsevier, 2003.

Oyinbo CA. Secondary injury mechanism in traumatic spinal cord injury: a nugget of this multiply cascade. *Acta Neurobiol Exp* 2011;**71**:281–299.

Panacek EA, Mower WR, Holmes JF, et al. Test performance of the individual NEXUS low-risk clinical screening criteria for cervical spine injury. *Ann Emerg Med* 2001;**38**:22–25.

Panczykowski DM, Tomycz ND, Okonkwo DO. Comparative effectiveness of using computed tomography alone to exclude cervical spine injuries in obtunded or intubated patients: meta-analysis of 14, 327 patients with blunt trauma. *J Neurosurg* 2011;**115**(3):541–549.

Parizel PM, van der Zijden T, Gaudino S, et al. Trauma of the spine and spinal cord: imaging strategies. *Eur Spine J* 2010;**19**:S8–S17.

Sabiston CP, Wing PC, Schweigel JF, et al. Closed reduction of dislocations of the lower cervical spine. *J Trauma* 1988;**28**:832–835.

Savic G, Bergstrom EM, Frankel HL, et al. Inter-rater reliability of the motor and sensory examinations performed according to American Spinal Injury Association standards. *Spinal Cord* 2007;**45**:444–451.

Scott TF. Nosology of idiopathic transverse myelitis syndromes. *Acta Neurol Scand* 2007;**115**:371–376.

Scott TF, Frohman EM, De Seze J, Gronseth GS, Weinshenker BG. Evidence-based guideline: clinical evaluation and treatment of transverse myelitis: report of the Therapeutics and Technology Assessment

Subcommittee of the American Academy of Neurology. *Neurology* 2011;77:2128–2134.

Shlamovitz GZ, Mower WR, Bergman J, et al. Poor test characteristics for the digital rectal examination in trauma patients. *Ann Emerg Med* 2007;50:25–33.

Sohn M, Culver DA, Judson MA, et al. Spinal cord neurosarcoidosis. *Am J Med Sci* 2014;347:195–198.

Stiell IG, Wells GA, Vandemhen KL, et al. The Canadian C-spine rule for radiography in

alert and stable trauma patients. *JAMA* 2001;286(15):1841–1848.

Tomycz ND, Okonkwo DO, Anderson PA. Closed skeletal reduction and bracing of cervical, thoracic, and lumbar spinal injuries. In Vaccaro AR, Fehlings MG, Dvorak MF (eds.) *Spine and Spinal Cord Trauma: Evidence-Based Management.* Thieme, 2011.

Traynelis VC, Marano GD, Dunker RO, et al. Traumatic atlanto-occipital dislocation: case report. *J Neurosurg* 1986;65:863–870.

Neuro-ophthalmology Emergencies

18

Matthew Brucks, Erik Happ, Randy Beatty, and Brent Rau

18.1 Introduction

The goal of this chapter is to provide a concise summary of the most common emergencies in neuro-ophthalmology. The chapter's focus is three main neuro-ophthalmic emergency topics: diplopia, pupil abnormalities, and acute loss of vision. The chapter concludes with other important topics that are not neurological in nature, but are important to diagnose immediately such as a retinal detachment or ruptured globe.

Many non-ophthalmologists feel uncomfortable operating a slitlamp in the ED and may therefore limit their interaction with patients complaining of eye problems. However, one can still obtain a focused history and perform a basic eye examination to accurately diagnose ophthalmic disease. The "three vital signs" of ophthalmology are vision, pupils, and pressure; these should be assessed on every patient presenting with an eye emergency. Extraocular motility and visual field testing provide additional helpful clues to diagnosis and can be easily performed at the bedside.

1. **Visual acuity (VA):** Ask the patient to wear their corrective lenses (e.g., glasses, contact lenses) and test each eye individually. Start with the Snellen VA chart. If the patient is unable to read the 20/400 line, ask them to count how many fingers you are holding up. If they cannot count fingers, check for hand-motion vision by waving your hand. If they cannot see hand motion, shine a bright light directly into the eye. If they cannot see light, then record vision as "no light perception." Vision that improves when looking through a pinhole indicates refractive error and is the expected vision of the patient while wearing corrective lenses.

2. **Pupils (P):** The pupil examination has an important role in evaluating the integrity of the afferent and efferent reflex pathways, which include the optic nerves, optic chiasm, optic tract, midbrain, and the third cranial nerve. Check for pupil symmetry, direct light response, and for a relative afferent pupillary defect.

Most doctors are familiar with the term PERRLA (Pupils Equal, Round, Reactive to Light and Accommodation), but arguably a more important aspect of the pupil examination is the relative afferent pupillary defect (RAPD). The presence of an RAPD indicates relative dysfunction of the optic nerve, even in situations where there is a normal direct pupil response and good VA.

A RAPD is tested using the *swinging flashlight test* in which a bright light is shone into one eye and observed for 3 seconds. During this time a normal pupil will constrict to light (direct response) followed by an escape (the pupil dilates slightly) and hippus (the pupil rhythmically constricts and dilates). The light is then *rapidly* swung to the opposite eye and observed for 3 seconds. The eye should demonstrate the same findings, i.e., pupil constriction followed by escape and hippus. The swinging flashlight test can be repeated back and forth multiple times until you are satisfied that the responses are equal. A RAPD is noted if one pupil dilates immediately without constriction each time the light is swung to that side. *See* Video 18.1 *for an example of an RAPD.*

Video 18.1 Relative Afferent Pupillary Defect (RAPD; Marcus–Gunn pupil). Video 18.1 can be accessed at http://www.cambridge.org/campbellkelly

---

3. **Intraocular pressure (IOP):** Measurement of the IOP should be a routine part of the eye examination, as elevated intraocular pressure often requires immediate treatment to prevent vision loss. When checking eye pressure using the tonopen, ensure the patient has first received a drop of proparicaine or tetracaine in the eye. Once the eye is comfortable, ask the patient to open both eyes and to fixate on an object in the distance so that they are less likely to squeeze their eyes as you measure the pressure. Place a protective cover over the tip of the tonopen and hold the tonopen in your dominant hand as you would a pencil. The nondominant hand gently elevates the patient's upper eyelid while the dominant hand can be used to retract the lower eyelid. *It is very important to ensure that your fingers are not putting pressure on the eyeball as you help to open their eye. For an accurate pressure measurement, ensure your fingers are pulling the eyelids against the orbital rim rather than pushing against the eyeball.*

4. **Extraocular motility (EOM):** With the patient facing straight ahead, have them fixate on your finger as you direct their eyes to each field of gaze, including the corners of the superior and inferior quadrants.

5. **Confrontational visual fields (CVF):** To test the patient's peripheral vision of the right eye, sit approximately 1 meter away from the patient. Close your right eye as the patient covers their left eye and instruct the patient to fixate on your open eye. Hold up a set number of fingers (1, 2, or 5) and slowly advance your hand from one quadrant of their visual field toward the center until they can state the correct number. Your hand should be midway between you and the patient so that you can estimate their peripheral vision against your own. Repeat for each quadrant of the visual field, as well as for the left eye.

18.2 Diplopia

In the assessment of diplopia, first determine if the diplopia is monocular or binocular. Binocular diplopia is secondary to a misalignment of the eyes (e.g., secondary to a cranial nerve palsy). Binocular diplopia is diagnosed by simply covering either eye and noting the subsequent elimination of diplopia. Monocular diplopia is secondary to a problem with how the eye refracts light, such as with certain cataracts or dry eye. It is diagnosed when the patient continues to complain of diplopia while only one eye is open and it resolves when looking through a pinhole or by covering the problematic eye.

The second part of the diplopia assessment is determining the direction of the doubled images. For instance, for patients complaining of diplopia despite seemingly full extraocular motility, ask them if the images are primarily side by side (horizontal diplopia) or if one is above the other (vertical diplopia). *Horizontal diplopia* is most likely a cranial nerve 3 or 6 palsy, while *vertical diplopia* likely represents a cranial nerve 4 palsy.

18.2.1 Third Nerve Palsy (CN3 Palsy)

Presentation: Binocular diplopia and ptosis, with or without pain.

Examination: The presence of a headache or periorbital pain is variable and is not helpful in establishing the cause of the third nerve palsy.

- a. **Complete, pupil-involving:** Complete ptosis, eye positioned down and out, and a dilated pupil that responds poorly to light.
- b. **Complete, pupil-sparing:** As above, but with normal pupillary function.
- c. **Partial:** Variable limitation of upward, downward, or adducting movements, ptosis, or pupillary function (response may be sluggish).

Differential diagnosis:

- a. **Complete, pupil-involving:** Aneurysm, intracranial mass, trauma.
- b. **Complete, pupil-sparing:** Ischemic, giant-cell arteritis (GCA).
- c. **Partial:** Any of the above causes.
- d. **CN3 palsy in children:** Postviral or post vaccination, ophthalmoplegic migraine.

Diagnostic testing: Rule-out GCA by history and labs if there is suspicion. Full neurologic examination. Blood pressure and blood glucose. *Immediate CNS imaging with contrast-enhanced CT/CTA is indicated for:*

- a. pupil-involving or partial CN3 palsies
- b. pupil-sparing palsy for patients with age <50 years, partial motility deficits, absence of vasculopathic risk factors, or if there are any additional cranial nerve or neurologic abnormalities.

Treatment: Treat the underlying abnormality.

- a. **Ischemic:** Antiplatelet therapy is usually provided for secondary prevention of stroke.
- b. **Symptomatic:** Patch one eye for short-term diplopia relief.

Disposition: Partial third nerve palsies require daily follow-up for 7 days as it may evolve into a pupil-involving palsy.

18.2.2 Fourth Nerve Palsy (CN4 Palsy)

Presentation: Binocular vertical diplopia.

Examination: The involved eye is higher, with deficient inferior movement when attempting to look down and in. Patient may tilt their head to the contralateral shoulder to eliminate diplopia.

Differential diagnosis: Trauma, vasculopathic. aneurysm, tumor, and GCA are rare.

Diagnostic testing: Rule-out GCA by history and labs if there is suspicion. Full neurological examination. Blood pressure and blood glucose. *MRI of the brain is indicated for:*

a. patients <45 years old with no history of trauma.

b. patients 45–55 years old with no vasculopathic risk factors or trauma.

Treatment: Treat the underlying disorder.

a. **Symptomatic:** Patch one eye for short-term diplopia relief.

Disposition: To be evaluated by a primary care physician for vascular risk factors and followed by ophthalmology to ensure recovery.

18.2.3 Sixth Nerve Palsy (CN6 Palsy)

Presentation: Binocular horizontal diplopia.

Examination: Deficient lateral movement of an eye (i.e., abduction deficit).

Differential diagnosis: Vasculopathic, trauma. Less commonly intracranial mass/pressure, stroke, or GCA.

Diagnostic testing: Rule-out GCA by history and labs if there is suspicion. Full neurological examination. Blood pressure and blood glucose. *MRI of the brain is indicated for:*

a. Patients <45 years old with no history of trauma; if MRI is negative, consider a lumbar puncture.

b. Patients 45–55 years old with no vasculopathic risk factors or trauma.

c. CN6 palsy with severe pain or other neurologic signs.

d. Any history of cancer.

e. Bilateral CN6 palsies.

Treatment: Treat the underlying disorder.

a. **Symptomatic:** Patch one eye for short-term diplopia relief.

Disposition: To be evaluated by a primary care physician for vascular risk factors and followed by ophthalmology to ensure recovery.

18.2.4 Multiple Ocular Motor Nerve Palsies (Cavernous Sinus Syndrome)

Presentation: Any combination of diplopia, eyelid droop, facial pain, or numbness.

Examination: Any combination of limited eye movement (third, fourth, or sixth nerve palsy); facial pain or numbness (fifth nerve palsy); ptosis and a small pupil (Horner syndrome); or a dilated pupil (third nerve palsy). May have proptosis, injected conjunctival vessels, and decreased vision.

Differential diagnosis: Arteriovenous fistula, cavernous sinus tumor, intracavernous aneurysm, mucormycosis, cavernous sinus thrombosis, or Tolosa–Hunt syndrome (idiopathic inflammation).

Diagnostic testing:

    a. History: vasculopathic risk factors, recent trauma, prior cancer, or severe headache.

    b. Examination: careful attention to pupils, extraocular motility, and resistance of the eye to retropulsion. Auscultate the eye to listen for an ocular bruit.

    c. Imaging: CT scan or MRI of the sinuses, orbit, and brain. CTA of the head.

    d. Labs: CBC with diff, ESR, ANA.

Treatment/disposition: Dependent on etiology and will require consultation from the appropriate service (neurosurgery, ENT, ID).

18.2.5 Other Causes of Diplopia to Consider

18.2.5.1 Thyroid Eye Disease

Presentation: Diplopia, periorbital pain or pressure, and possibly decreased vision.

Examination: Limited eye movement, upper eyelid retraction, proptosis, conjunctival chemosis/injection, and increased resistance to retropulsion. If the optic nerve is compressed there may be a RAPD, decreased VA, or decreased color vision. Can be unilateral or bilateral.

Differential diagnosis: Autoimmune thyroid disease. Eye findings may precede systemic disease.

Diagnostic testing:

    a. In the ED it is most important to assess for visual loss from optic neuropathy (see examination above).

    b. Imaging: CT orbits without contrast (extraocular muscle enlargement and increased fat volume).

Treatment: *For visual loss from optic neuropathy:*

    a. Treat immediately with prednisone 100 mg PO daily or solumedrol 1000 mg IV × 3 days.

Disposition: Requires immediate consult from ophthalmology to determine need for possible posterior orbital surgical decompression.

18.2.5.2 Nonspecific Orbital Inflammation (Orbital Pseudotumor)

Presentation: An explosive, painful onset that may involve a prominent red eye, double vision, "boggy" pink eyelid edema, or decreased vision.

Examination: Proptosis and/or restriction of motility, usually unilateral.

Differential diagnosis: Idiopathic, orbital cellulitis, thyroid eye disease, sarcoidosis, or malignancy.

Diagnostic testing: Vital signs (especially temperature), CBC with differential, ESR, blood sugar.

a. Imaging: CT scan orbits with contrast (thickened sclera, orbital fat, or lacrimal gland involvement, thickening of the extraocular muscles). CXR to rule-out sarcoidosis.

Treatment/disposition: Ophthalmology to initiate steroid treatment after excluding other causes of orbital inflammation (listed above).

18.2.5.3 Ocular Myasthenia Gravis

Presentation: Ptosis or diplopia that is variable throughout the day or worse with fatigue. May have systemic weakness, including dysphagia or dyspnea.

Examination: Ptosis, limitation of extraocular motility, possible systemic weakness. Pupil function is NOT affected.

Differential diagnosis: Myasthenia gravis may be limited to ocular findings.

Diagnostic testing: Assess for fatigability of ptosis by having the patient focus in upgaze on your finger for 1 minute and observe if the ptosis worsens. The icepack test involves covering the eyelid with an icepack for 5 minutes and observing for improvement of the ptosis. Test pupil function – should have normal response. Check breathing and swallowing function.

Treatment/disposition:

a. Difficulty swallowing or breathing: Urgent hospitalization for plasmapheresis, IVIg, and ventilatory support may be indicated.

b. Purely ocular: Follow-up with neurology or neuro-ophthalmology for treatment.

18.2.5.4 Orbital Wall Fracture with Muscle Entrapment

Presentation: Diplopia in the setting of recent orbital trauma.

Examination: Limited extraocular motility. Muscle entrapment will often result in an oculocardiac reflex; pain, nausea, and bradycardia. Periorbital ecchymosis or edema. Note: Children may have a "quiet" appearing eye (i.e., *white-eyed blowout*). Hypesthesia in the distribution of the infraorbital nerve.

Differential diagnosis: Diplopia can result from either extraocular muscle entrapment or orbital fat/septa impingement in the orbital bone fracture, as well as from severe orbital edema. It is rare for an orbital roof fracture to entrap a muscle.

Diagnostic testing: Imaging with CT orbits or CT maxillo-facial. If diagnosis of muscle entrapment is uncertain, forced duction testing is required. Look for associated ocular injury such as corneal abrasion, hyphema, or retrobulbar hemorrhage.

Treatment/disposition:

a. Surgical repair urgently: Pediatric patients in whom the inferior rectus is tightly trapped beneath a trapdoor fracture.

b. Surgical repair within 2 weeks:

1. Diplopia with limited upgaze or downgaze within 30 degrees of primary position with a positive forced duction test 7–10 days after injury.

2. Enophthalmos that exceeds 2 mm and is cosmetically unacceptable to the patient.
3. Large fractures involving >50% of the orbital floor, especially when associated with a medial wall fracture.

18.3 Pupil Abnormalities

18.3.1 Anisocoria: Difference in Pupil Size

Benign causes of anisocoria: Exposure to mydriatic or miotic agents, including eyedrops, scopolamine patches, pesticides, or certain weeds (e.g., Jimson weed).

The eyelid position and extraocular motility **must** be evaluated when anisocoria is present.

Try to determine which pupil is abnormal by comparing sizes in light and in dark. If the difference in size between the two pupils (i.e., anisocoria) is greater in one setting then the differential can be narrowed to the following:

The smaller pupil is the abnormal pupil: anisocoria is greater in a *dark room*.

1. **Horner's syndrome:** Associated with 1–2 mm ipsilateral ptosis and anhidrosis.
   a. **Differential diagnosis:** Brainstem infarct (e.g., lateral medullary syndrome), multiple sclerosis, lung apex tumor, internal carotid dissection (traumatic or spontaneous), migraine.
   b. History: Inquire about trauma, headaches, jaw or neck pain, other neurologic symptoms, history of cancer or tobacco use.
   c. Diagnostic testing: MRI/MRA of the brain and neck (especially if neck pain is present), CT of the chest to rule-out a mass.

The larger pupil is the abnormal pupil: anisocoria is greater in a *lit room*.

1. **Third cranial nerve palsy:** *Always* associated with diplopia and ipsilateral ptosis.
2. **Adie (tonic) pupil:** Typically a young woman. Pupil with minimal or no reactivity to light, and slow, tonic constriction with convergence. Convergence is tested by asking the patient to focus on a target in the distance and then to look at their own finger as it is brought closer toward their face. Routine follow-up with ophthalmology.
3. **Traumatic mydriasis or iritis:** Inquire about recent trauma, eye pain, redness, and photosensitivity.

18.4 Acute Vision Loss in Neuro-Ophthalmology

18.4.1 Monocular Vision Loss

18.4.1.1 Central Retinal Artery Occlusion (CRAO)

Presentation: Acute, painless loss of vision.

Examination: Afferent pupillary defect; pale retina with cherry-red spot; 80% of patients have VA of counting fingers or worse.

Differential diagnosis: Atherosclerosis-related thrombus/embolus, GCA.

Diagnostic testing: Rule-out GCA by history and then laboratory tests if there is suspicion. CBC, ESR, CRP, and fibrinogen.

Treatment:

1. The best chance for visual recovery requires treatment in less than 3 hours, and no more than 6 hours, from onset of vision loss.

2. "Conservative" measures such as reducing the IOP by ocular massage, IOP-lowering medications (e.g., acetazolamide 500 mg IV), hyperbaric oxygen, steroids, heparin, or aspirin have *not* been proven effective.

3. The role of thrombolytics is controversial. Two large reviews and several observational studies suggest that thrombolytics may improve the visual outcome with few complications in CRAO patients. However, methodological flaws in these studies, and the lack of a well-designed randomized controlled study, limit the conclusions that can be drawn from them. Yet, in a patient preference survey, about one-third of CRAO patients were willing to accept some risk of stroke or life-threatening complication to triple the chances of recovering 20/100 VA in an eye with CRAO. Despite the absence of a randomized clinical trial, there is now enough evidence to consider thrombolysis in patients seen within 3–6 hours of visual loss from CRAO. This treatment for selected patients should be discussed with the stroke and interventional radiology teams.

Disposition: Follow-up with ophthalmology to monitor monthly for signs of neovascularization.

18.4.1.2 Optic Neuritis

Presentation: Typically unilateral vision loss over hours to days. Pain with eye movement. Age 18–45 years. Women are affected more often than men by 3:1.

Examination: A RAPD is present unless it is bilateral optic neuritis; decreased VA; decreased color vision. Only one-third of patients will have a swollen optic nerve.

Differential diagnosis: Idiopathic, multiple sclerosis, neuromyelitis optica (NMO), or viral infection.

Diagnostic testing: MRI of the brain and orbits with gadolinium, fat suppression, and FLAIR sequencing. If associated myelitis, obtain an MRI of the spine to evaluate for NMO.

Treatment: Based on the Optic Neuritis Treatment Trial, treatment with IV steroids can reduce the initial progression to multiple sclerosis for 3 years. Steroid therapy increases the rapidity of visual return by 2 weeks but does not improve the final visual outcome. The choice of when to treat partially depends on MRI results:

1. MRI shows demyelination: The risk of developing multiple sclerosis is high (72% at 15 years). Methylprednisolone 250 mg IV q 6 h for 3 days, then prednisone 1 mg/kg/day PO for 11 days followed by taper.

2. MRI does not show demyelination: The risk of developing multiple sclerosis is low (25% at 15 years). Discussion with the patient about risks and benefits of steroid treatment.

3. Note: Low-dose oral prednisone as a primary treatment has historically been avoided because of increased risk of recurrence. However, if IV methylprednisolone is not readily available, the oral prednisone equivalent can be used (prednisone 1,250 mg daily for 3 days, followed by taper).

18.4.1.3 Nonarteritic Ischemic Optic Neuropathy (NAION)

Presentation: Sudden, painless loss of vision. Typically age 40–60 years.

Examination: A RAPD, decreased central vision, altitudinal visual field defect, pale disc swelling, flame-shaped hemorrhages, normal ESR.

Differential diagnosis: Risk factors include hypertension, diabetes, hyperlipidemia, tobacco use, anemia, and sleep apnea. There is no evidence of a thrombotic event.

Diagnostic testing: Check blood pressure and glucose, ESR, CRP, CBC, and fibrinogen. It is extremely important to inquire about signs and symptoms of GCA (see the next section on GCA), as the visual loss in GCA is much more severe and requires prompt treatment with steroids.

Treatment: Cardiovascular risk factor modification and observation. Consider daily aspirin to decrease the risk of contralateral eye involvement.

Disposition: Close follow-up with ophthalmology.

18.4.1.4 Arteritic Ischemic Optic Neuropathy (Giant-Cell Arteritis, GCA)

Presentation: Sudden, painless loss of vision. Occurs in patients >55 years old (average age 70 years). May have jaw claudication, scalp tenderness, headache, fatigue, weight loss, polymyalgia rheumatica (muscle and joint aches), or fever.

Examination: A RAPD; severe vision loss (often count fingers or worse); pale, swollen disc. ESR, CRP, and platelets may be markedly elevated.

Differential diagnosis: Large-vessel vasculitis.

Diagnostic testing: Immediate ESR, CRP, CBC, and fibrinogen.

Treatment: Methylprednisolone 250 mg IV q 6 h for 3 days, then prednisone 80–100 mg PO daily. A temporal artery biopsy can be performed while the patient is hospitalized.

Note: Treatment should be initiated immediately if there is suspicion of GCA, as the contralateral eye can become involved within days to weeks.

Disposition: Temporal artery biopsy should be scheduled within 1 week if GCA is suspected.

18.4.1.5 Other Causes of Optic Neuropathy

1. *Compressive lesions:* Intraorbital or intracanalicular tumors may not produce optic disc edema. They typically present with slowly progressive vision loss, RAPD, and decreased color vision. High suspicion if the eye appears proptotic. Orbital imaging with CT or MRI is required for the diagnosis. **Differential diagnosis** includes optic nerve sheath meningioma, optic nerve glioma, cavernous hemangioma, or thyroid eye disease.
2. *Inflammatory:* **Differential diagnosis** includes neuroretinitis (inquire about cat scratches or bites), syphilis, Lyme disease, and viruses.

3. *Hereditary*: Leber hereditary optic neuropathy (LHON) affects males age 10–30, presenting with acute, severe (<20/200), painless vision loss with a RAPD. May have a family history of males from the mother's side with similar vision loss. Associated with cardiac conduction abnormalities so order an EKG.
4. *Toxic*: Gradual, progressive, painless, bilateral vision loss, and decreased color vision. Methanol and ethylene glycol toxicity result in rapid onset of severe vision loss. Ethanol abuse is associated with malnutrition and deficiencies of vitamin B12, folate, and thiamine. Lead ingestion in children.

18.4.2 Binocular Vision Loss

18.4.2.1 Optic Disc Edema

Presentation: Transient, bilateral vision loss; headache; decreased VA and peripheral vision; tinnitus; may have double vision.

Examination: Bilateral swollen optic discs (blurred disc margins that obscure the blood vessels emanating from the optic disc), peripapillary retinal hemorrhages, dilated retinal veins. May have unilateral or bilateral sixth nerve palsies from increased intracranial pressure.

Differential diagnosis:

a. *Diseases that raise intracranial pressure:* Intracranial tumor, hydrocephalus, subdural/epidural hematoma, subarachnoid hemorrhage, arteriovenous malformation, brain abscess, meningitis, cerebral venous sinus thrombosis.

b. *Diseases that infiltrate the optic nerves:* Leukemia, sarcoid, TB, metastasis.

c. *Idiopathic:* Idiopathic intracranial hypertension (**IIH; pseudotumor cerebri**). Associated with obesity, oral contraceptives, tetracyclines, nalidixic acid, cyclosporine, steroid use, and vitamin A.

Diagnostic testing:

a. Check blood pressure and CBC. Full neurological examination.

Emergency MRI with gadolinium and MRV (to assess for cerebral venous sinus thrombosis).

b. If MRI is not available emergently, then CT head.

c. If normal imaging, the patient should have a lumbar puncture: Record the opening pressure and send the CSF for analysis (cell count, protein, glucose, Gram stain, culture, and sensitivity).

Treatment: Directed at the underlying cause of the increased intracranial pressure.

IIH (pseudotumor cerebri):

a. The treatment of choice is acetazolamide 250 mg PO QID initially, in addition to weight loss, and discontinuation of any causative medication. Other options include methazolamide, topiramate, and furosemide.

b. A neurosurgical device such as a lumboperitoneal shunt (LPS) or ventriculoperitoneal shunt (VPS) is indicated for intractable headaches and vision loss that are nonresponsive to medication.

   c. Optic nerve sheath decompression surgery can be considered if vision is threatened and headaches are only a minor component.

18.4.2.2 Visual Field Defects

Patients with intracranial pathology, such as pituitary tumors or cerebral infarctions, may complain of decreased vision despite having normal VA and pupil responses. It is important to check their peripheral visual fields to help identify the source of their vision loss.

1. Homonymous hemianopia: occipital lobe lesion.
2. Homonymous superior quadrantanopia: parietal lobe lesion.
3. Homonymous inferior quadrantanopia: temporal lobe lesion.
4. Bitemporal hemianopia: chiasmal lesion (e.g., pituitary adenoma, craniopharyngioma).

18.4.3 Nonorganic Vision Loss

Occasionally patients will be evaluated with vision loss that is not attributable to an organic lesion of the visual system. When a patient is malingering, they deliberately feign vision loss and history often reveals potential for secondary gain (e.g., lawsuits or worker's compensation). In conversion disorder, however, the patient does not control their visual symptoms, and they may not seem overly concerned about their vision loss (i.e., *la belle indifference*). Patients with conversion disorder often have histories of significant stress or traumatic events in their lives.

   Vision loss should not be attributed to nonorganic vision loss without the appropriate work-up to rule-out an organic problem. Check the VA, pupil responses, intraocular pressure, CVF, and obtain imaging of the brain and orbits when appropriate.

   For patients claiming significant vision loss (e.g., no light perception), there are tests that can raise suspicion for nonorganic vision loss:

1. Normal pupil response: Acute, severe monocular vision loss from any cause should result in a RAPD. If the pupil responses are symmetric, there is a high likelihood the vision loss is nonorganic.
2. Menace reflex: Cover the unaffected eye. Produce a threatening hand gesture toward the eye. An intact menace reflex indicates some degree of crude vision.
3. Mirror test: Rotate a mirror before the "blind" eye and observe for pursuit movements, which would indicate some vision.
4. Simple tests of proprioception: A patient who is truly blind can still neatly sign their name or touch their index fingers together. A malingerer may believe these tests to be vision-dependent and fail them.

18.4.4 Non-neuro-ophthalmologic Causes of Vision Loss

18.4.4.1 Acute Angle Closure Glaucoma

Presentation: Single or multiple episodes of acute vision loss associated with pain, red eye, photophobia, nausea/vomiting, or halos around sources of light.

Examination: Elevated IOP, conjunctival injection, corneal edema/haze, decreased vision, nonreactive mid-dilated pupil.

Differential diagnosis: Anatomically narrow angles. Rarely topiramate, intraocular tumor.

Diagnostic testing: Proceed to treatment.

Treatment/disposition: Call ophthalmology immediately.

   a. Definitive treatment: Laser peripheral iridotomy by ophthalmology.

   b. While awaiting ophthalmology, can attempt to reduce IOP with acetazolamide 500 mg IV, and topical timolol, brimonidine, and/or dorzolamide.

   c. Supportive care: Anti-nausea control, pain control.

18.4.4.2 Retinal Detachment

Presentation: Progressively enlarging shadow or curtain-like vision loss, may be preceded by new flashes of light or floaters. Usually in a patient with a history of high myopia (near-sighted), so inquire about the strength of their glasses' prescription or if there is a history of laser eye surgery.

Examination: In a complete retinal detachment, VA is usually <20/200. If the macula is still attached, the VA should be >20/200 with decreased peripheral vision. There is a decreased red reflex using the direct ophthalmoscope. Ultrasound of the eye shows detachment.

Differential diagnosis: High myopia, trauma, idiopathic.

Diagnostic testing: Ocular ultrasound.

Treatment: Call ophthalmology to discuss timing of follow-up. Most retinal detachments do not require overnight surgery.

18.4.4.3 Corneal Hydrops

Presentation: Sudden decrease in vision, pain, photophobia, and profuse tearing.

Examination: Inquire about a history of keratoconus, eye rubbing, and frequent change in glasses' prescription. Corneal edema appears like a cloudy cornea, may have a corneal scar.

Differential diagnosis: Keratoconus, post-LASIK surgery ectasia.

Diagnostic testing: Proceed to treatment.

Treatment: Cyclopentolate 1% TID, bacitracin ointment QID, sodium chloride 5% ointment BID, and glasses or eyeshield for those at risk for trauma.

18.4.4.4 Traumatic Hyphema

Presentation: History of blunt trauma, with pain and blurry vision.

Examination: Blood in the anterior chamber (between the cornea and iris).

Differential diagnosis/etiology: Blunt or penetrating trauma.

Diagnostic testing: First rule-out a ruptured globe. Check the IOP but avoid pushing too hard on the eye. Consider a CT scan of the orbits if an orbital fracture or intraocular foreign body is suspected. African American patients should be screened for sickle cell trait or disease.

Treatment: Children generally require admission for close observation, whereas adults can be treated as outpatients.

a. Bed rest with bathroom privileges, elevated head of bed, and an eye shield (not gauze). Discontinue blood thinners.

b. Eyedrops: atropine 1% TID, prednisolone acetate 1% QID.

c. For elevated IOP: Start with timolol 0.5% BID. If the IOP remains high and the patient does not have sickle cell, brimonidine 0.2% (avoid in children) and/or dorzolamide 2% TID can be added. If topical therapy fails, add acetazolamide 500 mg PO BID for adults.

d. Follow-up with ophthalmology the next day.

18.4.4.5 Ruptured Globe

Presentation: History of trauma, with pain, loss of vision, loss of fluid from the eye.

Examination: Severe subconjunctival hemorrhage, poor vision, irregular or "peaked" pupil, iris protruding from cornea. Note: Once the diagnosis is made, further evaluation of the eye should be deferred until the time of surgical repair.

Differential diagnosis: Blunt trauma, fall, and penetrating sharp object.

Diagnostic testing: Place an eye shield or paper cup over the eye for protection, and order a CT of the orbits to rule-out an intraocular foreign body.

Treatment:

a. Make the patient NPO, bedrest with bathroom privileges, pain and nausea control, systemic antibiotics (cefazolin or vancomycin and ciprofloxacin), and tetanus shot PRN.

b. Ophthalmology to evaluate the patient and schedule surgical repair.

Pearls and Pitfalls

- Three vital signs of ophthalmology should be documented: vision, pupils, and pressure.
- Diplopia, eyelid droop, facial pain, or numbness: consider cavernous sinus etiology and order CT, CTA, and/or MRI.
- Eye findings may precede systemic findings in autoimmune thyroid disease. Diplopia, periorbital pain, and vision loss with CT findings of muscle enlargement or fat excess require rapid consultation and steroids.
- Central retinal artery occlusion: acute monocular vision loss with pale retina and cherry-red spot. If within 3–6 hours of onset, *consider thrombolysis* with stroke and interventional radiology team consultations.
- *Pediatric patients* with entrapped inferior rectus muscle and infraorbital paresthesias from orbital floor fracture require *urgent consultation and surgery*. Most other orbital fractures can have delayed repair.

Bibliography

Beatty S. Non-organic vision loss. *Postgrad Med J* 1999;**75**:201–207.

Biousee V. Thrombolysis for acute central retinal artery occlusion: is it time? *Am J Ophthalmol* 2008;**146**(5):631–634.

Cugati S, Varma D, Chec C, Lee A. Treatment options for central retinal artery occlusion. *Curr Treat Options Neurol* 2013;**15**(1):63–77.

Kupersmith MJ, Frohman LP, Sanderson MC, et al. Aspirin reduces second eye anterior ischemic optic neuropathy. *Ophthalmology* 1995;102:104.

Morrow SA, Fraser JA, Day C, et al. Effect of treating acute optic neuritis with bioequivalent oral vs intravenous corticosteroids: a randomized clinical trial. *JAMA Neurol* 2018;**75**:690–696.

Wajda B, Begheri N, Calva C, Durrani A. *The Wills Eye Manual*. 6th ed. Lippincott Williams and Wilkins, 2012.

Chapter 19

Brain Tumors and Other Neuro-oncologic Emergencies

Tulika Ranjan and Charles J. Feronti

19.1 Introduction

Neuro-oncologic emergencies encompass a wide variety of complaints and can occur in patients with both CNS and non-CNS malignancies. The differential diagnosis for neurologic symptoms includes brain metastases, primary brain tumor, leptomeningeal disease, spinal cord compression, infection, and neurologic complications of cancer. The emergency physician must consider CNS tumors in their initial differential diagnosis of common chief complaints (e.g., headache, seizure, weakness), and deal with CNS emergencies in patients with established cancer diagnoses.

While any history of cancer is concerning, those with cancers of the lung or breast, or melanoma, are especially prone to brain metastasis. Lung cancer often metastasizes early in the disease process, whereas breast cancer is known for late metastasis to the brain. Brain metastasis can be expected in 10–30% of adults and a recently observed increasing incidence is likely due to the longer survival of cancer patients. Skull metastases are more common than parenchymal brain metastases (e.g., prostate and breast cancer).

Common neuro-oncologic emergencies can be broadly categorized as follows: altered mental status, focal neurologic deficits, seizure, stroke (hemorrhagic and ischemic), and spinal cord compression.

19.2 The Approach to Altered Mental Status in the Neuro-oncologic Patient

The approach to the cancer patient with altered mental status is similar to the general approach to undifferentiated altered mental status, with a few unique considerations. The emergency physician begins with a wide differential that is quickly and efficiently narrowed to one or more working diagnoses. Studies have shown that the etiology of altered mental status in this population is often multifactorial. Altered mental status, broadly speaking, encompasses a spectrum from disorientation and agitation to lethargy and coma.

19.2.1 Evaluation and Differential Diagnosis

Table 19.1 provides a broad differential for a neuro-oncologic patient presenting with altered mental status. In general, the emergency physician will work through a differential that considers structural causes (e.g., mass, edema), infectious processes (CNS or elsewhere), treatment-related effects (e.g., steroid psychosis), and metabolic derangements (e.g., electrolytes, fluid imbalance).

Table 19.1 Causes of altered mental status

Structural	Metabolic	Treatment-/toxin-related	Infectious
Tumor	Dehydration	Narcotics/sedatives	Meningitis
Vasogenic edema	Hypercalcemia	Steroids	Encephalitis
Hemorrhage	Renal failure	Antiseizure medications	Neutropenic fever
Hydrocephalus	Liver failure	Chemotherapeutics	Pneumonia
Stroke/seizures	Endocrine disorders	Radiation therapy	Urinary tract infection

Infection always needs to be considered in the evaluation of altered mental status. In addition to searching for common causes such as pneumonia or urinary tract infections, recent or remote CNS procedures, such as shunt placement, lumbar puncture, or tumor resection need to be assessed. With several existing sources for immunosuppression, namely steroid use and chemotherapy, opportunistic infections need to be considered as well.

19.2.2 Management

Because the altered patient's cooperation with the history and physical exam can be difficult, the physician is obligated to be liberal with testing when ordering laboratory and radiologic tests to narrow the differential. When available, the list of the patient's medications is very important as it may point to the possible causes of their altered mental status. Determine use of any controlled substance (e.g., opioids, benzodiazepines) and ensure that the patient is not wearing a transdermal narcotic patch.

Reasonable laboratory studies to consider include a complete blood count, comprehensive metabolic panel, urinalysis, and levels of medications that have a narrow therapeutic index, such as antiseizure medications (ASMs). Encephalopathy can often be attributed to hyponatremia or other electrolyte derangements. An arterial blood gas can assess for acidemia, hypoxia, and hypercarbia, all of which can be implicated in mental status changes. Imaging options include CT scans and MRI. The former is more readily available at most institutions and can serve as a screening test for structural lesions (e.g., tumor, abscess), hemorrhage, herniation, and hydrocephalus (Figure 19.1). MRI is more sensitive for characterization of tumor, recognizing small tumors and leptomeningeal disease, and providing better imaging of the cerebellum and brain stem lesions. However, MRI will involve the patient leaving the department for a longer period of time, which may pose a risk for decompensation in the altered or unstable patient.

19.3 Focal Neurological Deficit

Focal neurological symptoms due to brain tumors are usually progressive and subacute in nature. However, some tumors can present as a stroke or transient ischemic attack, and MRI scans may initially be mistaken for infarction due to restricted diffusion.

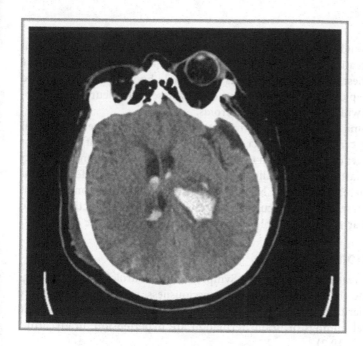

Figure 19.1 Intracerebral hemorrhage (thalamic) with evolving hydrocephalus.

19.3.1 Clinical Evaluation and Differential Diagnosis

The differential diagnosis for focal neurological deficit includes brain metastases, primary brain tumor, leptomeningeal disease, spinal cord compression, infection, and treatment-related toxicities. Patients with infection have a history of fever and other signs and symptoms of infections. Metabolic derangements and infection can exacerbate pre-existing neurological deficits.

Cerebral tumors can produce headache, papilledema, contralateral weakness, sensory loss, aphasia, neglect, dyspraxia, seizures, and visual field loss depending on their location. Aphasia likely localizes to the left hemisphere, whereas neglect typically localizes to the right. Cognitive and behavioral decline is typically seen with large subfrontal meningiomas or gliomas, occurring in about 20% of patients at diagnosis without focal neurological symptoms.

Brainstem tumors can cause ataxia, cranial nerve palsies (particularly third, fourth, and sixth) and symptoms of raised intracranial pressure due to hydrocephalus, usually caused by obstruction of the fourth ventricle. Dorsal midbrain infiltration or compression due to tumors may present with Parinaud's syndrome (vertical gaze palsy, convergence–retraction nystagmus, and light-near dissociation). Cerebellopontine angle tumors cause progressive unilateral hearing loss, facial sensory loss, and ataxia. Cavernous sinus syndrome (involving cranial nerves III–V [including V1, V2] and VI) can be caused by tumors, the most common being meningioma.

Paraparesis, urinary incontinence, and lower motor neuron findings indicate a process involving the spinal cord. Acute onset of multiple cranial nerve findings, radicular pain, and cauda equina syndrome may raise the suspicion for leptomeningeal disease.

19.3.2 Management

A CT scan of the head should be performed, followed by a brain MRI with or without contrast to determine the location of the tumor. Patients with suspected stroke should have an urgent CT scan. CT of chest, abdomen, and pelvis and a whole-body PET scan is needed for initial diagnostic work-up of newly diagnosed brain metastases. The neurologic symptoms can often be reversed with the initial use of steroids.

If primary CNS lymphoma is suspected, it is important to avoid administering steroids in the ED if possible, as it can adversely affect the pathological accuracy of the biopsy. Figure 19.2 shows MRI images of various brain tumors, including CNS lymphoma. Primary brain tumors such as glioblastoma are usually infiltrative in nature, with heterogeneous enhancement on MRI, whereas primary CNS lymphoma tends to have homogeneous enhancement. Brain metastases tend to occur at the gray–white matter junction due to the rich blood supply and narrow-diameter blood vessels where the metastatic cell lodges.

19.4 Brain Herniation

Brain herniation is a life-threatening emergency. Symptoms and neurologic findings suggestive of herniation include changes in the level of consciousness, papilledema, pupillary and eye movement irregularities, decorticate and decerebrate posturing, and projectile vomiting. Advanced clinical findings of brain herniation are hypertension, bradycardia, and the Cushing reflex (Table 19.2).

19.4.1 Management

If there are findings suggestive of herniation or increased intracranial pressure, the treatment should begin immediately to decrease the intracranial pressure. The patient should have a CT scan performed when stable. Emergency treatments to prevent

Table 19.2 Herniation syndromes

Herniation type	Motor	Eye findings	Respiration
Subfalcine	Contralateral leg weakness if anterior cerebral artery is compressed	Normal	
Uncal	Hemiparesis	Hutchinson pupil, unilateral fixed and dilated pupil and unilateral ptosis (third nerve)	
Diencephalic	Decorticate posturing	Small midpoint pupil reactive to light	Cheyne–Stokes
Midbrain	Decerebrate posturing	Midpoint fixed pupil	Hyperventilation
Tonsillar	No response to pain	Dilated and fixed pupil	Irregular or gasping

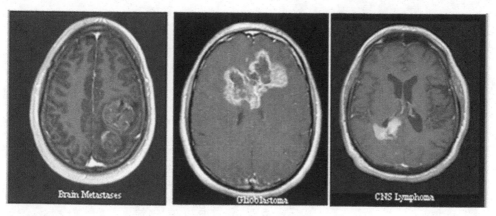

Figure 19.2 Brain MRI pattern in brain metastases (gray–white matter junction), glioblastoma (heterogenous enhancement), primary CNS lymphoma (homogeneous enhancement).

herniation are hyperventilation and administration of mannitol and steroids. Dexamethasone is helpful when increased intracranial pressures are secondary to intracranial tumor or leptomeningeal disease. With incipient brain herniation, dexamethasone is most commonly administered at an initial bolus dose of 40–100 mg intravenously then 40–100 mg/day. Solutions of 20–25% mannitol are administered intravenously at a rate of 0.5–2.0 g/kg over 20–30 minutes.

19.5 Neuro-oncologic Disorders Associated with Seizures and Status Epilepticus

19.5.1 Evaluation and Differential Diagnosis

The etiology of seizures in cancer patients may include structural, metabolic, infectious, and treatment-related causes (Table 19.3). In a review of 50 cancer patients presenting to an emergency center with seizures, 16% had seizures due to a new structural lesion and 52% had previously documented CNS lesions. Seizures commonly occur in patients with intracranial tumors, either due to metastatic disease or a primary brain tumor. Patients usually have a postictal phase that may last for 24 hours or longer. Clinical findings that suggest that a seizure occurred may include bruising or tongue bites, urinary or fecal incontinence, and increases in lactic acid levels and muscle enzymes.

After radiation treatment, especially stereotactic radiosurgery, patients can have increased vasogenic edema and subsequent neurologic symptoms, including seizures. These effects can last for months before stabilization of symptoms. The changes seen on brain MRI could be treatment effect (pseudo progression) rather than actual progression of tumor.

19.5.2 Management

Acute seizure management consists of three phases:

1. Assessment and supportive treatment: Attention to airway, breathing, and circulation take precedence. Measurement of vitals (cardiac monitoring, blood pressure

Table 19.3 Seizure etiology in cancer patients

Structural	Metabolic	Treatment-/toxin-related	Infectious
Tumor (primary/metastases)	Hyponatremia (SIADH)	Chemotherapy: carboplatin busulfan, carmustine (BCNU), cytosine arabinoside, methotrexate, vincristine	Intracranial infection
Increased vasogenic edema	Hypomagnesemia (0.8 mEq/L)	Antibiotics: imipenem	Meningitis
Elevated ICP	Anoxic encephalopathy	Aqueous iodinated contrast agents, hypocalcemia	
Hemorrhagic transformation of tumor		Other medication: hyperbaric oxygen, methylphenidate, ondansetron	
Stroke		Postradiation increase in vasogenic edema	

measurement, and pulse oximetry), laboratory studies (including complete blood count, basic metabolic profile, including calcium and magnesium, ASM levels, CK, liver function tests [LFTs]), and rapid finger stick glucose should be done emergently. A drug screen may also be indicated. Lumbar puncture may also be indicated depending upon the suspected seizure precipitant, condition of the patient, and findings on imaging. Screening head CT to evaluate for tumor progression, hemorrhage, or hydrocephalus should be done after stabilizing the patient. Long-acting neuromuscular blocking agents such as rocuronium, commonly used for rapid sequence intubation, can mask the motor manifestation of ongoing status epilepticus (SE) and therefore might require an EEG to rule-out ongoing status.

2. Initial pharmacologic therapy: Benzodiazepines are the first-line treatment for generalized convulsive SE. In addition, treatment with maintenance ASMs is recommended to prevent recurrence. For IV therapy, lorazepam is preferred and should be administered, up to 0.1 mg/kg IV at a maximum rate of 2 mg/minute. With lorazepam, allow 1 minute to assess its effect before deciding whether additional doses are necessary.

3. Maintenance therapy: Commonly used IV ASMs for loading are fosphenytoin (20 mg/ kg), valproate (20–40 mg/kg), and levetiracetam (2,000–4,000 mg). If the patient is enrolled in any clinical trial, an ASM that is not a CYP-450 inducer (e.g., levetiracetam) should be used. In patients who have ongoing seizure activity despite two initial doses of lorazepam or other benzodiazepines, consideration for potential continuous midazolam or propofol infusion should occur simultaneously with administration of the maintenance ASM. In this way the primary role of the nonbenzodiazepine ASM is to prevent recurrence rather than truncate the seizure. If IV access is not available, intramuscular (IM) midazolam is a good alternative for initial benzodiazepine therapy. Midazolam can be given at a dose of 10 mg IM, nasally, or buccally, for patients with a body weight >40 kg, and 5 mg for patients with a body weight of 13–40 kg. For IV therapy, lorazepam is preferred in adults; midazolam is preferred for IM, intranasal, or buccal therapy; and diazepam is preferred for rectal administration.

Continuous EEG monitoring is critical during the treatment of refractory SE. Once continuous infusion of midazolam, propofol, or pentobarbital has begun, continuous EEG monitoring is necessary to confirm that seizures have been adequately treated. For patients having continuing seizure activity despite ASM treatment, combination ASM therapy is required with complete sedation. These patients will require intubation, frequent clinical monitoring in an intensive care setting, and continuous EEG. Patients with seizure activities due to reversible medical causes should have correction of the reversible cause. These patients likely will not require long-term ASM therapy.

19.6 Neuro-oncologic Disorders Associated with Stroke

Several etiologies exist as possible mechanisms for stroke in cancer patients. Autopsy data have shown that 15% of cancer patients have evidence of cerebrovascular disease. Not all of these strokes, however, were clinically apparent during the patient's life. A large prospective registry followed over 327,000 cancer patients and their matched controls, and found the 3-month risk of stroke to be 5.1% in lung cancer patients vs 1.2% in controls. The risk attenuated over time and was eliminated by one year.

Table 19.4 Etiology of stroke in cancer patients

Intracranial hemorrhage	Cerebral infarction
Intraparenchymal hemorrhage	Atherosclerosis
Coagulopathy: *Thrombocytopenia* *Thrombocytopathia*	Intravascular coagulation
	Nonbacterial thrombotic endocarditis
Liver dysfunction	Vasculitis: *leukemia*
Drugs	Septic occlusion: *leukemia*
Disseminated intravascular coagulopathy	Tumor embolus: *lung cancer, myxoma*
Intratumoral bleed	Hyperviscosity: *lymphoma, myeloma*
Subdural hematoma	
	Venous occlusion
	Leukostasis: *leukemia*
Subarachnoid hemorrhage	
Venous sinus thrombosis: *leukemia*	Chemotherapy: *bevacizumab, mitomycin, bleomycin, platinum*

The etiology for stroke in cancer patients is diverse (Table 19.4). In addition to ischemic strokes, hemorrhagic strokes can occur secondary to metastasis, most commonly being lung, renal cell cancer, and melanoma. Finally, the coagulation changes in cancer patients can lead to disseminated intravascular coagulation, possibly complicated by a hemorrhagic stroke.

The hypercoagulability due to the cancer and its subsequent treatment often leads to thrombosis during the course of illness. Chemotherapy can damage vascular endothelium and also kill cells, which then spill their procoagulant substances. Cancer can directly damage vasculature as well. Finally, the multitude of infections that immunosuppressed patients are at risk of acquiring can lead to secondary strokes. Despite these unique causes of stroke, cancer patients still are most likely to have a stroke secondary to the traditionally taught risk factors, including hypertension, atrial fibrillation, diabetes, and tobacco use.

One such possibility resulting from hypercoagulability is nonbacterial thrombotic endocarditis (NBTE). Eighty percent of cases are due to advanced malignancy. Sterile vegetations of platelets and fibrin that adhere to heart valves can embolize throughout the body, including the brain. Lung cancer is a common source for NBTE. These vegetations have a variable rate of embolization to the brain, anywhere from 14% to 91%. Diagnosis is typically made via transesophageal echocardiography, which can identify vegetations but not distinguish infectious causes from NBTE.

19.6.1 Management

CT of the head can confirm intraparenchymal or intratumoral hemorrhage, subdural hematoma, or subarachnoid hemorrhage. Brain MRI with contrast can confirm acute stroke, which shows restricted diffusion in the ischemic area with dark ADC (apparent diffusion coefficient).

Some intracranial metastases are hemorrhagic in nature (melanoma) and the risk of intracranial bleeding increases with the use of strong anticoagulants (warfarin, enoxaparin, fondaparinux). Close follow-up and dose reduction is needed in those cases. Treatment for NBTE usually consists of heparin and consideration of valve replacement if the patient's prognosis is favorable.

19.7 Neuro-oncologic Disorders Associated with Back Pain and Spinal Cord Compression

The complaint of back pain must always include the consideration of spinal cord compression, especially in those with known or suspected malignancy. Vertebral metastasis is quite common, seen on autopsy in 90% of prostate cancer patients and 74% of breast cancer patients. Fortunately, metastatic epidural spinal cord compression (MESCC) does not occur as often, but can still lead to significant morbidity (Figure 19.3). Timely diagnosis is essential to preserving function. Consequences of a missed MESCC include paralysis, bowel or bladder dysfunction, as well as the subsequent complications of being bedridden (e.g., pulmonary embolism, decubitus ulcer, pneumonia).

19.7.1 Evaluation and Differential Diagnosis

As with any ED patient complaining of back pain, the physician must consider a broad differential diagnosis and be attuned to red flags in the history and physical examination that demand further evaluation. The frequent chief complaint of musculoskeletal back pain

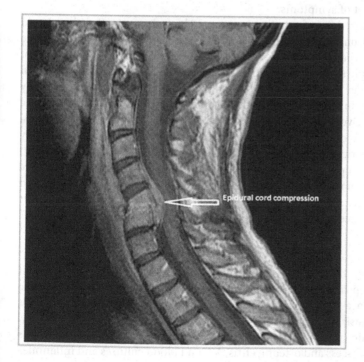

Figure 19.3 Epidural spinal cord compression at C5–C6 due to a metastasis.

Table 19.5 Red flags of back pain

History	Physical
Active/remote malignancy	Motor weakness (especially bilateral)
Unintentional weight loss, fatigue	Urinary retention or bowel/bladder incontinence
Pain at night	Fever
Progressive pain and/or unrelieved by rest	Sensory deficits
Chronic steroid use	Spinal process tenderness

can lead one to quickly dismiss the complaint as non-urgent. Broadly speaking, the emergency physician must consider traumatic, vascular, infectious, and malignant etiologies, and document their absence. Tumors to the spine can be both primary and metastatic, making it important to document that there is no history of cancer. The vast majority of metastases will be to the bony spine (up to 98%) and only rarely to the spinal cord.

Despite the long list of malignant lesion types, the important point is to initially consider the possibility of MESCC. Be especially concerned with a history of breast, lung, and prostate cancers, as they are the most frequent causes of spinal metastasis. Lymphoma and multiple myeloma are also common sources of MESCC. Twenty percent of MESCC cases are the initial manifestation of malignancy, so a pre-existing cancer diagnosis is not needed to consider this entity in the differential diagnosis. The spread to the spine is primarily via the hematogenous route. Pathologic fractures can also lead to direct cord compression and rapid onset of symptoms.

Table 19.5 briefly lists the red flags from the history and physical examination that should be asked of these patients. Concerning findings are progressive pain and pain that is worse when lying down. Abrupt changes in this pain level may indicate the development of a pathologic fracture. The physical examination should focus on a few key areas that can alert the physician to pathology more concerning than simple musculoskeletal pain. As many of these tumors can localize to the thoracic vertebral column, percussion over the thoracic spine may elicit tenderness. Over 60% of patients present with weakness at time of diagnosis, suggesting early diagnosis is often critical to preserve motor function. Lower extremity weakness is usually symmetric in these patients, but occasionally they will present with unilateral motor signs and symptoms. A digital rectal examination can confirm the presence of adequate rectal tone, and an assessment of saddle anesthesia can be performed. Bowel and bladder dysfunction happen late in the disease, and usually consist of urinary retention. Gait assessment is important in cancer patients; new ataxia warrants a work-up to exclude MESCC.

19.7.2 Management

Once a patient is suspected of having a dangerous lesion in the spinal column, be it infectious or MESCC, empiric treatment and movement toward confirmation of the diagnosis need to occur in a timely fashion. Unfortunately, studies show that there is a significant delay in diagnosis for many of these patients, leading to increased morbidity. Obtain early, aggressive pain control so that an accurate exam can be obtained. Infectious concerns, such as epidural abscess and osteomyelitis, warrant blood cultures and inflammatory markers (erythrocyte sedimentation rate and C-reactive protein). It should be noted that these cannot exclude the possibility of infection, but are helpful in a cancer patient, who often cannot mount a fever or leukocytosis. Plain films should be ordered of the spine and they are often abnormal. CT scan sensitivity for MESCC is only 66%, compared with the 93% with a contrast-enhanced MRI, making MRI the test of choice. The MRI should cover the complete spine, as the physical exam can be misleading when attempting to identify the level involved. CT myelography is an option in patients in whom MRI is contraindicated. In addition to physical examination issues, multilevel disease has been found in almost half of patients, so liberal multilevel imaging of the spine should be considered. The most important prognostic factor is the level of motor function at the time of treatment initiation, so time is of the essence.

Initial medical management in suspected MESCC is systemic steroids, unless contraindicated. The exact dose has not been agreed upon due to the side effects seen with high-dose steroids. Clinical practice guidelines recommend an intravenous bolus of 10 mg of dexamethasone to reduce edema, followed by an inpatient daily regimen, with a goal of improving ambulatory status. Consider a higher dose of 100 mg in patients with a dense paraparesis, realizing the adverse events that can result from high-dose steroids. These side effects can include hyperglycemia, psychosis, and increased risk of opportunistic infections.

For patients in whom MESCC is found, a decision as to the next step should be made via a multidisciplinary approach, including neurosurgery and radiation oncology. A 2005 randomized controlled trial and subsequent guidelines recommend anterior decompressive surgery plus postoperative radiotherapy over radiotherapy alone for a select group of these patients. Surgery in this select group of patients leads to more ambulatory patients and patients ambulating for a longer period of time. Other surgical options include vertebroplasty to help with pain, and laminectomy as another means of decompression. If these services are not available at the treating institution, timely transfer needs to occur. If radiation is used for patients who are not surgical candidates, it is directed at a level above and below the lesion to prevent epidural spread. Certain malignancies are unfortunately resistant to radiation, and they include melanoma and renal cell carcinoma.

Pearls and Pitfalls

- Eye findings vary based on the type of brain herniation syndrome.
- Carefully review medication lists in cancer patients who present to the ED with altered mental status.
- Patients without tonic-clonic activity can have subclinical SE with altered mental status.
- Use caution when using anticoagulants for stroke or DVT/PE in brain tumor patients.
- Consider spinal cord compression in cancer patients with back pain.
- Back pain that is worse when lying down or at night is a red flag for pathology and malignancy-related disease.

Bibliography

Bauer KA. Nonbacterial thrombotic endocarditis. Available at: www.UpToDate.com.

Behl D, Hendrickson AW, Moynihan TJ. Oncologic emergencies. *Crit Care Clin* 2010;26(1):181–205.

Casazza BA. Diagnosis and treatment of acute low back pain. *Am Fam Physician* 2012;**85**(4):343–350.

Dearborn JL, Urrutia VC, Zeiler SR Stroke and cancer: a complicated relationship. *J Neurol Transl Neurosci* 2014;**2**(1):1039.

Giglio P, Gilbert MR. Neurologic complications of cancer and its treatment. *Curr Oncol Rep* 2010;**12**(1):50–59.

Grisold W, Oberndorfer S, Struhal W. Stroke and cancer: a review. *Acta Neurol Scand* 2009;**119**(1):1–16.

Khan UA, Shanholtz CB, McCurdy MT. Oncologic mechanical emergencies. *Emerg Med Clin North Am* 2014;**32**(3):495–508.

Loblaw, DA. Mitera G, Ford M, et al. Updated systematic review and clinical practice guideline for the management of malignant extradural spinal cord compression. *Int J Radiat Oncol Biol Phys* 2011;**84**(2):312–317.

Navi BB, Reiner AS, Kamel H, et al. Association between incident cancer and subsequent stroke. *Ann Neurol* 2015;**77**(2):291–300.

Newton, HB. Neurologic complications of systemic cancer. *Am Fam Physician* 1999;**59**(4):878–886.

Tuma R, DeAngelis LM. Altered mental status in patients with cancer. *Arch Neurol* 2000;**57**(12):1727–1731.

Wen PY. Overview of the clinical manifestations, diagnosis, and management of patients with brain metastases. Available at: www.UpToDate.com.

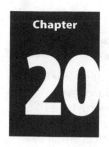

Peripheral Nerve and Neuromuscular Disorders

George A. Small, Sandeep Rana, and Mara Aloi

20.1 Guillain-Barré Syndrome

20.1.1 Introduction

Guillain-Barré syndrome (GBS) is an acquired neuromuscular disorder that presents as rapidly progressive weakness and numbness, usually in an ascending fashion. The underlying pathophysiology is monophasic inflammatory immune-mediated demyelinating polyneuropathy that in many cases is triggered by viral illnesses, usually a few weeks prior to the onset of the syndrome. The majority of cases are in young adults, although it can occur in pediatric and elderly age groups. GBS should be considered in the differential diagnosis of new-onset rapidly progressing weakness in an otherwise healthy individual.

20.1.2 Emergency Presentation

GBS is typically heralded by diffuse paresthesias, myalgias, and cramps ("charley horse"), at times associated with back pain. This is followed by weakness that makes walking and climbing stairs difficult. In most cases there is ascending (i.e., distal to proximal) spread of weakness, although variants are not uncommon. Cranial nerves are frequently involved, producing facial diplegia, and on occasion difficulty chewing and swallowing. On examination, muscle stretch reflexes are absent or hypoactive. Despite patient complaints of paresthesias, examination typically reveals minimal loss of sensory modalities. In up to two-thirds of patients there is involvement of the autonomic nervous system, which manifests as labile blood pressure, cardiac arrhythmias, and bladder or bowel dysfunction.

The disease may vary in severity. In some patients the weakness remains mild throughout the course of illness, although in other patients the weakness rapidly progresses to quadriplegia. Up to one-third of patients with GBS develop weakness of respiratory muscles and require intubation with ventilator support. The weakness rarely progresses beyond 4 weeks, with maximal weakness usually occurring by 7–14 days.

Well-known variants of GBS include Miller–Fisher syndrome, which is characterized by a triad of ophthalmoplegia, ataxia, and areflexia. In this syndrome there is minimal to no weakness. Bickerstaff brainstem encephalitis is another rare variant in which patients present with ophthalmoparesis, gait ataxia, hyperreflexia, and encephalopathy. Other rare variants have been reported, some with a regional pattern of weakness or isolated dysautonomia.

20.1.3 Emergency Evaluation and Differential Diagnosis

In the early phase of the illness, ancillary testing may not be helpful and diagnosis may have to be made on clinical presentation and ruling out other disorders that can mimic

295

Table 20.1 Diagnostic criteria for typical GBS

Features required for diagnosis	Features strongly supporting the diagnosis	Features making the diagnosis doubtful
Progressive weakness in both arms and legs Areflexia	Paresthesias in legs and arms Myalgias, back pain Relative symmetry of symptoms Progression of symptoms over days to 4 weeks Absent or mild sensory findings Cranial nerve involvement, particularly facial diplegia Autonomic dysfunction Absence of fever at onset of symptoms Elevated CSF protein with <20 WBCs/mm^3 Typical nerve conduction studies and electromyography	Distinct sensory level Early and severe bladder or bowel dysfunction Persistent asymmetry of clinical findings Progression of symptoms beyond 4 weeks More than 50 WBCs/mm^3 in CSF CPK >3–5 times normal

GBS (Table 20.1). After the first week, CSF analysis can be helpful in supporting the diagnosis as it typically reveals elevated protein without leukocytosis, referred to as albumin-cytological dissociation. The extent of protein elevation varies, although extremely high values (i.e., greater than 2.5 g/L) should raise suspicion for cord compression. Pleocytosis in CSF should prompt testing for Lyme disease, HIV, neoplasia, sarcoid, and other diseases.

Blood counts, chemistry profile, and other laboratory tests do not enhance the diagnosis of GBS, but are indicated to rule-out other associated conditions. Creatine kinase (CPK) levels may be mildly elevated in GBS, but levels beyond 3–5 times normal should raise the possibility of a myopathic disorder (Table 20.1).

Usually by the second week of symptom onset, nerve conduction studies can reveal abnormalities that can be helpful in supporting the diagnosis. Typical findings on nerve conduction studies that support the presence of a demyelinating polyneuropathy include prolonged distal latencies, conduction blocks with abnormal temporal dispersion, and slowed conduction velocities.

20.1.4 Management

Good supportive care is paramount to achieving a favorable outcome. Respiratory status is assessed with periodic vital capacities. Elective intubation is considered when vital capacity is below 15 mL/kg. Manifestations of dysautonomia (i.e., labile blood pressure, cardiac dysarrhythmias) are treated aggressively. Patients with severe weakness should receive prophylaxis for deep vein thrombosis. Good nutritional support and bladder care can decrease morbidity.

Two forms of immunomodulating therapy, namely intravenous immunoglobulins (IVIg) and plasmapheresis, have been shown in double-blind controlled studies to be effective in shortening the disease course. Either one can be used to treat patients when they are presenting within 2 weeks of illness. It may be reasonable to treat beyond 2 weeks particularly when the weakness is progressing. Corticosteroids have not been shown to be beneficial in altering the course of GBS and should not be used as they may cause complications and thereby worsen the outcome.

Causes of death in patients with GBS include unrecognized respiratory failure, complications of ventilator use, pulmonary infections (usually nosocomial), cardiac arrhythmias, and pulmonary embolism.

20.2 Peripheral Neuropathy

20.2.1 Introduction

The hallmarks of peripheral neuropathy, which forms one subgroup of peripheral nervous system disorders, are weakness and altered sensation. Pain can variably be a part of the process, as can asymmetry. These patients come to the ED when they are distressed due to rapid symptom progression or when significant pain, speech, swallowing, and breathing are involved. Occasionally, when peripheral neuropathies affect the nerves to the bulbar muscles, double vision and/or facial weakness can be the presenting signs.

In order to best characterize the type of peripheral neuropathy, one must localize the process within the peripheral nervous system:

1. Nerve roots including the dorsal nerve roots (sensory), ventral nerve roots (motor), or both.
2. Dorsal and ventral nerve roots combine to form mixed nerves that end in a plexus.
3. Peripheral nerves travel from the plexus to either the end organs of muscle or primary sensory afferent neurons that provide the sensation of touch, proprioception, or even possibly temperature appreciation. Disorders affecting peripheral nerves can be as serious as GBS or as relatively less serious as irritating mononeuropathy, such as carpal tunnel syndrome.
4. The major motor neuron disease is known as "Lou Gehrig disease" (amyotrophic lateral sclerosis [ALS]). Historically, this is not considered a peripheral neuropathy, but in actuality it is a pure motor radiculopathy and therefore is included in this chapter.

20.2.2 Evaluation

The exacerbation of a peripheral neuropathy can result in a transition from normal breathing to hypoventilation, hypercarbia, and hypoxemia requiring intubation and mechanical ventilation. In addition, the inability to manage oropharyngeal secretions can result in panic, prompting an ED evaluation. It is very important to determine whether the patient's respiratory effort is becoming fatigued. Unlike patients with traditional COPD from smoking, hypercarbia is generally not seen in patients with neuromuscular weakness; hypercarbia can occur when patients with peripheral nerve causes of dyspnea begin to decompensate. The forced vital capacity and negative inspiratory force are the best quantitative measures of ventilatory muscle function and therefore, by extension, phrenic nerve function. A forced vital capacity <15 mL/kg or a negative inspiratory force of <15 mm Hg likely suggests the need for assisted ventilation. The normal forced vital capacity in the average-sized individual is 65 mL/kg. Aspiration of oropharyngeal contents, even saliva alone, can occur due to phrenic nerve problems or GBS, the more common causes of peripheral nerve problems requiring elective intubation.

In addition, autonomic symptoms or signs may occur in patients with peripheral nervous system problems, such as mild or malignant arrhythmias, significant blood pressure changes, and lightheadedness.

20.2.3 Focused Examination of the Peripheral Nervous System Strength Testing

Strength testing is done to assess the power of muscles and the distribution of any weakness, whether it is proximally predominant, distally predominant, mixed, or when there is an asymmetric presentation. These findings aid in the differential diagnosis of peripheral nerve causes of weakness. Brief testing of shoulder abduction, elbow flexion and extension, wrist flexion and extension, hip flexion and extension, knee flexion and extension, and ankle movements usually suffices during the initial presentation. Symmetrical weakness that is diffuse and proximal with intact reflexes may suggest a more myopathic or neuromuscular junction process. Absent reflexes diffusely suggests a peripheral nerve process. Common peripheral neuropathies present with distally predominant weakness with loss of ankle reflexes and preservation of more proximally related reflexes such as those from the biceps or patellae. Asymmetrical weakness may suggest more of a problem at the root level, such as occurs with herniated discs or a motor neuropathy multiplex from an autoimmune process or a traumatic process of the brachial plexus.

20.2.4 Sensory Testing

The presence of numbness or paresthesias (spontaneous abnormal sensations), or dysesthesias (spontaneous painful sensations), suggests that the primary process is not at the level of the neuromuscular junction or muscle, but is clearly a problem in the peripheral nervous system (e.g., peripheral neuropathy). Myopathies do not cause numbness or tingling, although they can cause aching. Sensation carried by large-diameter nerves can be tested using a tuning fork and also by assessing position sense of the small joints of the toes or the larger knee joints to determine whether there is a large-fiber sensory neuropathy. Sensory loss in a focal distribution of one or several nerve roots may also aid in the differential diagnosis of the patient's peripheral nervous system process.

20.2.5 Reflexes

Diseases of the brain and spinal cord generally cause increased reflexes. Peripheral neuropathies generally cause absent or decreased reflexes. If an increased reflex is found in the distribution of a peripheral nerve to a muscle that is weak, it is highly unlikely to be from a peripheral nerve process. Muscle stretch reflex loss that is asymmetrical suggests a radicular or mononeuropathic process. Abnormal reflexes such as the Hoffmann sign or the Babinski response are not seen in peripheral nervous system problems. The key is to localize the pathological process to a group of peripheral nerves and expeditiously triage the patient.

20.2.6 Differential Diagnosis and Management

1. Disorders involving nerve roots.

    a. Radiculopathic pain radiating into a dermatomal distribution of a given nerve root with or without associated weakness or sensory loss helps to localize the lesion to a particular nerve root.

2. Disorders of mixed nerves.

    a. Plexopathy. The brachial plexus and lumbosacral plexus are intertwined areas of a variety of nerve roots coming together to form peripherally named nerves. Autoimmune disorders, diabetes, trauma, and spontaneous hemorrhage into these areas are common causes of the various plexopathies. The pattern of weakness can suggest the region of the plexus involved: upper lumbosacral plexus, lower lumbosacral plexus, upper brachial plexus, or lower brachial plexus.

    b. Brachial plexus. The most common causes of brachial plexopathy are trauma, radiation effect, or cryptogenic. Upward shoulder displacement causes lower brachial plexopathy and downward shoulder displacement causes upper brachial plexopathy. Shoulder and neck traumas tend to cause the well-known "stingers," known to a variety of athletes. Idiopathic brachial plexopathy is also referred to as Parsonage–Turner syndrome. It is likely an autoimmune process that can occur following viral infections, vaccination, post-trauma/surgery, or without obvious precipitant. It presents as acute onset of severe pain followed by weakness in the proximal arm that typically develops over the course of 1–2 weeks. On many occasions the weakness of the arm is associated with winging of the scapula. Treatment generally requires more observation and physical therapy than specific medical therapy. It is largely a diagnosis of exclusion. It generally improves within 12 months with the above-mentioned therapies.

    c. Lumbosacral plexus. The lumbosacral plexus is particularly vulnerable to acute hemorrhage in patients who are on warfarin or thrombin inhibitors and can present with significant pain radiating from the pelvis into the thigh. Also, poorly controlled diabetics tend to be subject to nerve infarction within the lumbosacral plexus, causing severe weakness and pain in the general distribution of the femoral nerve, generally improving with time. The proper management and localization of both brachial plexopathy and lumbosacral plexopathy has been greatly aided by advanced imaging that has come to the fore within the last 20 years.

3. Disorders of peripheral nerves.

    a. Polyneuropathy. Polyneuropathies generally are symmetrical, resulting in distal weakness and numbness. Findings of weakness, distal sensory loss, and hypo- or areflexia are the rule. Acute presentation of severe peripheral neuropathy in GBS can result in respiratory failure 20% of the time, and is supported most specifically by EMG testing and spinal fluid analysis.

    b. Mononeuropathy. Mononeuropathies, as the name suggests, cause abnormal primary motor, sensory, or mixed dysfunction in the distribution of a peripheral nerve. The most common cause is compression of a nerve in the carpal tunnel, causing significant pain in the lateral volar surface of the hand with or without weakness. In all peripheral neuropathies, a history of diabetes, particularly diabetes that is not controlled, tends to "prime" nerves for damage due to the vasculopathy occurring within small blood vessels in the peripheral nervous system in such patients. Mononeuropathy multiplex refers to multiple mononeuropathies occurring fairly simultaneously and is distinguished from radiculopathy by the inclusion of peripheral nerves that are innervated by more than one nerve root. Rheumatologic diseases tend to predispose people to such disorders. The most common peripheral neuropathy above the neck is that of Bell's palsy, creating significant and variable muscle weakness either unilaterally or bilaterally that includes mainly the muscles of the cheek and periocular area, but also of the brow, distinguishing it from an upper motor neuron process such as stroke. Hyperacusis and altered taste sensation can also occur. This type of facial weakness, which can occur abruptly or over several days, is generally treated with a short course of steroids and 5–7 days of an antiviral therapy. Protecting the cornea by using lubricating eye drops and an eye patch and judicious consultation with an ophthalmologist for any ocular concerns are in the best interests of the patient.

A variety of other peripheral nervous system dysfunctions can mimic peripheral neuropathy, particularly those causing neuromuscular junction or muscle disease, and will be discussed in another chapter.

20.3 Myasthenia Gravis

20.3.1 Introduction

Myasthenia gravis (MG) is the most common primary disorder of neuromuscular transmission and one of the well-understood autoimmune diseases. It causes variable weakness, diplopia, and speech and swallowing difficulty, and may progress to respiratory failure if inappropriately managed. In MG, autoantibodies against the postsynaptic acetylcholine receptors at the myoneural junction of skeletal muscle are released, resulting in a reduction in the number of functional receptors. Serologic testing for these antireceptor antibodies is not readily available and may not be conclusive; therefore, its role is limited in the emergent management of myasthenic patients. ED evaluation is based on the recognition of the symptoms and signs of exacerbations or of medication complications.

The prevalence of MG is estimated to be 14–20 per 100,000 persons, but may be higher due to underdiagnosis. There is a bimodal distribution of the disease, with young women and older men being most commonly affected. Most patients with MG are over the age of 50. Rare variants do occur in neonates and children. Mortality for those affected approached 75% in past years but is now less than 5% due to more timely diagnosis of the disorder and subsequent crises and more effective therapies. Complete remission is possible in some cases.

20.3.2 Classification

According to the Myasthenia Gravis Foundation of America Clinical Association, MG may be divided into the following five classes:

Class I: ocular involvement alone; all other muscle strength is normal (10%).
Class II: mild generalized weakness, with or without ocular muscle weakness.

IIa: affects limb and axial muscles more than oropharyngeal muscles.

IIb: weakness most pronounced in oropharyngeal muscles; limb and axial muscles less affected.

Class III: moderately severe generalized weakness, which may include ocular muscles.

IIIa: affects limb and axial muscles more than oropharyngeal muscles.

IIIb: weakness most pronounced in oropharyngeal muscles; limb and axial muscles less affected.

Class IV: patients with group III disease who progress to severe weakness despite optimal medical therapy.

Class V: severe weakness resulting in impending respiratory failure, defined by the need for emergent intubation and ventilatory support.

20.3.3 ED Evaluation

The majority of patients present to the ED with an established diagnosis of MG. On rare occasions, a patient may present with undiagnosed disease, typically with complaints of specific muscle weakness that is worsened by exercise and improves with rest. Approximately 30% of patients present with progressive proximal upper and/or lower extremity weakness manifested as difficulty rising from a seated position or combing one's hair. Weakness is usually less severe in the morning because acetylcholine stores have been replenished during sleep. Many patients will also have bulbar weakness, or weakness of the oropharyngeal and facial muscles. Dysarthria, fatigue with chewing, hypophonia, and dysphagia may be presenting complaints. Drooling occurs when pharyngeal muscle weakness impairs normal reflex swallowing mechanisms. Ocular symptoms are primarily limited to ptosis and diplopia due to extraocular muscle dysfunction. This can be the initial presenting complaint in up to two-thirds of patients. Patients may report that these symptoms are worse after activities that require sustained use of the eyes, such as reading, television viewing, or computer use. In up to 15% of cases, patients present exclusively with ocular muscle weakness. Loss of visual acuity, a change in mental status or level of alertness, muscle pain, and any pupillary changes suggest alternative diagnoses. If physical examination is normal by the time the patient presents to the ED, attempt to provoke specific muscle weakness by sustained use of the affected muscle (e.g., sustained upward gaze may cause ptosis to develop).

In patients known to have MG, it is crucial to determine whether the patient's weakness is due to a myasthenic crisis or a cholinergic crisis because treatment will be different for each.

Myasthenic crisis: This is usually seen within the first 2 years of diagnosis. The presenting complaint is progressive weakness. Conditions such as thyroid disease, pregnancy, menstruation, emotional distress, and exposure to bright sunlight may worsen the disease, but infectious processes, such as upper respiratory tract infections and other viral or bacterial illnesses, are more likely to be the inciting factor for disease exacerbations. The symptoms of MG may also be worsened by medications, including beta-blockers, calcium-channel blockers, haloperidol, and antibiotics, particularly aminoglycosides and fluoroquinolones. These patients will require supplemental acetylcholinesterase inhibitor (AChI) medications.

Cholinergic crisis: This is due to overmedication with AChI agents, with excessive acetylcholine causing muscle weakness and muscarinic symptoms such as excessive salivation, muscle fasciculations, bradycardia, abdominal cramping, and urinary urgency. Treatment includes atropine and the cessation of AChI medications.

The most ominous presentation of MG is subtle, progressive respiratory failure due to diaphragmatic and intercostal muscle weakness. Agitation, diaphoresis, and increased respiratory rate frequently occur prior to shortness of breath. This is a classic presentation of restrictive lung disease. Abnormal arterial blood gases do not reliably predict the need for mechanical ventilation. A careful physical examination and assessment of respiratory function using objective tests, including measurement of vital capacity (VC) and negative inspiratory force (NIF), can help to identify patients with impending respiratory failure. A VC <20 mL/kg or a NIF <20 cmH$_2$O are signs of significant respiratory weakness, and mechanical ventilation should be considered. If these tests are not readily available in the ED, a bedside test to assess respiratory muscle strength can be done by having the patient count to 20 in a single breath. Inability to do so signifies weakness.

20.3.4 Differential Diagnosis

Several other diagnoses can present with progressive weakness, in a similar fashion to MG. These include:

- GBS and the *Miller–Fisher variant* of GBS, covered above. Lack of muscle stretch reflexes, ataxia, and normal CSF cell counts with high CSF protein levels distinguish these conditions from MG.
- ALS. Key aspects of ALS, including muscle atrophy, fasciculations, and vague, nonlocalizable fatigue are absent in MG.
- *Hypokalemia* and *myxedema* can be ruled out quickly with readily available laboratory testing. Note that some degree of thyroid dysfunction seen in up to 10% of myasthenic patients is not the primary cause of their weakness.
- *Botulism.* Caused by a toxin that affects the presynaptic neuromuscular junction and decreases the release of acetylcholine. Botulism may present with ptosis, but affected patients will manifest pupillary dilatation unreactive to light, helping to distinguish MG from botulism. A history of ingestion of poorly canned foods may be the only way to reliably distinguish the two entities when pupillary function is normal.
- *Polymyositis* also presents with progressive muscle weakness but laboratory abnormalities such as elevated creatine kinase, liver enzymes, and erythrocyte sedimentation rate are not seen in MG.
- *Multiple sclerosis* (MS) will also have a variable course and presentation, but the following more strongly suggest MS: (1) optic neuritis presenting with vision loss and eye pain; (2) nystagmus; and (3) painful, electric shock-like sensations radiating down the back (Lhermitte's sign).
- *Chronic meningitis* associated with carcinoma, sarcoidosis, or Lyme disease may be difficult to distinguish from MG. Spinal fluid analysis in MG is normal and is frequently diagnostic in these other conditions.

- *Brainstem stroke* can present with altered mental status, ptosis, diplopia, and pupillary abnormalities. MRI with diffusion-weighted imaging can reliably distinguish acute brainstem stroke from MG.

20.3.5 Diagnostic Testing

Tensilon test: A useful tool for the management of myasthenic patients in the ED is the edrophonium (Tensilon) test, which may help to differentiate a cholinergic crisis from a myasthenic crisis and to guide subsequent therapy. A short-acting AChI with a rapid onset of action, edrophonium prevents enzymatic degradation of acetylcholine, prolonging its presence at the neuromuscular junction and interaction with muscle cell receptors, thereby allowing improved muscle contraction. Appropriate monitoring and readily available resuscitative equipment are required before any Tensilon test. Atropine should be drawn up in a separate syringe ready at the bedside before administering edrophonium. A test dose of 2 mg edrophonium should be administered intravenously, with the patient monitored for both improvement of muscle weakness and for the appearance of any adverse effects. Improvement of ptosis or ophthalmoparesis should be seen within 1–2 minutes. This effect is transient and may last only 15 minutes. If no improvement is observed, subsequent doses of 2 mg can be given every 1 minute to a maximum of 10 mg. Lack of response to the maximum dosage of edrophonium indicates that the patient's weakness is not due to MG. Increased weakness or the development of excessive muscarinic symptoms after edrophonium administration identifies a patient in cholinergic crisis. Relative contraindications to the use of edrophonium include advanced age, cardiac diseases, and asthma. Side effects due to the muscarinic effects of edrophonium can occur and include bradycardia, abdominal cramps, and urinary urgency. Wheezing due to bronchospasm can result, especially in patients with underlying asthma or COPD. Respiratory failure can develop in those already in cholinergic crisis. Atropine should be given in the event that overwhelming muscarinic side effects develop. Cardiac monitoring is important throughout the entire test because of possible bradyarrhythmias and asystole. This test is often done by consultants in a monitored environment rather than in the ED.

Ice pack test: Another diagnostic tool that is readily available in any ED is the ice pack test. The utility of this modality is based upon the electrophysiologic finding that neuromuscular transmission improves with cooling. In a patient presenting with prominent ptosis of presumed MG, placement of an ice pack over a closed eyelid for 2 minutes should result in improvement. A sensitivity of up to 77% has been reported. This may be a more attractive choice if edrophonium is considered too risky for a particular patient.

In patients with exclusively ocular symptoms, rule-out a mass lesion with MRI of the brain and orbits.

20.3.6 Management

20.3.6.1 Airway Management

Airway evaluation and management is of vital importance when treating a myasthenic patient in the ED. The potential for respiratory depression and aspiration is great.

Ideally, at-risk patients are identified before respiratory failure and emergent endotracheal intubation is required. As outlined above, objective respiratory function tests can help to identify seemingly well-appearing patients before they tire and decompensate to respiratory failure. Beta-agonist bronchodilators (albuterol) and inhaled anticholinergic medications (ipratropium) may improve respirations and bronchospasm due to excessive cholinergic effects. Suctioning is performed when copious oropharyngeal secretions are present.

Noninvasive ventilation (NIV): NIV may prevent intubation in some patients since it enhances airflow, alleviates the work of breathing, and prevents airway collapse and atelectasis. In some studies, patients treated initially with NIV required fewer days of ventilatory support and had shorter ICU stays. A trial of BiPAP should be considered in patients with mild to moderate respiratory distress without significant tachypnea or hypercarbia.

Endotracheal intubation: Over 20% of patients in myasthenic crisis will require intubation in the ED. If intubation is deemed necessary, medications for rapid sequence intubation should proceed but with some alterations to the choice and dose of medications used. Due to the relative lack of functioning ACh receptors, succinylcholine, a depolarizing paralytic agent, may have less predictable results in the myasthenic patient. Moreover, paralysis may be prolonged. Rapid-onset nondepolarizing neuromuscular blocking agents (NMBAs) such as rocuronium are the agents of choice to induce paralysis in these patients. Myasthenic patients are relatively sensitive to NMBAs, so 50% of the standard dose is recommended (0.5–0.8 mg/kg for rocuronium). A prolonged recovery period from neuromuscular blockade should be expected. Nasotracheal intubation has a limited role in the airway management of these patients since they will likely require an extended period of intubation.

20.3.6.2 Supportive Measures

Fever should be aggressively controlled as high temperatures worsen muscle strength by impairing neuromuscular transmission. The presence of fever indicates that an infectious process may be responsible for the myasthenic exacerbation. An appropriate evaluation for active infection is indicated and includes a chest radiograph and urinalysis. In keeping with the mandate to "first do no harm," it is important to avoid iatrogenic complications unique to the myasthenic patient population. It is crucial to remember that antibiotics such as fluoroquinolones and aminoglycosides can worsen neuromuscular transmission and should be avoided in patients with MG. Limit the use of sedatives and narcotic agents because of their respiratory depressant effect. The use of low-osmolality IV contrast is associated with a significant increase in MG-related symptoms, usually seen within 1 day of contrast administration. If absolutely required for diagnostic purposes, an admission to the hospital should be considered. Most patients with exacerbations of MG require admission to the hospital because of the variable course of the disease. All patients with airway compromise require ICU admission. Those patients with infectious processes, especially pneumonia, should be admitted.

20.3.7 Therapy

Once the patient has been stabilized, emergent consultation with a neurologist should be sought in order to guide further therapy. The Tensilon test may be carried out as outlined above in the hospital. Thymectomy results in some degree of clinical improvement in the majority of patients and may even induce remission of the disease in up to 60% of cases. It has been proposed as the treatment of choice for all patients with thymoma and should be considered for post-pubescent patients without thymoma but who have generalized myasthenia. Improvement of symptoms and disease remission is 2–3 times more likely after a thymectomy.

Pearls and Pitfalls

- Decreased or absent muscle stretch reflexes are hallmarks of GBS. If reflexes are brisk, the diagnosis should be questioned.
- Weakness in GBS occurs over days, although in some severe cases the progression of weakness can occur over hours.
- In patients with GBS, the respiratory function should be monitored closely, with serial measurements of vital capacities. Decisions regarding elective intubation should not be based on blood gas abnormalities as these occur late in the disease process.
- CSF evaluation can be normal in the first week of GBS, followed by elevation in protein level without leukocytosis.
- Corticosteroids are not indicated for treatment of GBS.
- Peripheral reflexes (ankle) are lost before proximal (knee and biceps) reflexes in peripheral neuropathies.
- Diseases of the brain and spinal cord generally cause increased reflexes while peripheral neuropathies generally cause absent or decreased reflexes.
- Hoffmann sign and Babinski response are not seen in peripheral nervous system problems.
- Differentiate ptosis in botulism from myasthenia gravis by pupils being dilated and nonreactive in botulism.
- Rapid sequence intubation in myasthenic patients should include use of a nondepolarizing agent such as rocuronium rather than depolarizing agents such as succinylcholine to improve reliable result and prevent prolonged paralysis.

Bibliography

Abbott SA. Diagnostic challenge: myasthenia gravis in the emergency department. *J Amer Acad Nurse Practition* 2010;**22**:468–473.

Alshekhlee A, Miles JD, Katirji B, Preston DC, Kaminski HJ. Incidence and mortality rates of myasthenia gravis and myasthenic crisis in US hospitals. *Neurology* 2009;**72**:1548–1554.

Blichfeldt-Lauridsen L, Hansen BD. Anesthesia and myasthenia gravis. *Acta Anaesthesiol Scand* 2012;**56**:17–22.

Deymeer F, Gungor-Tuncer O, Yilmaz V, et al. Clinical comparison of anti-MuSK- vs anti-AchR- positive and seronegative myasthenia gravis. *Neurology* 2007;**68**:609–611.

Golnik KC, Pena R, Lee AG, Eggenberger ER. An ice test for the diagnosis of myasthenia gravis. *Ophthalmology* 1999;**106**:1282.

Jaretzki A, Barohn RJ, Ernstoff RM, et al. Myasthenis gravis: recommendations for clinical research standards: Task force of the medical scientific advisory board of the Myasthenia Gravis Foundation of America. *Neurology* 2000;**55**(1):16–23.

Kearsey C, Fernando P, D'Costa D, Ferdinand P. The use of the ice pack test in myasthenia gravis. *J R Soc Med Sh Rep* 2010;**1**:14.

Larner AJ, Thomas DJ. Can myasthenia gravis be diagnosed with the "ice pack test"? A cautionary note. *Postgrad Med J* 2000;**76**:162–163.

Mandawat A, Kaminski HJ, Cutter G, et al. Comparative analysis of therapeutic options used for myasthenia gravis. *Ann Neurol* 2010;**68**(6):797–805.

Mehndiratta MM, Pandey S, Kuntzer T. Acetylcholinesterase inhibitor treatment for myasthenia gravis. *Cochrane Database Syst Rev* 2014;**10**:006986.

Movaghar M, Slavin ML. Effect of local heat versus ice on blepharoptosis resulting from ocular myasthenia. *Ophthalmology* 2000;**107**(12):2209–2214.

Pascuzzi RM. The edrophonium test. *Semin Neurol* 2003;**23**(1):83–88.

Somashekar DK, Davenport MS, Cohan RH, et al. Effect of intravenous low-osmolality iodinated contrast media on patients with myasthenia gravis. *Radiology* 2013;**267**(3):727.

Takanami I, Abiko T, Koizumi S. Therapeutic outcomes in thymectomied patients with myasthenia gravis. *Ann Thorac Cardiovasc Surg* 2009;**15**(6):373–377.

Wendell LC, Levine JM. Myasthenic crisis. *Neurohospitalist* 2011;**1**(1):16–22.

Movement Disorders

Susan Baser, Timothy Leichliter, Donald Whiting, and Michael Oh

21.1 Introduction

Movement disorders are rarely medical emergencies or reason for evaluation in the emergency department (ED). However, they may be seen, and range from the familiar parkinsonism and drug-induced dystonia to rare disabling hemiballism secondary to a stroke. Movement disorders are typically a sign of an underlying neurological or nonneurological disorder, rather than the primary diagnosis. They can be strange in appearance and are often misdiagnosed as being hysterical or psychiatric in origin. In the ED, movement disorders are diagnosed based on a history and physical examination, with relatively few contributions from laboratory and radiographic studies.

Movement disorders are classified as either hypokinetic (diminished movement) or hyperkinetic (uncontrollable movement) disorders. Characteristics of various movement disorders are discussed in this chapter, with an emphasis on drug-induced movement disorders, which commonly present to the ED. This chapter ends with a section on deep brain stimulation therapy and complications, which is becoming increasingly utilized for various movement disorders. Complications can arise from this type of surgery and may be evaluated in the ED.

21.2 Evaluation of Movement Disorders

21.2.1 History

Important characteristics of movement disorders include onset, duration or temporal nature, location, and particular body parts, as well as exacerbating or mitigating factors. History should include whether the symptoms are present at rest, with sustained posture, with movement, or only during the execution of specific tasks. Possible association to environmental factors, toxins, and medication use must be determined. Family, social, and psychiatric history should be reviewed. In a pediatric patient, evidence of premature birth, prenatal injury, or behavioral problems is important. The use of psychotropic medications or antiemetics needs to be ascertained.

21.2.2 Physical Examination

Evaluation in the ED begins as soon as the patient is viewed, either walking back to the exam room, on a stretcher, or as soon as the physician walks into the room. Airway, breathing, and circulation remain the initial assessment. Movement disorders are evaluated with careful neurological examination, with accurate characterization of the abnormalities.

This characterization is best assessed by observation. This is accomplished first by observation of the patient's head, neck, trunk, and limbs. Eye movements, tone, and fine coordination are more subtle details giving clues to the diagnosis. Gait is extremely important in evaluating subtle findings (weakness, ataxia, shuffling) that may be otherwise missed. Radiographic imaging is of limited use in movement disorders. Some movement disorders occur acutely from a focal structural lesion such as stroke. Typically they are present in a localized body area or follow a "hemi-distribution." Urgent brain imaging can be helpful following the acute onset of symptoms with a focal distribution of findings.

21.2.3 Classification of Movement Disorders

Movement disorders can be classified into two categories based on phenomenological features, clinical pharmacology, and neuropathology (Table 21.1):

1. hypokinetic movement disorders
2. hyperkinetic movement disorders

Descriptive features of individual movement disorders are summarized in Table 21.2. Chorea, athetosis, and ballism are appropriately viewed as part of the spectrum of involuntary movements with a common pathophysiology.

21.3 Hypokinetic Movement Disorders

21.3.1 Parkinsonism

21.3.1.1 Characteristics

Parkinsonism is a syndrome associated with deficient dopamine innervation or dopamine effect within the striatum (caudate and putamen). The cardinal features are tremor, rigidity, akinesia or bradykinesia, and postural instability (Table 21.3). Symptoms and findings are often asymmetrical, with onset on one side of the body. Other symptoms and patient complaints include incoordination, notably with fine motor tasks, loss of facial expression, and loss of voice amplitude (hypophonia). Historical features often useful include difficulty with initiating or halting movement, especially getting in and out of chairs, and history of micrographia.

Table 21.1 Classification of movement disorders

Hypokinetic movement disorders	Hyperkinetic movement disorders
Parkinsonism	Dystonia
Parkinson's disease	Chorea
Other neurodegenerative diseases	Athetosis
Stiff-person syndrome	Ballism
	Tics
	Tremors
	Myoclonus

Table 21.2 Features of movement disorders

Parkinsonism	Tremor (resting), rigidity ("cogwheel"), akinesia/bradykinesia, postural instability
Stiff-person syndrome	Extreme muscle stiffness and rigidity, painful muscle spasms, exaggerated startle response
Dystonia	Involuntary, sustained muscle contractions, twisting and repetitive movements, abnormal postures
Chorea	Continuous flow of involuntary movement, motor impersistence
Ballism	Large-amplitude flinging, flailing movements
Tics	Brief, sudden, stereotyped repetitive movements or vocalizations
Tremors	Involuntary, rhythmic, sinusoidal movements of head, limbs, or voice
Myoclonus	Brief, rapid jerks or shock-like movements, usually of limbs

Table 21.3 Cardinal features of Parkinson's disease

Tremor – typically resting tremor, 4–6 Hz frequency

Rigidity – "cogwheel" in nature

Akinesia/bradykinesia

Postural instability – leading to poor balance and falls

The primary differential diagnosis is idiopathic Parkinson's disease, drug-induced parkinsonism, and rare neurodegenerative disorders involving the basal ganglia, including the family of neuroferritinopathies (PKAN), Fahr's disease (idiopathic basal ganglia calcification), and Wilson's disease. Medication history of exposure to any antipsychotic, antiemetics, and some antihypertensives that can interfere with dopaminergic neurotransmission must be documented.

21.3.1.2 Management

Drug therapy with dopamine replacement and/or dopamine agonists provides excellent symptomatic relief for several years. Generally after extended periods of time and increased dosages of medications, many patients develop marked fluctuations in response to therapy, with periods of complex involuntary movements called dyskinesias. Decreasing medication doses or lengthening the dosing interval can improve choreic dyskinesias.

Nausea is the most common side effect of these medications; however, orthostatic hypotension is more problematic as it can lead to syncope and falls prompting ED visits. All medications used in the treatment of Parkinson's disease can cause altered mental status. Many patients with Parkinson's disease can manifest varied pain symptoms such as muscle spasms, cramps, and burning paresthesias. Severe localized pain, chest pain, or abdominal pain in the patient with Parkinson's disease can cause confusion in the evaluation of these patients. Respiratory distress secondary to ventilatory dyskinesias could also be difficult to accurately diagnose and treat. The discontinuation of dopamine replacement therapy can cause a neuroleptic malignant syndrome, which is a medical emergency (see Chapter 25). Abruptly stopping medications must be avoided in patients with Parkinson's disease.

21.3.2 Stiff-Person Syndrome

21.3.2.1 Characteristics

The clinical hallmark of stiff-person syndrome (SPS) is an extreme degree of muscle stiffness and rigidity. The persistent nature of these signs may lead to fixed spinal deformities, such as a pronounced lumbar or cervical lordosis. This is thought to be due to the simultaneous contraction of opposing paraspinal muscle groups. The onset of stiffness and rigidity in the axial muscles, either lumbar or cervical, is insidious and generally progresses slowly over time to involve proximal limb muscles. There may be considerable pain in a symmetric fashion, and volitional movements become difficult. Paroxysmal autonomic dysfunction, characterized by transient hyperpyrexia, diaphoresis, tachypnea, tachycardia, pupillary dilatation, and arterial hypertension, has been described and may result in sudden death.

An autoimmune process was originally postulated to underlie SPS since the disorder often occurred in conjunction with a variety of autoimmune diseases. Circulating anti-GAD (glutamic acid decarboxylase) antibodies are present in approximately 60% of patients with SPS. These antibodies can be reliably detected using a commercially available radio-immunoassay. Additional autoantibodies not targeted to GAD, but which bind to the surface of GABAergic neurons, have been identified in association with anti-GAD antibodies in the sera of patients with SPS.

21.3.2.2 Management

Benzodiazepines are generally considered the optimal initial therapy for patients with SPS. Alternative therapies include baclofen, a GABA$_B$ receptor agonist drug, as monotherapy or added to the benzodiazepine. Immunosuppressive therapy including glucocorticoids or IVIg can be tried in patients who are not responsive to other medical therapies.

21.4 Hyperkinetic Movement Disorders

The hallmark of hyperkinetic movement disorders is the intrusion of involuntary movements into the normal flow of motor acts. Hyperkinetic movement disorders include dystonia, chorea, hemiballism, tics, tremors, and myoclonus. A specific hyperkinetic movement disorder may have features of multiple of these overlapping disorders.

21.4.1 Dystonia

21.4.1.1 Characteristics

Dystonia can refer to a symptom, a sign, or a disorder. Dystonia is defined as a movement disorder characterized by sustained or intermittent muscle contraction causing abnormal and often repetitive movement, postures, or both. Dystonic movements are typically patterned and twisting, and may be tremulous. They are often worsened by voluntary action and can be associated with overflow muscle activity.

Dystonia is one of the most frequently misdiagnosed neurological conditions. It can be misinterpreted as a psychiatric or hysterical condition because of the patient's bizarre

Table 21.4 Differential diagnosis of dystonia

Neurodegenerative disease – Parkinson's disease, Wilson's disease, other degenerative disorders of the basal ganglia and midbrain

Structural neurological diseases – posterior fossa tumor, syringomyelia, Arnold–Chiari malformation, herniated cervical disc

Structural musculoskeletal diseases – muscular or ligamentous absence, laxity, or injury, bony spinal abnormalities, cervical soft tissue lesions

Labyrinthine disease

Traumatic brain injury, stroke

Focal seizure

Encephalitis

Acute reaction to drug, medication, toxin

movements and postures, the finding of "action-induced dystonia," diurnal fluctuations, and frequent effectiveness of various sensory maneuvers. The differential diagnosis of dystonia is broad (Table 21.4).

21.4.2 Specific Dystonia

Idiopathic Torsion Dystonia (Dystonia Musculorum Deformans). Most common among Ashkenazi Jews, this is usually an autosomal dominant trait with variable penetrance. This is the most common childhood-onset primary dystonia.

Focal Dystonia. Focal dystonia refers to the involvement of a specific part of the body (e.g., writer's cramp). A primary dystonia that begins in adulthood is usually focal (e.g., spasmodic torticollis). Torticollis can mimic a variety of orthopedic and neurological disorders that are important to recognize in the ED (Table 21.4).

Blepharospasm/Oromandibular Dystonia/Meige Syndrome. Blepharospasm (blinking that progresses to clonic and then tonic closure of the eyelids) is the second most common focal dystonia, either isolated or associated with oromandibular dystonia (abnormal mouth movements). Blepharospasm–oromandibular dystonia syndrome is commonly referred to as Meige syndrome.

Torticollis. Torticollis refers to cervical dystonia producing abnormal neck postures. Specifically, torticollis is rotation of the neck, with anterocollis, retrocollis, and laterocollis referring to neck movements in specific directions.

Secondary Dystonia. Secondary dystonias are a consequence of underlying metabolic disorders, degenerative processes, or structural lesions. Sudden onset, presence of dystonia at rest, rapid progression, or an unusual distribution such as hemidystonia in an adult suggest secondary dystonia. Hemidystonia suggests a focal lesion such as a mass, infarction, or hemorrhage of the basal ganglia and should prompt urgent radiographic imaging.

21.4.2.1 Management

Anticholinergic medications are frequently successful in ameliorating dystonia. Botulinum toxin is an effective therapy for treating some types of focal dystonias. The patient with torticollis due to an orthopedic or neurosurgically treatable disorder is referred to the appropriate specialist. Treatments of drug-induced acute dystonia are reviewed in Section 21.5.

21.4.3 Chorea

21.4.3.1 Characteristics

Chorea, a Greek term for dance, consists of involuntary irregular, rapid, jerky movements without rhythmic pattern, randomly distributed with a flowing "dance-like" quality that involves multiple body parts. Athetosis (writhing movement) and ballism are part of the spectrum of chorea and appear to share a common pathophysiology, usually involving the striatum or subthalamic nucleus. Unlike primary dystonia, these movements are regarded as symptoms of an underlying neurological disorder.

Chorea can be a presenting symptom of a variety of conditions (Table 21.5). The most commonly encountered chorea, although not typically a presenting complaint in the ED, is L-dopa-induced chorea/dyskinesia in patients with parkinsonism. Other underlying causes include systemic lupus erythematosus, primary antiphospholipid antibody syndrome, and rarely multiple sclerosis. Structural lesions, including stroke and intracranial hemorrhage, can induce chorea and these are the most common causes of hemichorea/hemiballism. Pregnancy can also lead to chorea, known as chorea gravidarum, and should be evaluated in the ED and may require a consult to obstetrics and neurology services.

21.4.4 Sydenham's Chorea

Sydenham's chorea is a form of autoimmune chorea preceded by group A *Streptococcus* infection, typically rheumatic fever. Sydenham's chorea occurs several months after the onset of acute streptococcal infection and usually affects patients 5–15 years of age, girls more frequently than boys. There appears to be a familial prevalence, suggesting hereditary susceptibility. It tends to occur abruptly, worsens over 2–4 weeks, and usually resolves spontaneously in 3–6 weeks. Measurement of antistreptolysin-O titers can help physicians to detect recent streptococcal infection. However, Sydenham's chorea can occur 6 months after the streptococcal infection, and measurements of antistreptolysin-O and antistreptokinase antibody concentrations obtained later may not be helpful.

21.4.5 Huntington's Disease

Huntington's disease is a hereditary neurodegenerative disorder characterized by chorea, incoordination, dementia, and numerous psychiatric problems. Huntington's disease is the most common choreiform neurodegenerative disorder.

Patients with Huntington's disease are evaluated in the ED for complications of the disease that require immediate care. These patients are at a much higher risk of suicide than the average population and suicide attempts are a major concern. Other symptoms associated with the disease are swallowing dysfunction, poor balance and coordination leading to frequent falls, severe dysarthria, dysphasia, dementia, and loss of ambulation. The dopamine receptor

Table 21.5 Causes of chorea

Hereditary causes

Huntington's disease

Wilson's disease

Benign familial chorea

Neuroacanthocytosis

Porphyria

Ataxia-telangiectasia

Tuberous sclerosis

Autoimmune or inflammatory causes

Antiphospholipid antibody syndrome

Behcet's disease

Celiac disease

Hashimoto encephalopathy

Polyarteritis nodosa

Primary CNS angiitis

Sarcoidosis

Sjögren's syndrome

Sydenham's chorea

Systemic lupus erythematosus

Cerebrovascular causes

Arteriovenous malformation

Intracerebral hemorrhage

Ischemic stroke

Moyamoya disease

Post-pump chorea

Drugs and toxic causes

Dopaminergic agents

Phenytoin

Lithium

Amphetamines

Oral contraceptives

Alcohol intoxication or withdrawal

Carbon monoxide

Manganese

Toluene

Table 21.5 (cont.)

Infectious causes

AIDS

Creutzfeldt–Jakob disease

Encephalitis

Meningitis/tuberculous meningitis

Malaria

Progressive multifocal leukoencephalopathy

Metabolic causes

Hepatic failure

Hyperthyroidism

Hypo/hypercalcemia

Hypo/hyperglycemia

Hypo/hypernatremia

Hypomagnesemia

Hypoparathyroidism

Polycythemia vera

Neoplastic causes

Basal ganglia involvement

Paraneoplastic

antagonist haloperidol is the medication most frequently used to control symptoms in Huntington's disease. Dopamine-depleting agents such as tetrabenazine can also be effective.

21.4.6 Ballism

Ballism is characterized as uncontrollable, rapid, large-amplitude proximal flinging movements of the limbs. Unilateral involvement is termed hemiballism, whereas rare bilateral involvement is called biballism. Typically, the face is spared. Hemiballism is an extreme form of hemichorea and is part of the spectrum that includes chorea and athetosis. It can occur from lesions in parts of the basal ganglia and the thalamus.

The most common cause of hemiballism is stroke, generally lacunar infarct or intracranial hemorrhage, affecting the subthalamic nucleus. Hemiballism occurs most frequently in individuals over 60 years of age with risk factors for stroke. Dopamine-blocking agents such as haloperidol are the most effective drug therapy.

21.4.7 Tics

Tics are characterized by intermittent, sudden, repetitive, stereotyped movements (motor tics) or sounds (vocal tics) and are the most common movement disorder. Tics can be

Table 21.6 Classification of tics

Primary tic disorders	Secondary tic disorders
Tourette's syndrome	Infections – encephalitis, Creutzfeldt–Jakob disease
Transient motor or phonic tics (<1 year)	Drugs – stimulants, antiseizure medications, antipsychotics
Chronic motor or phonic tics (>1 year)	Toxins – carbon monoxide poisoning
Huntington's disease	Developmental – intellectual disability, static encephalopathy, autism, pervasive developmental disorder
Neuroacanthocytosis	Other – head trauma, stroke, neurodegenerative conditions, chromosomal abnormalities
Primary dystonia	

abrupt and fast, or slow and sustained. Tics can result from contraction of only one group of muscles, causing simple tics, which are brief, jerk-like movements or single, meaningless sounds. Complex tics result from a coordinated sequence of movements. Tics can be suppressed temporarily, and often wax and wane in type, frequency, and severity. Disorders associated with tics are listed in Table 21.6.

The most well-known tic disorder is Gilles de la Tourette's syndrome. Tourette's syndrome is a disorder characterized by childhood onset of motor and vocal tics. Both types of tics are required for the diagnosis, although they need not occur concurrently. Obsessive compulsive disorder and attention deficit hyperactivity disorder are strongly associated with Tourette's syndrome. Tics tend to worsen in adolescents and abate in adults. Medications used to treat tics range from alpha-2 agonists to dopamine antagonists. Selective serotonin reuptake inhibitors such as fluoxetine are widely used to treat obsessive compulsive disorder, including that which is associated with Tourette's syndrome.

21.4.8 Tremors

Tremors are defined as involuntary, rhythmic, and roughly sinusoidal movements. There are multiple types of tremors, including resting, postural, kinetic, and task-related tremors. Resting tremor is one of the cardinal features of Parkinson's disease, whereas action tremors are more typical of essential tremor. Physiological tremor is a normal phenomenon due to the viscoelastic properties of joints in limbs. All tremors, regardless of underlying etiology, can be made worse because of anxiety, fatigue, or stress, as well as other factors (Table 21.7).

Parkinson's disease tremor is characterized as a resting tremor. Many patients notice this tremor when mentally distracted and also notice, at least early in the course, that changing position or even just thinking about the tremor seems to make it stop. It is typically a 4–6 Hz tremor. Mental distracting maneuvers tend to help bring out a resting tremor.

Essential tremor is characterized by postural and kinetic tremor with no identifiable cause or neurological findings. It has a more variable frequency than the typical resting tremor and Parkinson's disease. Patients typically complain of difficulty with eating, writing, and drinking. A useful diagnostic maneuver is to have the patient drink from a cup of water. Drinking alcohol tends to improve this type of tremor, whereas it tends to have no effect on the resting tremor of Parkinson's disease.

Table 21.7 Conditions that can enhance tremors

Mental state – anxiety, stress, fatigue, excitement, anger, nervousness

Physiologic – hypoglycemia, hyperthyroidism, pheochromocytoma, fever/illness

Medications – neuroleptics, lithium, corticosteroids, beta-adrenergic receptor agonists, calcium channel blockers, valproic acid, thyroid hormones, tricyclic antidepressants

Ingested – caffeine, nicotine, monosodium glutamate, ethanol

Table 21.8 Features of patients with psychogenic tremors

Multiple undiagnosed, vague complaints

Absence of significant findings on physical examination or imaging studies

Presence of secondary gain – pending compensation or litigation

Fluctuations in symptoms, body parts affected, severity

Symptoms improve or resolve with mental or physical distraction

Employment in the healthcare field

History of psychiatric illness

Orthostatic tremor is a rare but frequently misdiagnosed condition. It occurs more frequently in women, and the onset is typically in the sixth decade. It manifests as tremor of the legs triggered by standing and tends to get better with the onset of walking.

Cerebellar or Holmes tremor is a common consequence of injury to the cerebellum or its outflow pathways. This type of tremor can have resting, postural, and kinetic components associated with ataxia, dysmetria, and other signs of cerebellar dysfunction.

Psychogenic tremor is the typical hysterical movement disorder. Careful observation of the patient with psychogenic tremor reveals marked fluctuation of the tremor. Inconsistencies during the exam tend to give clues to the physician (Table 21.8).

21.4.9 Myoclonus

Myoclonus is defined as brief, very rapid, sudden, and shock-like jerks that involve anything from the very small muscles to the entire body. These movements can be caused by active muscle contractions (positive myoclonus) or lapses in posture (negative myoclonus). Myoclonus is a descriptive term and not a diagnosis.

There are four broad categories of myoclonus, including physiological, essential, epileptic, and symptomatic.

Physiological myoclonus occurs in normal people and includes hypnic jerks, anxiety-induced myoclonus, exercise-induced myoclonus, and hiccups.

Essential myoclonus is likely a hereditary disorder, which begins at a young age and generally has a benign course.

Epileptic myoclonus occurs in the setting of a seizure disorder and is a component of several different epileptic syndromes. Myoclonus can occur as a component of a seizure or is the sole manifestation of a seizure.

Symptomatic myoclonus refers to syndromes associated with an identifiable underlying disorder. This can result from metabolic derangements such as uremia, hepatic encephalopathy, hypercapnia, and hypoglycemia, and usually produces multifocal, arrhythmic myoclonic jerks predominantly affecting the face and proximal musculature. This is generally in the setting of mental status changes and resolves as the encephalopathy is corrected.

Posthypoxic myoclonus resulting from global cerebral hypoxia from any cause occurs in two forms. Transient rhythmic myoclonic jerks can appear immediately following the hypoxic injury and while the patient is comatose. This signifies a very poor prognosis. The second clinical form is delayed posthypoxic myoclonus, known as Lance–Adams syndrome, which is observed in patients during recovery from coma following cerebral hypoxic injury.

Asterixis, or negative myoclonus, was described originally in patients with hepatic encephalopathy; however, it is now known to occur in numerous other metabolic or toxic disorders. Asterixis can occur in the recovery phase of general anesthesia, with sedative or antiseizure medication (ASM) drug administration, and in normal drowsy individuals.

Management of symptomatic myoclonus is based solely on the treatment of the underlying condition. The myoclonic jerks improve as the underlying condition improves. In certain situations valproic acid and clonazepam are effective in treating symptomatic myoclonus. Physiological myoclonus does not require specific treatment. Although rare, intractable myoclonus can cause hyperthermia, hyperkalemia, hyperuricemia, systemic hypotension, and renal failure secondary to rhabdomyolysis.

21.5 Drug-Induced Movement Disorder

The cause-and-effect relationship between the drug and the movement disorder is poorly understood, but pre-existing CNS pathology likely predisposes to the development of movement disorders.

There are many medications that have a tendency to cause movement disorders. The most common medications include ASMs, neuroleptics, stimulants, oral contraceptives, antihistaminics, and antidepressants.

21.5.1 Antiseizure Medications

Toxicity of phenytoin and carbamazepine can lead to cerebellar signs. These include nystagmus, dysarthria, and ataxia. Asterixis and spontaneous myoclonic jerks are common in the toxicity of phenytoin, phenobarbital, primidone, and carbamazepine. Chorea and dystonia can be observed with ASM use and are usually secondary to chronic use of multiple ASMs concurrently. Approximately 20–25% of patients taking valproic acid have a postural tremor that is similar to essential tremor or enhanced physiologic tremor.

21.5.2 Neuroleptic Agents

There are five major categories of movement disorders associated with the use of neuroleptic medications. These are: (1) acute dystonic reactions, (2) akathisia, (3) drug-induced parkinsonism, (4) tardive disorders, and (5) neuroleptic malignant syndrome.

1. *Acute dystonic reactions* tend to occur within 96 hours of initiation of therapy 95% of the time. Acute dystonic reactions typically involve cranial or truncal musculature. Children tend to have more generalized involvement, particularly of the trunk and extremities. Acute dystonic reactions are the most common cause of oculogyric crisis, which consists of forced conjugate eye deviation upward or laterally, often accompanied by extension or lateral movements of the neck, mouth opening, and tongue protrusion. These reactions typically follow a variable course, with symptoms lasting from minutes to hours and can be difficult to diagnose in the ED because the abnormal movements can subside or fluctuate spontaneously.

   Acute dystonic reactions have a familial tendency and are more common in children, young males, and in relatives of patients with idiopathic torsion dystonia. Females aged 12–19 years are more prone to metoclopramide-induced acute dystonic reaction. A history of these reactions with neuroleptic therapy is an indicator for future risk. Cocaine abuse increases the risk of neuroleptic-induced acute dystonic reaction. The risk of developing an acute dystonic reaction increases with the potency of the neuroleptic agent and occurs more frequently with parenteral neuroleptic use than with oral medications. These reactions resolve spontaneously when the offending drug is withheld. The duration of symptoms depend on the half-life of the drug that caused the reaction.

   Treatments of acute dystonic reactions typically include anticholinergic agents such as benztropine, and parenteral administration of these medications can control the signs and symptoms of an acute dystonic reaction quickly. Following the initial dose, maintenance doses of benztropine should be continued for 7–14 days to prevent recurrence. Alternatively, diphenhydramine can also be used.

2. *Akathisia* is a subjective sensation of restlessness commonly associated with the inability to remain seated. Abnormal limb sensation, inner restlessness, dysphoria, and anxiety are the commonly described symptoms associated with akathisia. Discontinuing the offending agent and use of amantadine may help treat the symptoms.

3. *Drug-induced parkinsonism* can be caused by several different medications, including neuroleptic medications, antinausea medications, and antihypertensive agents. The features of drug-induced parkinsonism are generally indistinguishable from those of idiopathic Parkinson's disease. In addition to these signs, rhythmic, perioral, and perinasal tremor mimicking a rabbit chewing, termed rabbit syndrome, is typical. Treatment is removal of the offending agent, and if necessary using typical anti-parkinsonian medications.

4. *Tardive dyskinesia* presents as involuntary, stereotypical movements involving oral, facial, neck, trunk, and axial muscles. It tends to occur following prolonged use of neuroleptic medications and occurs in about 20% of patients treated with these drugs. Tardive dyskinesia is often precipitated or worsened when the dose of the neuroleptic is reduced or the drug is withdrawn. Increasing age increases the risk of developing tardive dyskinesia. Treatment typically includes amantadine, dopamine-blocking medications (haloperidol), or dopamine-depleting medications (tetrabenazine).

5. *Neuroleptic malignant syndrome* is reviewed in Chapter 25.

21.5.3 Stimulants

Dextroamphetamine, methylphenidate, pemoline, and cocaine are all stimulant (dopaminomimetic) drugs with peripheral and central actions. Chorea, oral facial dyskinesia, stereotyped movements, dystonia, and tics are associated with these medications.

21.5.4 Oral Contraceptives

Chorea is the most frequently experienced movement disorder caused by the use of oral contraceptives in otherwise healthy young females. The unilateral distribution of chorea suggests the possibility of pre-existing basal ganglia pathology. Symptoms generally abate within a few weeks following the discontinuation of the contraceptive.

21.5.5 Antihistaminics

The use of H1 antihistamine medications is associated with the development of oral facial dyskinesia, blepharospasm, tic-like movements, dystonia, and involuntary, semipurposeful movements of the hands. The use of H2 antihistamine medications is associated with the development of postural and action tremor, dystonic reactions, parkinsonism, confusion, and cerebellar dysfunction. The movement abnormalities induced by these agents are generally short-lived and resolve after the offending medication is discontinued.

21.5.6 Antidepressants

The use of monoamine oxidase inhibitors is associated with tremors and less often with myoclonic jerks. Tricyclic antidepressants such as amitriptyline and nortriptyline can cause choreiform movements infrequently, particularly oral facial dyskinesia.

21.6 Deep Brain Stimulation Therapy

21.6.1 Overview

Deep brain stimulation (DBS) has become a widely accepted therapy for movement disorders, including Parkinson's disease, essential tremor, and dystonia. As DBS becomes increasingly ubiquitous, knowledge of the adverse effects and complications related to stereotactic DBS surgery or stimulation effects will help guide management of patients with implanted DBS systems. Unlike other patients with movement disorders, evaluation of DBS patients in the ED requires an understanding of the particular issues that may affect this unique patient population. As alluded to earlier in the chapter, patients with movement disorders that present to the ED typically do not need an exhaustive battery of laboratory and radiographic testing. However, patients with implanted DBS systems are exceptions to this rule and may benefit from blood work and radiographic imaging (x-rays and CT scans) due to the presence of indwelling hardware. Adverse events that require evaluation in the ED include those related to: (1) surgery, (2) hardware, or (3) stimulation.

21.6.2 Surgery-Related Complications

21.6.2.1 Hemorrhage/Venous Infarction

Characteristics

Intracerebral hemorrhage (ICH) is the most feared consequence of stereotactic neurosurgery, with rates ranging from 0.6% to 3.3%. As part of routine postoperative care following DBS surgery, most neurosurgeons obtain a noncontrast head CT to ensure proper electrode placement and to exclude intracerebral hemorrhage. However, a negative CT scan after initial electrode placement does not preclude hemorrhage from occurring in a delayed fashion, especially venous infarction. Whereas the vast majority of patients with ICH following DBS are asymptomatic, most large series report symptomatic hemorrhage rates of 0.7–1.2% and rarely occur at the level of the stereotactic target but instead along the electrode trajectory. Hemorrhage can manifest clinically as an altered sensorium, decrease in the level of arousal, subtle changes in personality, seizures, or focal neurologic deficits, including hemiparesis. In the case of venous infarction with hemorrhage, these deficits may present several days after surgery, especially after an initial negative head CT following DBS electrode placement.

When a patient who has undergone DBS electrode placement presents with any subtle neurologic findings as described above, a noncontrast CT scan is warranted to rule-out intracerebral hemorrhage as a cause for their clinical presentation. Radiographically, intra-cerebral hemorrhage can be in any of the intracranial compartments, including epidural, subdural, subarachnoid, intraparenchymal, or intraventricular, caused by electrodes as they traverse along their trajectory to reach their intended target. In the case of venous infarcts, hemorrhage occurs as a result of injury to small cortical veins at the time of surgery that were either sacrificed to allow for electrode placement or not accounted for on preoperative planning. Age, pre-existing hypertension, number of electrode passes, and trans-sulcal or transventricular approaches are known risk factors for precipitating ICH.

Management

Most ICH is managed conservatively, without the need for surgical intervention. Strict control of blood pressure, prophylactic ASMs when appropriate, and admission to the ICU for serial neurologic assessments is generally the mainstay of therapy. Patients with small hemorrhages generally have an excellent outcome with resolution of their symptoms over time.

21.6.3 Cognitive/Behavioral Problems

Characteristics

Cognitive or behavioral effects are common after DBS surgery, and the vast majority of them are temporary in nature. Postoperative delirium following electrode placement may occur in anywhere from 8% to 22% of patients and may be related to advanced age, disease duration, as well as a pre-existing history of delirium. In addition, anticholinergic medica-tions as well as missed doses of medications (e.g., dopaminergic drugs for Parkinson's disease) may also play a role.

Management

Paramount to management of postoperative delirium in DBS patients is identifying obvious causes (urinary tract infection, hemorrhage, etc.) and instituting appropriate treatment, including hospital admission if necessary. If no obvious cause for delirium or mental status changes can be identified, then a multidisciplinary approach and use of neuroleptic medica-tions may be warranted in the short term until symptoms resolve.

21.6.4 Hardware-Related Complications

21.6.4.1 Loss of Efficacy/Hardware Malfunction

As with all implanted devices, DBS systems are also subject to malfunction, which is most often clinically apparent by loss of DBS efficacy. Symptom "rebound" (see below) is most often due to battery failure; however, other etiologies including lead fracture, lead migration, and extension cable fracture all may be the source of loss of clinical efficacy. In instances where the patient's pre-existing motor symptoms recur in an abrupt onset, the DBS programmer should be called to interrogate the system and check impedances of all contacts to ensure integrity of the entire system. In addition, plain radiographs of the skull and chest should be taken to ensure continuity of the DBS leads and extension cables and to ensure there is no kinking or fracture of either that could contribute to hardware failure. If the radiographs are nondiagnostic and impedances are within a normal range, work-up of other causes of symptom rebound, including infection, should be excluded. In rare cases operative intervention may be necessary to switch the extension cables and/or intracranial leads.

21.6.4.2 Infection

Characteristics

Infection rates following DBS are variable, depending on the institution, with ranges of 1–15%. Management of infections following DBS are particularly important because of the continuity of the system with the intracranial compartment. Thus, any superficial infection of the scalp or pulse generator pocket must be addressed vigilantly due to the potential for development of an intracranial abscess. As stated in other sections, infections can manifest in a number of ways, including superficial wound dehiscence with drainage, fevers, altered mental status, loss of efficacy, and exacerbation of dyskinesias, among others.

Management

It should be noted that while the pulse generator pocket is more likely a source of wound infections in DBS surgery compared to cranial wound infections (up to three times as common), the management is quite different. In the former case, removal of the pulse generator with irrigation and debridement is the mainstay of therapy. Long-term intravenous antibiotics after the pulse generator is removed may salvage the remaining hardware, including the intracranial leads, to allow for stimulation to resume once the infection has cleared. In contrast, cranial wound infections are best managed by removal of the entire system.

21.6.5 Stimulation-Related Complications

21.6.5.1 Motor Symptoms

In contrast to both surgical and hardware-related complications, most stimulation-related adverse effects are transient and generally reversible with adjustment of DBS programming parameters (voltage, pulse width, frequency). Stimulation-related complications may include both motor and nonmotor effects. Motor effects encompass dyskinesias, chorea/ballism, gait disturbances, dysarthria, and hypophonia. In cases of excessive dyskinesias, stimulation parameters may need to be adjusted and dosage of oral medications (e.g., levodopa) reduced over many weeks to find a balance between stimulation efficacy and adverse effects. Most stimulation-related motor adverse effects are reversible with programming adjustments; however, persistence of excessive dyskinesias after thorough medication and stimulation parameter changes should prompt a work-up for underlying infection or other causes. Whereas speech problems prior to DBS typically do not benefit from stimulation, the settings used for optimal tremor control may sometimes induce dysarthria and exacerbate hypophonia. If this is the case, reducing the voltage, changing the configuration of stimulating electrodes, or decreasing stimulation from high- (>100 Hz) to lower-frequency (<100 Hz) stimulation may alleviate symptoms.

Motor symptoms may also manifest as a "rebound" of the patient's pre-existing symptoms prior to DBS implantation. There is abundant evidence that DBS reduces the amount of medications regardless of the underlying movement disorder. The magnitude of efficacy of DBS for motor symptoms parallels the "rebound" effects seen in cases of battery failure. Any patient with a movement disorder (essential tremor, Parkinson's disease, or dystonia) who presents with an exacerbation of their disease process should have evaluation of their pulse generator and system by an experienced DBS programmer. In addition, hardware malfunction or kinking (see the previous section) may also result in symptom rebound and should be thoroughly investigated.

21.6.5.2 Nonmotor Symptoms

Nonmotor adverse effects of stimulation are primarily due to current spread to surrounding neural structures and elements of the limbic system. These effects include feelings of "unpleasantness," paresthesias, and behavioral effects, including depression or mania. Depression in Parkinson's disease patients is common and may lead to suicidal attempt/ideation, and while controversial, DBS may slightly increase this risk. When a patient with DBS presents with severe depression or suicidal ideation, inpatient admission is warranted to allow for a thorough assessment of lead location (using radiographic imaging as necessary), stimulation parameters, and medications. Pseudobulbar affect including mood-incongruent laughing or crying may also follow stimulation changes and can be addressed with stimulation adjustments. In all cases of mood-related effects, efforts should be made to contact the neurosurgeon who performed DBS for evaluation of the system, a movement disorders specialist for thorough assessment of medications, and a psychiatric consultant for further evaluation and treatment. Inpatient admission may be necessary for a multidisciplinary approach to address mood-related complaints, as they may be multifactorial in nature.

21.6.6 Emergency DBS

While DBS is generally performed in an elective fashion, patients with primary or secondary dystonia may present with dystonic storm (status dystonicus [SD]), which is a life-threatening disorder. Dystonic storms may be precipitated by trauma or infection, and result in an exacerbation of the underlying dystonia, resulting in painful, hyperkinetic muscle spasms that may lead to respiratory failure, hyperthermia, rhabdomyolysis, renal failure, and even death. In addition, as DBS has become more common in treating patients with dystonia, those with unilateral DBS systems for dystonia may also present with dystonic storm in cases of a battery failure. In effect, SD may be clinically similar to neuroleptic malignant syndrome or serotonin syndrome. The low incidence of SD makes an approach to managing the condition challenging; however, oral medications such as tetrabenazine and pimozide may be used in conjunction with intravenous medications such as propofol and midazolam.

All patients suspected of having SD should have an emergent neurosurgery consult and be admitted to the ICU for supportive care and sedation, with endotracheal intubation if necessary due to the high risk for respiratory compromise. Treatment includes the use of intravenous midazolam and propofol as well as intrathecal baclofen. In patients in whom these measures are ineffective and in whom symptoms continue for an extended period of time, DBS of the globus pallidus may be effective.

Pearls and Pitfalls

- Movement disorders resulting from an acute event such as a stroke, requiring emergent imaging studies, are rare but commonly present as an acute onset of focal or "hemi-distribution" abnormal movements.
- Acute changes in patients with Parkinson's disease are rarely related to the disease itself and are commonly medication-induced or signs of infection or metabolic disturbance.
- Many movement disorders lead to impaired postural reflexes and are a common cause of falls presenting to the ED.
- Acute dystonic reactions may present to the ED as a new onset of painful muscle spasms. These are usually caused by medication, such as neuroleptics, making a good medication history essential.
- The most common cause of chorea evaluated in the ED is L-dopa-induced chorea or dyskinesia in a patient with Parkinson's disease.
- Transient tic disorder is common in children, with an estimated prevalence of 5–24% in school-age children. Treatment is not necessary unless these tics are injurious or stigmatizing to the patient.
- Abrupt discontinuation of dopamine replacement therapy in Parkinson's disease can cause neuroleptic malignant syndrome.
- The increasing usage of deep brain stimulation in patients with Parkinson's disease, essential tremor, and dystonia is leading to new ED visits. The complications will likely require a multidisciplinary approach to address.

Bibliography

Carlson JD, Neumiller JJ, Swain LD, et al. Postoperative delirium in Parkinson's disease patients following deep brain stimulation surgery. *J Clin Neurosci* 2014;**21**(7): 1192–1195.

Fenoy AJ, Simpson Jr RK. Risks of common complications in deep brain stimulation surgery: management and avoidance. *J Neurosurg* 2014;**120**:12.

Jankovic J, Tolosa E (eds.) *Parkinson's Disease and Other Movement Disorders*. Urban and Schwarzenberg, 1987.

Kurlan R (ed.) *Treatment of Movement Disorders*. JB Lippincott, 1995.

Mariotti P, Fasano A, Contarino MF, et al. Management of status dystonicus: our experience and review of the literature. *Mov Disord* 2007;**22**(7):963–938.

Morishita T, Foote KD, Burdick AP, et al. Identification and management of deep brain stimulation intra- and postoperative urgencies and emergencies. *Parkinsonism Relat Disord* 2010;**16** (3):153–162.

Pepper J, Zrinzo L, Mirza B, Foltynie T, et al. The risk of hardware infection in deep brain stimulation surgery is greater at impulse generator replacement than at the primary procedure. *Stereotact Funct Neurosurg* 2013;**91**(1):56–65.

Sillay KA, Larson PS, Starr PA. Deep brain stimulator hardware-related infections: incidence and management in a large series. *Neurosurgery* 2008;**62**(2):360–366.

Solimena M, Folli F, Denis-Donini S, et al. Autoantibodies to glutamic acid decarboxylase in a patient with stiff-man syndrome, epilepsy, and type I diabetes mellitus. *N Engl J Med* 1988;**318**(16):1012.

Teive HA, Munhoz RP, Souza MM, et al. Status dystonicus: study of five cases. *Arq Neuropsiquiatr* 2005;**63**: 26–29.

Watts R, Koller W (eds.) *Movement Disorders: Neurologic Principles and Practice*, 2nd ed. McGraw-Hill, 2004.

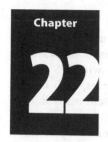

Chapter 22

Multiple Sclerosis

Thomas F. Scott and Omar Hammad

22.1 Introduction

Multiple sclerosis (MS) is a common disorder, characterized by inflammatory lesions of the CNS (brain and spinal cord), affecting approximately 0.15% of the population in the United States. The disease has a peak incidence in the third and fourth decades of life, typically presenting in this age group as relapsing–remitting disease (RRMS). Patients with RRMS present to the emergency department (ED) with acute exacerbations of their illness, as well as "pseudorelapses" relating to concomitant illness, often febrile. Good recovery from attacks is typically seen following the initial attacks. Attack frequency decreases with time, but many patients begin to accumulate permanent disability within the first decade after onset. In patients over 40 years of age, the disease presents commonly as a slow primary progressive illness (PPMS). Approximately 10–15% of patients have PPMS. Patients with PPMS present to the ED with commonly occurring problems associated with their illness such as pain and spasticity, and with acute worsening neurological symptoms caused by infection (often of the urinary tract) and other illnesses (i.e., pseudorelapse).

MS is diagnosed primarily from clinical data (obtained through history and physical exams) and "paraclinical" laboratories (MRI primarily, and sometimes CSF examination). Other possible causes of presenting signs and symptoms must be ruled out. The criteria developed by the Schumacher panel in 1965 are the most widely used clinical guidelines for the diagnosis of MS. According to these guidelines, a patient must exhibit neurological abnormalities attributable to the CNS involving two or more areas (primarily white matter), and two or more episodes of associated dysfunction must occur, each lasting more than 24 hours. Alternatively, a stepwise progression of neurological disability over a 6-month period or more can qualify a patient for the diagnosis. Several additional diagnostic tests can be used to help establish the diagnosis of MS and rule-out other disorders. Nonspecific tests for inflammatory disorders that can mimic MS are generally used to help establish the initial diagnosis (sedimentation rate, serum IgG levels, autoantibody testing). CSF testing might include IgG index, oligoclonal bands, and routine cell counts, glucose, and protein. In difficult-to-diagnose cases, evoked potential studies are employed. Interpretation of MRI scanning, showing a classic shape and distribution of lesions, is not only the mainstay of the laboratory evaluation, but is essential to verify the diagnosis. A classic-appearing MRI, with several rounded lesions, is considered sufficient for a high suspicion of the diagnosis in the classic presenting clinical settings. In 1983, a new set of diagnostic criteria were elaborated that included the use of these tests and characterized patients as having either probable or definite MS. Over the past few decades newer criteria have been proposed and refined, retaining the basic principles of separation of lesions in time and space, often accompanied by evolving lesions seen on MRI.

22.2 Pathophysiology

The primary pathological event in MS lesion development is an immune-mediated destruction of the neuronal myelin sheath, often resulting in axonal transection. Some scattered remyelination takes place, but this is probably of minor importance following MS attacks. Inflammatory perivenular lesions are composed mainly of T lymphocytes, with macrophages present during acute lesion development. Wallerian degeneration of many injured neurons ultimately leads to cerebral and spinal cord atrophy. Lesions of MS may be present throughout the white matter of the CNS, but they have a predilection for the optic nerve, periventricular white matter, spinal cord, and brainstem. Based on pathological or immunological criteria, it is often difficult to differentiate between lesions of MS and other demyelinating diseases such as neuromyelitis optica (Devic's disease), acute transverse myelitis (ATM), and encephalomyelitis. Differentiation between MS and these rarer entities is achieved primarily on a clinical, not a histopathological, basis. An increasing appreciation for cortical demyelination and gray matter atrophy has evolved as part of the basic pathology of MS, creating an emphasis on looking beyond cerebral white matter.

22.3 Evaluation and Management

The inflammatory lesions of MS can affect any part of the CNS, including the optic nerves, resulting in a wide variety of presenting symptoms. The first symptoms of MS are commonly weakness, paresthesias, visual loss, incoordination, vertigo, and sphincter impairment. Onset of symptoms occurs most typically over days, but stroke-like onset may evolve over minutes to hours. Symptoms referable to MS involving the spinal cord commonly present in an asymmetrical fashion (i.e., partial transverse myelitis). Lhermitte's sign (electric-like sensations radiating up and down the spine, often exacerbated by neck flexion) is commonly observed. A "sensory-level" or hemi-spinal cord syndrome (Brown–Sequard) may also be observed. Other presenting symptoms include speech disturbance, a wide variety of pain syndromes, including radicular pain, and transient acute nonpositional vertigo. Psychiatric manifestations of MS include depressive illness, manic-depression (observed much less frequently), and psychosis (observed rarely). Other "clinically isolated syndromes" at presentation include optic neuritis (about one-quarter of cases at presentation) and brainstem syndromes such as internuclear ophthalmoplegias (INOs).

22.3.1 Neurological Examination

The neurological examination of patients with MS may be normal, minimally abnormal, or markedly abnormal. Focused testing of cranial nerve function, strength, coordination, gait, and sensation, and an evaluation for pathological reflexes are important. It is best to record corrected visual acuity with a Snellen chart and to determine whether optic disc (i.e., nerve head) pallor exists. Assessment for red desaturation is carried out by asking the patient to view a red object with each eye in an alternating fashion and indicate any subjective change in depth of color. A decrease in perception of the color red in one eye suggests impairment of vision in that eye. The typical visual field loss in optic neuritis is a central scotoma. Occasionally, a junctional defect (a small temporal area of field loss opposite a more severe and generalized field loss) may be observed. Rarely, altitudinal defects, arcuate defects, or peripheral visual loss are noted. Disc swelling is present in up to 10% of patients with MS during acute optic neuritis, and sometimes optic disc pallor from an old asymptomatic injury is observed. An afferent pupillary defect (Marcus–Gunn pupil) is often found. INO is a classic finding in patients with MS.

22.3.2 Common Presentations and Differential Diagnosis

22.3.2.1 Optic Neuritis

The onset of MS is heralded by a bout of optic neuritis in about 25% of patients with MS, and about 50% of patients with MS eventually develop optic neuritis. Typically, optic neuritis is associated with pain either preceding, during, or following the onset of visual loss. The pain is often accentuated with eye movement, and the eye may be tender. The onset of visual loss can be sudden but is more often gradual over one or more days, especially when progressing to blindness. Visual problems are described initially as blurred vision or a sensation of looking into a fog. The differential diagnosis for optic neuritis primarily includes anterior ischemic optic neuropathy, viral papillitis, and central retinal artery occlusion (Table 22.1). Anterior ischemic optic neuropathy is unlikely to occur in young patients and is associated with risk factors for arterial disease. Central retinal artery occlusion is generally a disorder of the elderly and is associated with a pale retina and a cherry-red spot in the macula. MRI at the time of presentation with optic neuritis can identify those at increased risk for achieving a diagnosis of MS, and can help rule-out other optic neuropathies.

22.3.2.2 Stroke-Like Syndromes

The most important and difficult diagnostic decisions made in the ED involve distinguishing the acute onset of RRMS from symptoms due to CNS ischemia. Although several episodic or multifocal CNS disease processes can resemble MS, stroke is the most common alternative cause of acute focal or multifocal neurological dysfunction in young people, approaching the incidence of MS. An apoplectic onset of MS is rare, and this is the most important historical feature distinguishing the two processes. Clinical features suggesting a single lesion in the CNS favor a diagnosis of stroke in the acute setting. The presence of risk factors associated with stroke is sought, as is a complete review of systems to assess for features of connective tissue disease or coagulopathy. A history of migraine or "complicated" migraine is sought in patients with acute or rapidly evolving deficits, because complicated migraine can mimic a transient ischemic attack or acute MS symptoms. However, a prominent headache component is unusual in MS and is more commonly associated with complicated migraine or stroke.

22.3.2.3 Primary Progressive Multiple Sclerosis

Primary progressive multiple sclerosis (PPMS) presents a different set of differential diagnoses than RRMS. It occurs primarily in patients over 40 years of age, and is as common as RRMS among patients who are newly diagnosed after 55 years of age. Patients are affected primarily in the lower extremities with weakness and spasticity, and occasionally signs of cerebellar dysfunction are also observed. These patients are typically evaluated in an outpatient setting and rarely present to the ED for their initial evaluation. Spinocerebellar degenerative syndromes are the most difficult to distinguish from this form of MS. Insidious spinal cord compression due to cervical stenosis is also an important condition to consider in the differential diagnosis.

Table 22.1 Differential diagnosis for new-onset MS categorized by neuroanatomical presentation of a hemispheric or brainstem focal lesion

Mass lesion

Cerebrovascular event

  Ischemic stroke

  Intracerebral hemorrhage

Hemispheric or brainstem multiple lesions

  Neoplastic (multifocal primary or metastatic)

  Infectious (abscess)

  Cerebrovascular

    Cardioembolic (consider subacute bacterial endocarditis and atrial lesions)

    Coagulopathies (often resulting in cardiac emboli)

    Vasculitis/connective tissue diseases

    Moyamoya disease

Spinal cord lesion

  Acute transverse myelitis (acute transverse myelopathy)

  Ischemic injury/vascular malformation

  Mass lesion

  Connective tissue disease/sarcoidosis/vasculitis

Ocular onset

  Amaurosis fugax/vascular

  Papilledema

  Viral papillitis

Spinal cord and ocular combined

  Devic's disease (neuromyelitis optica)

  Vasculitis/sarcoidosis/connective tissue disease

  Metastatic disease

Spinal cord and brain

  Encephalomyelitis

  Vasculitis/sarcoidosis/connective tissue disease

  Metastatic disease

22.3.2.4 Myelopathy

An urgent evaluation for spinal cord compression by a mass lesion is necessary when signs of acute or subacute spinal cord dysfunction are present. If a compressive lesion is not found by MRI or myelography, ATM and MS are considered as possible causes of myelopathy. These conditions are often identified by the increased signal observed in the spinal cord on T2-weighted MRI (Figure 22.1). MS presenting as a spinal cord lesion is

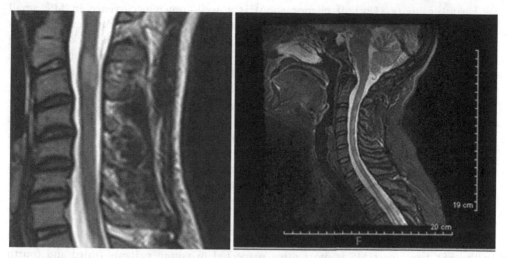

Figure 22.1 Idiopathic ATM (left) and mild partial myelitis as a presentation for MS (right).

much more likely to be associated with asymmetrical motor and sensory signs. In ATM, a sensory level is almost always present, motor findings are symmetrical, and sphincter dysfunction is also usually present. Urinary retention requiring bladder catheterization is common.

22.4 Associated Syndromes

Fatigue is a very common symptom in patients with MS. Symptoms associated with fatigue are often mistaken for depression in patients with MS. Because many patients who have MS also have anxiety, an initial misdiagnosis of a somatoform condition or depression is common. When evaluating patients with fatigue, consideration is given to thyroid function, electrolyte imbalance, hematological abnormalities, and connective tissue disease. New and established MS patients are prone to many brief but repetitive episodic syndromes such as trigeminal neuralgia pain, which may occur up to several times per day. Paroxysmal attacks of motor or sensory phenomena can occur with demyelinating lesions in various locations. They are likely caused by ephaptic transmission of nerve impulses at sites of previous or acute disease activity (symptoms do not necessarily indicate a true exacerbation of MS). Dystonic spasms are correlated with thalamic lesions. The dystonia is characterized by painful tonic contractions of muscles of one or two (ipsilateral) limbs, trunk, and occasionally the face. Brainstem lesions may cause paroxysmal diplopia, facial paresthesia, ataxia, and dysarthria. Spinal lesions cause a variety of painful sensations such as "the MS hug," in addition to the classic Lhermitte's sign. Other common syndromes include recurrent vertigo and Uhthoff's phenomenon, typically caused by overheating. Events may be triggered by movement, heat, or other sensory stimuli. These paroxysmal attacks often respond to low doses of antiseizure medications (ASMs) such as carbamazepine and valproic acid and frequently remit after weeks or months, often without recurrence. Other ASMs such as gabapentin, tiagabine, and oxcarbazepine have been used in small case studies. Less frequently used medications include benzodiazepines, baclofen, acetazolamide, ibuprofen, and bromocriptine.

Heat sensitivity (Uhthoff phenomenon) is a well-known occurrence in MS; small increases in the body temperature can temporarily worsen current or pre-existing signs and symptoms. This phenomenon is presumably the result of conduction block developing in central pathways as the body temperature increases. Symptom worsening can result from passive heat exposure, exercise, or a combination of heat exposure and increases in metabolism. Both physical and cognitive functions can be impaired by heat exposure, impacting overall patient safety and performance of routine activities of daily living. Symptom worsening is commonly seen after a hot shower or sunbathing. In sensitive patients, fluctuations in circadian body temperature from the morning to the afternoon can illicit changes in symptoms. Typically, deficits caused by increases in temperature are reversible by removing heat stressors and allowing subsequent cooling. Cooling strategies can include cold showers, applying ice packs or regional cooling devices, and drinking cold beverages.

22.5 Other Conditions

In the ED, new-onset MS is most often suspected in young patients (third and fourth decades of life) with acute or subacute neurological dysfunction. The differential diagnosis includes causes of stroke in young patients, which include cardiac emboli, coagulopathies (e.g., antiphospholipid antibody syndrome), and connective tissue diseases (e.g., vasculitis and other vasculopathies associated with systemic lupus erythematosus, periarteritis nodosa). Encephalomyelitis is a monophasic, often postinfectious disorder resembling MS in its histopathology and MRI findings, and is considered in the differential diagnosis of MS (Table 22.1). Lyme disease is also a consideration in the differential diagnosis of MS; Lyme disease mimicking MS but lacking other features suggestive of Lyme disease is uncommon. Sarcoidosis involving the CNS can be exceedingly difficult to distinguish from MS when systemic signs are absent; however, the prevalence of CNS sarcoidosis is very low. A "rheumatological review of systems" is helpful in determining initial laboratory testing, with special attention to the presence of rash, arthralgias, sicca syndrome, dry cough, and venous thrombosis.

22.6 Ancillary Tests

MRI or, less optimally, CT of the brain (without and with contrast), when available, provides the most comprehensive assessment in the ED. Neuroimaging assists in differentiating MS from mass lesions, infections, or strokes. MRI is a sensitive test for demonstrating lesions due to MS and is fairly specific for diagnosing MS in young patients (Figure 22.2).

MRI is much more sensitive in detecting MS than is CT scanning. Although often useful, abnormalities of CSF analysis, such as oligoclonal bands and elevated IgG concentration, are nonspecific and can be seen in other inflammatory and noninflammatory disorders. Evoked potential studies are generally done electively and also provide relatively nonspecific information concerning lesions of the optic nerve, spinal cord, and brainstem. A concise battery of rheumatological screening tests, including antinuclear antibody testing, erythrocyte sedimentation rate, Lyme titers, angiotensin-converting enzyme level (sarcoidosis), and SS-A and SS-B autoantibody titers (Sjögren's disease), is especially relevant when the patient's review of systems suggests the possibility of a rheumatological or a collagen vascular disorder. A complete blood count, including

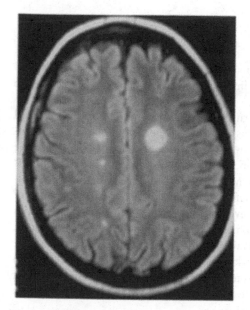
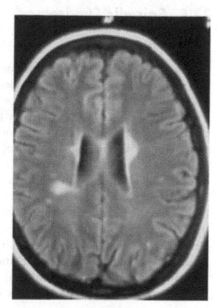

Figure 22.2 T2-weighted MRI scan showing typical globular periventricular white matter lesions.

platelets, and a coagulation profile are important in assessing possible hematological or coagulation defects. If lumbar puncture is considered to be required in the emergency setting for suspected MS, CSF findings in acute phases of MS include a slightly increased protein level, a mild lymphocytosis, and a normal glucose level. Test results for oligoclonal bands and other abnormalities of CSF immunoglobulins are not immediately available in the ED. Oligoclonal IgG bands are present in the CSF but not in the plasma in up to 95% of patients with MS.

22.7 Management

Patients with RRMS who experience an acute exacerbation of their illness present with either recurrence or worsening of old symptoms, or entirely new neurological symptoms. Although the long-term benefit of intravenous or oral corticosteroids is questionable in the treatment of acute relapses, many patients are "steroid-responsive," and the use of corticosteroids should be strongly considered in this group of patients. The role of corticosteroids in the treatment of chronic MS remains more controversial. However, corticosteroids are widely used and given either intravenously at high doses over a period of several days or orally in moderate or high doses over variable periods of time. Decisions about the use and dosing of corticosteroid therapy are made in conjunction with a neurologist. Immunosuppressive therapy with cyclophosphamide, azathioprine, or methotrexate in special situations is also considered, although the efficacy of these agents remains inconclusive. The first medications clearly shown to reduce the attack frequency in RRMS were interferon beta-1b, interferon beta-1a, and glatiramer acetate; these medications also appear to decrease accumulation of disability. More recently approved medications include natalizumab, fingolimod, teriflunimide, dimethlyfumerate, alemtuzimab, and ocrelizumab.

22.8 Episodic Syndromes

22.8.1 Disposition

Patients with new neurological symptoms or signs referable to one or more areas of the CNS by history and examination are considered for admission to the hospital for a comprehensive diagnostic evaluation (Figure 22.3).

Inpatient evaluation is based on the severity of symptoms and the overall clinical condition. Patients with mild symptoms such as paresthesias and numbness can be considered for outpatient evaluation. Many patients with an established diagnosis of MS require hospitalization with an acute loss of ambulation, deterioration of swallowing function, or other disabling effects of an acute exacerbation. Many patients require initiation or adjustment of medications for management of specific symptoms such as spasticity, bladder dysfunction, or psychiatric disturbance. Acute severe flexor spasms of the lower extremities may be managed effectively as above with benzodiazepines, baclofen, or other medications. Urinary tract infections are common in patients with moderately advanced MS and may be associated with lethargy and exacerbation of weakness or spasticity. Bladder catheterization for urinary retention is frequently required. An urgent psychiatric consultation is prudent in cases of suicidal depression or psychosis. A search for coexisting diseases is undertaken,

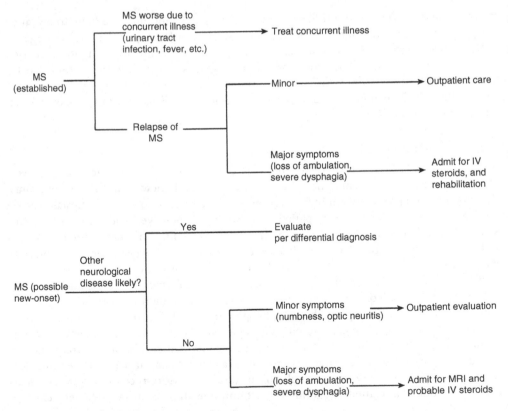

Figure 22.3 Multiple sclerosis management flowchart.

especially in patients with a recurrence of previous neurological symptoms; underlying infections often are responsible for this condition even in the absence of new CNS inflammation due to MS.

Pearls and Pitfalls
• Patients must have two bouts of neurological dysfunction referable to the CNS, or one bout plus an evolving MRI, to be considered for the diagnosis of RRMS.
• Patients should have experienced at least six months of progressive or stepwise neurological dysfunction to be considered for the diagnosis of PPMS.
• Emergency physicians should attempt to review briefly the neurological history of patients presenting with established MS before treating new or acute problems. Causes of neurological dysfunction other than MS must be considered.
• In patients with poorly documented history, minimal neurological findings, or other equivocal factors contributing to a possible diagnosis of MS, documentation of an MRI scan consistent with the diagnosis of MS is the single most helpful factor.

Bibliography

Davis SL, Wilson TE, White AT, Frohman EM. Thermoregulation in multiple sclerosis. *J Appl Physiol* 2010;**109**:1531–1537.

Humm AM, Beer S, Kool J, et al. Quantification of Uhthoff's phenomenon in multiple sclerosis: a magnetic stimulation study. *Clin Neurophysiol* 2004;**115**:2493.

Matthews WB (ed.) *McAlpine's Multiple Sclerosis.* Churchill Livingstone, 1991.

Poser CM, Paty DW, Scheinberg L, et al. New diagnostic criteria for multiple sclerosis: guidelines for research protocols. *Ann Neurol* 1983;**13**:227–231.

Poser C, Presthus J, Horstal O. Clinical characteristics of autopsy-proved multiple sclerosis. *Neurology* 1966;**16**:791.

Selhorst JB, Saul RF. Uhthoff and his symptom. *J Neuroophthalmol* 1995;**15**:63.

Schumacher GA, Beebe G, Kibler RF, et al. Problems with experimental therapy in multiple sclerosis: report by the panel on evaluation of experimental trials of therapy in multiple sclerosis. *Ann NY Acad Sci* 1965;**122**:552–568.

Chapter 23

Hydrocephalus and Shunt Evaluation

Kristen Stabingas, Diana J. Jho, Raj Nangunoori,
Alexander K. Yu, and Jody Leonardo

23.1 Introduction

Hydrocephalus is an extremely common neurological condition encountered in the emergency department (ED). The condition is characterized by symptomatic inability to drain or resorb CSF, resulting in pressure build-up within the brain. Hydrocephalus can result from both congenital and acquired etiologies, many of which can respond to shunting. The symptoms of hydrocephalus are classically due to an increase in intracranial pressure (ICP); however, normal- or low-pressure variants can occur. Hydrocephalus can result from a blockage within the ventricular system ("obstructive") or outside the ventricular system ("communicating"), thereby impairing CSF absorption into the cerebral venous sinuses. Hydrocephalus may also be caused by failure of CSF to be absorbed secondary to abnormalities in the brain parenchyma itself.

23.2 Hydrocephalus and Shunting

For the past 50 years, the mainstay of treatment for hydrocephalus has been shunting, a surgical procedure performed under general anesthesia in which CSF is diverted from the ventricular system to another body compartment by placement of a small drainage catheter. The catheter is then tunneled to an anatomical space of absorption which is usually (and preferentially) the peritoneum due to its high absorption capacity. Alternative recipient sites (pleural cavity, atrium of the heart, gallbladder, and ureter) are sometimes utilized if the peritoneum is unavailable (infection, adhesions).

Hydrocephalus is a particularly challenging pathology, which can be encountered in both pediatric and adult patients. The presenting symptoms may vary and the histories of hydrocephalic patients are often complex. While it may be tempting to treat all cases of hydrocephalus and shunt failure similarly, understanding the differences in etiology (Figure 23.1) will help to direct ED management appropriately.

23.3 Etiologies of Hydrocephalus

Depending on age, hydrocephalus can be congenital or acquired (Table 23.1). Congenital hydrocephalus can be associated with a wide spectrum of underlying pathology, including Chiari malformations (specifically Chiari II associated with hydrocephalus and myelomeningocele), Dandy–Walker malformation, primary aqueductal stenosis, hydranencephaly, and germinal matrix hemorrhage of the preterm newborn. Hydrocephalus can also be acquired secondary to intrauterine or postpartum infection or following a brain tumor resection. Rarely, hydrocephalus may be due to excessive CSF production, which can be seen with choroid plexus papilloma tumors. In adults, hydrocephalus is

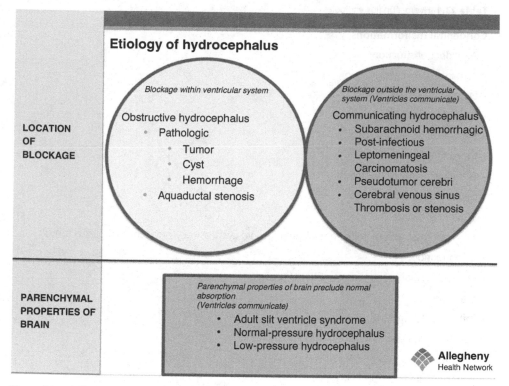

Figure 23.1 Differences in the etiologies of hydrocephalus.

typically acquired following trauma, tumor, infection, intracranial hemorrhage, or sub-arachnoid hemorrhage. Regardless of etiology, CSF diversion has become the gold standard of therapy.

23.4 Shunt Components

While a number of shunt systems currently exist on the market, the components are consistent. A shunt commonly includes three parts: an intraventricular catheter, a regulatory valve, and a distal catheter. Most shunts inserted in clinical practice today also include an additional sampling chamber, known as a reservoir. A reservoir not only allows for CSF sampling via needle puncture, but also provides vital information on shunt patency and ICP, and can be used to evaluate for infection. A collection of x-rays, known as a shunt series, can help the physician determine the manufacturer of the system implanted, the configuration of the shunt apparatus, and the setting of the shunt valve in programmable systems (Figure 23.2). A shunt series typically involves a radiographic image of the skull, the chest, and the abdomen, allowing physicians to visually trace the catheter from the ventricle to its termination.

In its simplest sense, a shunt valve is a mechanical device that regulates CSF flow. Most modern-day valves are one-way differential pressure valves driven by the pressure difference between the ventricular system and the absorption site. Each valve has an inherent manu-facturer-specific mechanism that regulates flow at a set threshold. Most modern-day

Table 23.1 Hydrocephalus etiologies

Congenital malformations

- Aqueduct obstruction
- Arnold–Chiari malformation
- Dandy–Walker syndrome
- Benign intracranial cysts
- Vein of Galen aneurysms
- Craniofacial anomalies
- Germinal matrix hemorrhage

Acquired causes

- Tumors and cysts

  Posterior fossa, pineal, third ventricle (e.g., colloid cyst), astrocytoma, choroid plexus tumor
- Inflammation

  Meningitis, granulomatous conditions/sarcoid
- Infections
- Intracranial hemorrhage
- Cerebral sinus thrombosis or cerebral sinus stenosis
- Pseudotumor cerebri
- Low-pressure hydrocephalus
- Normal-pressure hydrocephalus (NPH)

systems also include an antisiphon device that prevents excessive flow (or "siphoning") as a result of gravitational hydrodynamics when a patient is upright.

The development of programmable valves, which can be adjusted to increase or decrease CSF egress, revolutionized hydrocephalus management. Programmable valves can be adjusted with handheld tools utilizing magnetic forces to modify the internal mechanics of the valve, thereby increasing or decreasing flow. Skull x-rays (AP and lateral views) can be used in conjunction with the manufacturer's reference materials to identify which system is implanted, as well as the current setting.

23.5 Clinical Presentation

The most challenging part of managing hydrocephalus is the clinical recognition of shunt malfunction. Inevitably, a majority of shunts fail (30–40% by the first year, and 80–90% by 10 years). In pediatric patients with hydrocephalus it is unlikely that they will progress to adulthood without at least a single shunt revision. Pediatric shunt failure may present as headache, irritability, nausea, vomiting, abdominal pain, drowsiness, lethargy, or even an increase in seizure frequency. Children with recurrent shunt malfunctions often present with a similar constellation of signs and symptoms indicative of shunt failure, whereas older children often identify with some degree of certainty that their shunt system may be failing. In infants, parents often play a pivotal role in identifying shunt malfunction, especially

(a)

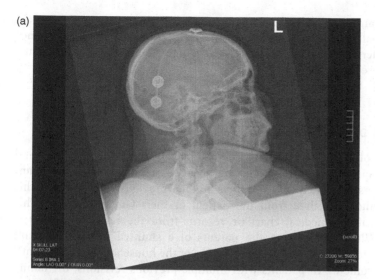

Figure 23.2 Lateral skull x-ray (left) and anterior–posterior view chest/abdominal x-ray (right) demonstrating an intact ventriculoperitoneal shunt system.

(b)

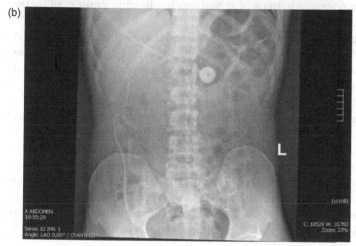

when they have witnessed similar clinical deterioration before. Fever, irritability, and vomiting are nonspecific signs and often present in viral illnesses. However, if the interview of the patient or parents does not convincingly provide evidence of a viral etiology of their symptoms, investigation of the shunt system becomes mandatory. Clinical findings suggestive of shunt malfunction include drowsiness, lethargy, pupillary changes or cranial nerve palsies, Parinaud's syndrome (paralysis of upward gaze), and a bulging fontanelle. Other brainstem signs, including respiratory dysfunction (ataxia or arrest), syncope, and heart rate variability, can all be secondary to increased ICP. In infants with shunted hydrocephalus, shunt malfunction may simply present as increasing head circumference (occipitofrontal circumference [OFC]). Ultimately, any time shunt malfunction is suspected, it is critical to investigate.

23.6 Evaluation

23.6.1 History and Physical Examination

The key to evaluation of any patient (pediatric or adult) is a thorough history and physical examination. Special attention should be given to when and why the shunt was placed, prior revisions, and whether or not the shunt has previously failed. While this information may be difficult to elicit from the patient or their family, obtaining this information by review of the medical chart or records from the referring facility is extremely important. When interviewing the parents of a shunted pediatric patient, focus should be directed toward whether other members of the household or the patient's school have recently become ill. In patients with multiple previous revisions, the family and patient may be able to refer to a pattern of symptoms implicating shunt malfunction that should not be dismissed.

An assessment of frequency of bowel movements is integral as severe constipation may manifest clinically as a distal shunt obstruction. Finally, pediatric patients that develop psychomotor or developmental milestone regression may do so secondary to an insidiously developing shunt malfunction.

The physical examination should focus on the patient's level of consciousness as well as a thorough neurological examination, including cranial nerve examination, motor strength examination, and testing of gait when appropriate. Neuro-ophthalmological signs such as cranial nerve (CN) palsies of III, IV, and VI or the presence of papilledema on fundoscopic examination may precede other symptoms of shunt malfunction. In addition, the course of the shunt from the scalp through the soft tissues of the neck into its final destination should be visually assessed by the examiner to ensure no areas of erythema, subcutaneous fluid tracking around the shunt tract, tenderness, erosion, or exposed hardware. In infants, measuring their OFC and comparing it with their prior head circumferences can also be an indirect measure of shunt functionality.

In peritoneal shunts, a focused abdominal examination should be performed to identify tenderness, guarding, or discomfort. Palpation of the abdominal wall can identify an extraperitoneal loculation or pseudocyst. Peritoneal signs such as severe abdominal pain or diffuse rigidity may indicate an abdominal abscess, which can track up the catheter and lead to meningitis with unusual bacterial species. If an abdominal infection is suspected, a CT of the abdomen should be performed to confirm the diagnosis and a neurosurgical consult should be placed immediately for externalization or removal of the shunt system. Primary abdominal issues such as small bowel obstruction, ileus, appendicitis, and diverticulitis may affect an intact shunt system by elevating abdominal pressures and preventing the normal outflow of CSF into the peritoneal cavity. For shunts terminating in the pleural space, auscultation of the lungs should be performed to rule-out pleural effusions. Above all, it is important to look at the overall clinical picture to ensure that the main causative factor for shunt failure is appropriately addressed.

23.6.2 Shunt Evaluation

Once a thorough history and physical examination have been obtained, attention should be focused toward the shunt system itself. As with any physical examination, inspection is the first step. The entire shunt system should be inspected for areas of swelling, erythema, or exposed hardware. Craniotomy scars and skull defects not only give clues to shunt location, but also to prior cranial surgeries. Distended scalp veins, bulging fontanelles, or swelling around the shunt site can indicate elevated ICP and shunt failure. The distal tubing can usually be followed visually in children, but may not be as obvious in adults. Inspecting the entire course of the tubing is important to identify any areas of underlying discontinuity, perforation, or abscess. Swelling at the distal insertion site indicates fluid tracking up the catheter due to an underlying obstruction.

Palpation of the shunt system allows the assessment of any gaps or irregularities between components of the shunt. The presence and location of reservoirs and pumping chambers can often be identified by palpation alone. A "floating reservoir" may indicate a disconnection with an associated CSF leak. The distal catheter should be traced as far as possible to assess for kinks, discontinuation, swelling, or warmth.

Manual evaluation can help to determine the patency of the shunt but should only be performed under the supervision of the neurosurgical team due to the individualized nature and varying composition of each system. However, manual evaluation can sometimes help the neurosurgeon predict whether shunt failure is due to a proximal or distal occlusion of the system. For example, in some shunt configurations, while manually occluding the shunt proximally, depressing the pumping chamber should eject CSF distally while preventing the refill of the chamber. Easy compression implies that the distal components of the system are patent. Difficulty compressing or high resistance indicates that the distal tubing is blocked or under pressure. When the manual occlusion of the shunt is released, the pumping chamber should quickly refill with CSF from the ventricles. If the chamber remains depressed or fills slowly, the proximal catheter may be partially or completely occluded. An audible "click" may be heard when the valve is compressed, indicating incompetence of the valve.

A shunt tap is a sterile bedside technique performed by neurosurgical practitioners for assessment of shunt system function as well as CSF sampling. A 23-gauge butterfly needle is percutaneously inserted into either the reservoir or a tapping chamber. If spontaneous CSF flow is noted in the needle, an opening pressure is obtained and CSF can be sampled for analysis. If spontaneous flow is absent, this indicates a proximal obstruction with a positive predictive value of 93%. If the opening pressure is elevated with brisk CSF flow from the proximal catheter, an occlusion in the shunt valve or distal catheter is suspected. In this case, draining a larger volume of CSF may act as a temporizing measure in cases of impending herniation (please see Chapter 16). Once CSF has been collected, a closing pressure is measured and documented. CSF should be sent for a stat Gram stain, aerobic and anaerobic cultures, cell count with differential, protein, and glucose. Of note, CSF cultures should be held in the laboratory for 14 days to rule-out a cutibacterium infection (previously *proprionobacterium acnes*), which can cause an indolent infection in shunted patients.

A radionuclide shuntogram, utilizing technetium 99m diethylenetriaminepentaacetic acid (Tc-99 m DTPA) or iohexal (240 mg I/mL), is a radiographic examination that can provide vital details about shunt patency. Similar to a shunt tap, a reservoir or pump chamber is accessed for confirmation of spontaneous CSF flow from the proximal catheter. Once accessed, a small volume of the radionuclide tracer is injected into the shunt system and serial images of the cranium, chest, and abdomen (or alternative terminus) are obtained. The rate of complete clearance of the injected indicator is monitored and free peritoneal spillage should be identifiable in patients with functioning shunt systems. The time of clearance ranges from 9 to 20 minutes, depending on the techniques used. Valve malfunction may be indicated by contrast material reflux from the reservoir into the ventricular system or if the radionuclide does not empty from the shunt system spontaneously. If free peritoneal spillage is not observed, peritoneal obstruction of the distal catheter should be suspected, whereas abnormal pooling in the peritoneum may indicate a pseudocyst or loculation. If the radionuclide or contrast cannot be cleared with pumping of the shunt, a complete distal catheter obstruction is present.

23.6.3 CT and MRI

Imaging studies provide valuable information about shunted patients and should be obtained as soon as shunt malfunction is suspected. In addition to plain-film x-rays (shunt series), CT scans and MRI are considered the gold standard for intracranial evaluation. Current practice relies heavily on neuroimaging as it provides a noninvasive and rapid evaluation of shunt integrity in emergent situations. One of the most valuable aspects of radiographic shunt evaluation is the potential to detect and predict ventricular behavior as assessed on cranial imaging during previous presentations. Changes in morphology of a given patient's ventricular system in the setting of shunt malfunction are often consistent and predictable.

CT features that are helpful in making the diagnosis of hydrocephalus, especially in the setting of shunted hydrocephalus, are global enlargement of the lateral ventricles, outward bowing of the third ventricle, and the emergence of pronounced temporal horns (Figure 23.3). Transependymal edema, or periventricular "blurring," may be visible around the periphery of the ventricular system, which should not be confused with white matter change of small-vessel disease. Longstanding, untreated hydrocephalus can classically result in "copper beaten skull," which describes the prominence of convolutional markings on the inner table of the cranial vault. The convolutional markings are the result of gyral imprints against the skull secondary to raised ICP. Conversely, in the setting of chronic shunting, the process is reversed and a thickened calvarial vault, termed "hyperostosis cranii ex vacuo," can develop as a result of low ICP.

MRI is an effective alternative to CT with the benefit of limiting exposure to ionizing radiation. Radiation exposure is of paramount concern in the pediatric population, prompting many healthcare systems to implement a rapid-sequence MRI protocol as an alternative to standard CT in cases of suspected shunt malfunction. In addition to disproportionate prominence of the ventricles, MRI features of hydrocephalus include pronounced periventricular FLAIR signal (Figure 23.4), partially empty sella turcica, increased fluid along the optic nerves, and elevation of the optic disc.

While the diagnostic value of neuroimaging cannot be overstated, it is important to acknowledge that the diagnosis of shunt failure is not always straightforward. Longstanding hydrocephalus can result in accelerated brain atrophy, which can make

(a)

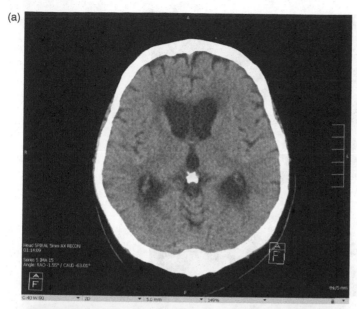

Figure 23.3 CT axial views demonstrating hydrocephalus; lateral/third ventricular enlargement (left) with pronounced temporal horns (right).

(b)

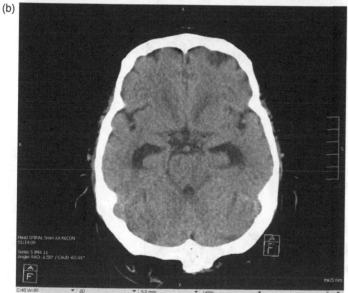

ventricular size a less reliable indicator of a failing shunt. In shunt-dependent patients, especially those shunted from birth, the development of "slit ventricle syndrome" (SVS) may complicate the radiographic diagnosis of shunt failure. Although poorly understood, SVS is thought to develop after multiple cycles of ventricular enlargement and decompression. These recurrent changes in ventricular size cause the system to lose compliance, which hinders its ability to enlarge with increased ICP. SVS patients

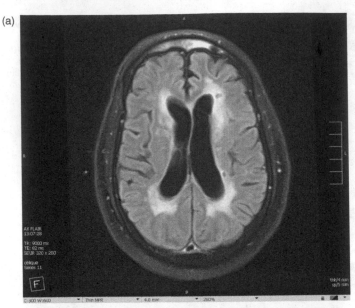

(a)

Figure 23.4 MRI axial views with periventricular FLAIR signal indicative of transependymal flow.

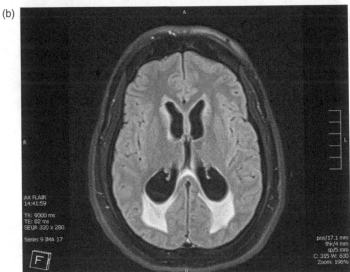

(b)

presenting in shunt failure may have the clinical signs and symptoms of intracranial hypertension, yet imaging will show small, slit-like ventricles with an intact shunt system.

Hydrocephalus and shunt failure can be fatal conditions when left untreated; however, it is of equal importance to recognize the clinical and radiographic signs of shunt over-drainage. Although ventricular shunt systems are regulated through a mechanical valve, there is a potential to drain CSF quicker than the body can

(a)

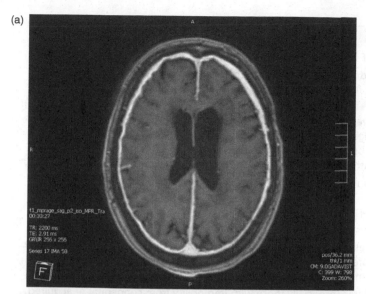

Figure 23.5 MRI axial (a) and coronal (b) views demonstrating diffuse pachymeningeal enhancement in the setting of longstanding ventriculoperitoneal shunt associated over-drainage.

(b)

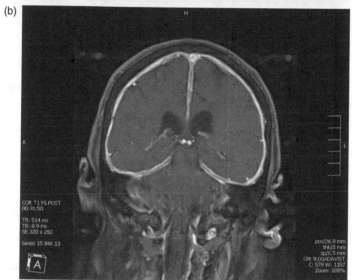

produce it. In these cases, patients will often present with classic positional head-aches that are exacerbated when upright and alleviated when supine. Increasing the shunt valve setting (which correlates with a decrease in CSF egress) will often relieve the symptoms. However, shunt over-drainage can lead to ventricular collapse and subsequent tearing of extra-axial blood vessels, with development of subdural hema-tomas or hygromas. Radiographic clues to over-drainage include distended dural venous sinuses as well as diffuse pachymeningeal enhancement (Figure 23.5).

Pearls and Pitfalls

- Expect up to 30% of shunts to fail in one year and 80% within 10 years.
- Shunt failure in children can present with generalized symptoms. Specific findings suggestive of shunt failure include lethargy, pupillary or cranial nerve changes, and bulging fontanelle.
- Shunt failure in children or adults who are known to be shunt-dependent (i.e., the shunt was placed prior to the age of two, precluding the normal development of the arachnoid granulation, which absorbs CSF resulting in dependence on the shunt to drain CSF) may result in coma or death. Immediate attention and neurosurgical consultation are imperative.
- Ask older children and adults if previous shunt malfunction mimics the current symptoms.
- Always visualize and palpate the entire shunt tubing course for swelling, erythema, or drainage.
- Programmable valves require specific tools necessary to change the settings. There are different manufacturers of programmable valves; each manufacturer produces their own unique programming device.
- Constipation in children, especially those with immobility from congenital or acquired disease processes, can cause distal shunt occlusion.

Bibliography

Bartynski WS, Valliappan S, Uselman JH, Spearman MP. The adult radiographic shuntogram. *AJNR Am J Neuroradiol* 2000;**21**(4):721–726.

Browd SR, Ragel BT, Gottfried ON, Kestle JR. Failure of cerebrospinal fluid shunts: part I. Obstruction and mechanical failure. *Pediatr Neurol* 2006;**34**(2):83–92.

Browd SR, Gottfried ON, Ragel BT, Kestle JR. Failure of cerebrospinal fluid shunts: part II. Overdrainage, loculation, and abdominal complications. *Pediatr Neurol* 2006;**34**(3):171–176.

Chiewvit S, Nuntaaree S, Kanchaanapiboon P, Chiewvit P. Assessment lumboperitoneal or ventriculoperitoneal shunt patency by radionuclide technique: a review experience cases. *World J Nucl Med* 2014;**13**(2):75–84.

Dewey RC, Kosnik EJ, Sayers MP. A simple test of shunt function: the shuntogram. *J Neurosurg* 1976;**44**:121–126.

Di Rocco C, Caldwell M. Surveillance of CSF shunt function. In Di Rocco C (ed.) *The Treatment of Infantile Hydrocephalus*. CRC Press, 1987.

Hayden PW, Rudd TG, Shurtleff DB. Combined pressure-radionuclide evaluation of suspected cerebrospinal fluid shunt malfunction: a seven-year clinical experience. *Pediatrics* 1980;**66**(5):679–684.

Khan AA, Jabbar A, Banerjee A, Hinchley G. Cerebrospinal shunt malfunction: recognition and emergency management. *Br J Hosp Med (Lond)* 2007;**68**(12):651–655.

Masinda AJ, Guazzo EG. Blocked ventriculoperitoneal shunt causing raised intracranial pressure diagnosed by prominent sinus pericranii. *J Clin Neurosci* 2009;**16**(12):1686–1687.

Ouellette D, Lynch T, Bruder E, et al. Additive value of nuclear medicine shuntograms to computed tomography for suspected cerebrospinal fluid shunt obstruction in the pediatric emergency department. *Pediatr Emerg Care* 2009;**25**(12):827–830.

Rekate HL. Shunt revision: complications and their prevention. *Pediatr Neurosurg* 1991;**17**(3):155–162.

Rocque BG, Lapsiwala S, Iskandar BJ. Ventricular shunt tap as a predictor of proximal shunt malfunction in children: a prospective study. *J Neurosurg Pediatr* 2008;1(6):439–443.

Savoiardo M, Solero CL, Passerini A, Migliavacca F. Determination of cerebrospinal fluid shunt function with water-soluble contrast medium. *J Neurosurg* 1978;49:398–407.

Sekhar LN, Moossy J, Guthkelch AN. Malfunctioning ventriculoperitoneal shunts. Clinical and pathological features. *J Neurosurg* 1982;56(3): 411–416.

Thompson EM, Wagner K, Kronfeld K, Selden NR. Using a 2-variable method in radionuclide shuntography to predict shunt patency. *J Neurosurg* 2014;121(6):1504–1507.

Vassilyadi M, Tataryn ZL, Matzinger MA, Briggs V, Ventureyra EC. Radioisotope shuntograms at the Children's Hospital of Eastern Ontario. *Childs Nerv Syst* 2006;22 (1):43–49.

Vernet O, Farmer JP, Lambert R, Montes JL. Radionuclide shuntogram: adjunct to manage hydrocephalic patients. *J Nucl Med* 1996;37(3):406–41.

Chapter 24

Post-Arrest Neurologic Resuscitation

John O'Neill and James P. Valeriano

24.1 Introduction

The management of unresponsive post-cardiac arrest patients has been an area of much controversy and research. Interventions during the arrest, particularly no-pause cardiopulmonary resuscitation (CPR) and the advent of the automated external defibrillator have placed patients in a better position to respond to post-resuscitative measures. The initiation of post-arrest therapeutic hypothermia protocols, now referred to as targeted temperature management (TTM), has resulted in significant improvement in the number of neurologically intact survivors. Post-arrest care is centered on TTM, but includes a series of protocolized steps that define the measures to be taken to optimize outcome in these patients. Post-arrest care is the fifth and final link in the American Heart Association's out-of-hospital chain of survival.

Post-arrest care crosses over several medical environments. Cardiac arrests may occur outside of the hospital, in the Emergency Department (ED), in the operating room, or on various medical wards. Creating a system that can coordinate care of these patients in an organized manner is essential in providing optimal care.

Cardiac arrest patients can be categorized by type of arrest: asystolic, pulseless electrical activity (PEA), and ventricular fibrillation/ventricular tachycardia (Vfib/Vtach). The patients are also dichotomized into in-hospital and out-of-hospital arrests. Arrests can be associated with trauma, recent surgery, toxic ingestion, and medical illnesses.

24.2 Indications for Protocolized Temperature Management

All patients who experience a cardiac arrest and are subsequently not able to follow commands should be considered for post-cardiac arrest protocolized care. Patients with severe medical illnesses, trauma, or surgical causes of arrest may require additional interventions to attempt to identify an underlying cause of the arrest that may exclude patients from a post-arrest protocol. Evidence for TTM in these patients is lacking; however, some benefit may result from protocolized management especially with a higher target temperature of 36°C rather than 33°C.

Current evidence most strongly supports the use of a TTM protocol in patients with an out-of-hospital cardiac arrest (OHCA) with an initial rhythm of Vfib or pulseless Vtach. Evidence for a TTM protocol for non-Vfib/Vtach arrest and in-hospital cardiac arrest (IHCA) is sparse and the results are mixed.

Despite the evidentiary differences in efficacy and outcomes regarding the different types of arrests, the American Heart Association and American College of Cardiology (AHA/ACC) guidelines combine their recommendation together as a Class I, level of evidence

Table 24.1 The European Resuscitation Council TTM Guidelines.

- TTM is recommended for adults after OHCA with an initial shockable rhythm who remain unresponsive after ROSC (return of spontaneous circulation) (strong recommendation, low-quality evidence).
- TTM is suggested for adults after OHCA with an initial nonshockable rhythm who remain unresponsive after ROSC (weak recommendation, very low-quality evidence).
- TTM is suggested for adults after IHCA with any initial rhythm who remain unresponsive after ROSC (weak recommendation, very low-quality evidence).

C expert opinion. The European Resuscitation Council guidelines are more complex and reflect the current level of evidence (Table 24.1).

The strongest evidence for improved clinical outcomes is in out-of-hospital Vfib/Vtach arrests. Using this as a guide, patients who do not fall strictly into this category but have similar features may benefit as well. A patient admitted with chest pain and awaiting a stress test who has a Vfib/Vtach arrest would be someone who should be strongly considered for a post-arrest protocol. Similarly, a patient who chokes on a hot dog, has a brief PEA arrest, and has return of circulation once the airway is secured would also be a good candidate. A third case is a patient who is shot in the thigh, has a PEA arrest that responds well to CPR and rapid transfusion, the source of bleeding is corrected, the vitals stabilize, but the patient does not follow commands. Patients who are otherwise well before the arrest who have a sudden correctable cause of the arrest should be strongly considered for a post-arrest protocol. As more evidence becomes available, there should be more clarity in choosing which patients are most likely to respond to a post-arrest protocol.

24.3 Pre-hospital

In the past, many emergency medical systems had incorporated administration of chilled intravenous (IV) fluids into the post-arrest protocol. Evidence has shown that despite these measures improving time to target temperature, neurological outcomes are not improved and the likelihood of pre-hospital arrest and pulmonary edema is increased. Industry has produced several devices that are designed to cool patients in the pre-hospital setting. None of these devices is supported by evidence of improved outcomes. The lack of efficacy of early cold fluids and the evidence supporting a target temperature of 36°C has caused the theory behind TTM to change from rapid induction of hypothermia to that of fever prevention.

Pre-hospital airway management in cardiac arrest is a complex issue. The time devoted to placement of the airway, the time to arrive at a receiving hospital, and the hemodynamic condition of the patient can all affect the final outcome of the patient. There is preclinical animal evidence that supraglottic airways (SGA) (laryngeal mask airway, etc.) may obstruct cerebral blood flow during CPR. Large studies have been performed with conflicting results when comparing SGAs with endotracheal intubation (ETI). A large meta-analysis concluded that overall ETI patients have better outcomes than SGA patients. Bag valve mask (BVM)-only ventilation is associated with improved outcomes when compared with ETI or SGA according to a large recent study. This result should not imply that ETI or BVM is better for all patients, but that there are many factors that must be considered in choice of airway placement.

24.4 Emergency Department

Post-arrest care continues in the ED. The issues to be addressed by the emergency team are airway and ventilator management, hemodynamic monitoring/interventions, initiation of TTM, and deciding the patient's disposition, be it to transfer the patient, to activate the catheterization team, or to admit the patient to an ICU.

24.5 Airway/Ventilator Management to Protect the Brain

Upon receiving a comatose patient the first priority is to ensure the airway is secure. Patients who continue to be comatose after ROSC and who are not intubated should have a definitive airway placed. Patients with an SGA should be evaluated for early replacement. Endotracheal tubes should be evaluated for proper positioning.

Ventilator management for post-arrest patients is similar to that of other critically ill individuals. Both hypocapnia and hypercapnia are associated with worse outcomes. Patients with a concurrent metabolic acidosis should have their carbon dioxide target adjusted accordingly, as the presence of this metabolic derangement is a worse prognostic factor than hypocapnia. Blood gas measurements should be temperature-corrected to ensure accuracy of the pCO_2 being reported.

Management of oxygen levels in post-arrest patients focuses on avoiding hypoxia and then avoiding hyperoxia. Hypoxia can lead to continued anoxic injury and contribute to poor neurological outcome. Hyperoxia may be associated with reperfusion injury and should be avoided as well. The current AHA/ACC guidelines recommend the practical approach of avoiding hypoxia by using a target of 100% oxygen saturation initially and when a stable accurate saturation can be reliably measured, titrate down and maintain an oxygen saturation greater than 94%. This approach avoids hypoxia while the patient is unstable or can't be well monitored and allows the physician to quickly decrease oxygen delivery to avoid reperfusion injury. Pulse oximeters may be affected by poor perfusion or finger/nail coloration. Blood gases, including those temperature-corrected, may not be as accurate as the clinician desires. Targeting a range that doesn't get too close to the inflection point in the oxygen dissociation curve (paO_2 of 90 mm Hg) while avoiding a paO_2 >120 mm Hg seems reasonable.

Ventilator humidifiers and warmers have not been a practical impediment in getting a patient to target temperature. The decision to manage a patient's temperature should not alter plans to humidify or warm the air delivered. Decompressing the stomach via an oro- or nasogastric tube may improve venous return, especially if an SGA or BVM has been used for a prolonged period of time.

24.6 Hemodynamic Monitoring for Neuroprotection Post-Arrest

Recommendations for blood pressure management in post-arrest patients are difficult to make as these patients may have varying degrees of dysfunction in multiple aspects of hemostasis. Vasodilation, reduced cardiac output, and oncotic pressures may play varying roles in different patients. While data are sparse, avoiding renewed hypotension is a goal. There is no target number for mean arterial pressure or systolic pressure that has been clearly shown to be superior. Adrenal insufficiency, hypothermia-associated diuresis, lactic acidosis, and the patient's baseline status should all be considered. A systematic review showed that while higher blood pressure and the avoidance of hypotension were associated with improved outcomes, there was too much heterogeneity in the studies to recommend any specific target. There are no clear-cut recommendations regarding post-arrest blood pressure management that would apply specifically to post-arrest patients. Cerebral perfusion pressure is the difference between the mean arterial pressure (MAP) and the intracranial pressure (ICP). Increased ICP that may be induced by brain edema should be considered when setting blood pressure goals for the patient; a MAP of 65 mm Hg may not be adequate.

Other markers for hemodynamics have been proposed such as monitoring urine output and central venous pressure. Cold diuresis, an increase in urine output that is thought to occur due to therapeutic hypothermia itself, may not be as important as first thought.

Ionotropic medications can be used to increase cardiac output, but may drop the MAP and should be monitored closely. In addition, vasopressors cause vasoconstriction that may exacerbate the cause of the arrest (e.g., acute myocardial infarction). Balloon pumps and other devices may be used to support pressure as well as extracorporeal membrane oxygenation (ECMO), which has the added benefit of providing excellent temperature control.

24.7 Emergent Cardiac Catheterization

There has been increasing, albeit observational, evidence that emergent catheterization and percutaneous coronary intervention leads to better outcomes in post-arrest patients. Patients with cardiac arrest, especially those with ST elevations on post-arrest EKG, are exceedingly likely to have coronary artery disease and are very likely to have a culprit lesion. A substantial minority of cardiac arrest patients without ST elevations or those suffering a PEA arrest still have coronary artery disease and culprit lesions. Patients have a survival benefit from early catheterization even when a culprit lesion is not found and no intervention takes place. The timing of the catheterization, differentiating emergent and early strategies, has been discussed and in at least one study the strategies have been shown to be equivalent.

There are controversies surrounding the eligibility of cardiac arrest patients as candidates for early percutaneous coronary interventions due to economic factors. Catheterization lab outcome results are publicly reported and may be tied to compensation from insurers and may be publicly reportable. The catheterization labs' mortality rate can affect their funding. Centers may have incentives to avoid unresponsive cardiac arrest patients who have a <50% survival rate. A small number of these patients can skew a center's mortality data and make it appear to be performing much worse than it really is. This can influence resources and public perception of the center that can place further stress on the center in its mission to serve the public.

In order to make best use of the catheterization lab's resources, it is reasonable to try to risk-stratify patients to see which are most likely to survive and to benefit from emergent catheterization. Patients who initially present in category IV (deep coma with loss of most or all brainstem reflexes) in the Pittsburgh Post Cardiac Arrest Category scale were found to have a low overall survival rate and no significant difference in survival with or without emergent catheterization. A more nuanced, though more complex, approach is proposed by Rab et al. A series of 11 factors are to be considered in consultation among the care providers to help determine which patients are best suited for emergent catheterization (Table 24.2). Each factor alone should not be considered an absolute contraindication, but as an

Table 24.2 Eleven factors to consider before post-arrest cardiac catheterization

1. STEMI on post-arrest EKG
2. Likely noncardiac cause of arrest such as drug overdose, respiratory failure, trauma
3. Unwitnessed
4. Initial rhythm non-VF/VT
5. No bystander CPR
6. >30 min to ROSC
7. Continued need for CPR
8. pH <7.2
9. Lactate >7
10. Age >85
11. Dialysis patient

individual data point in making a global decision. The first factor, the presence of STEMI (ST segment elevation myocardial infarction) on the EKG, makes the patient more likely to have a culprit lesion, but doesn't have a strong effect on potential neurologic outcome. The presence of a likely noncardiac cause such as a drug overdose, respiratory failure, or trauma may significantly decrease the likelihood of finding a culprit lesion as well. The next nine factors are used to determine the likelihood of survival and good neurologic outcome.

These factors imply a prolonged or inadequate response to resuscitation or pre-existing conditions that make the patient unlikely to survive the anoxic insult brought on by a cardiac arrest. The utility in listing and enumerating these factors is that these provide objective data to the subjective argument between physicians as to whether a patient is likely to benefit from cardiac catheterization. Unfortunately, this list of factors is not associated with a simple numerical cutoff after which point a patient should or should not be deemed eligible. Furthermore, the relative risk of each factor is not equivalent. A 32-year-old with a brief arrest after a heroin overdose may only score a 1 and be a reasonable person to not take for emergent catheterization, whereas a young dialysis patient who had a PEA arrest might be someone that may be appropriate for intervention.

While this scoring system focuses mostly on markers for neurologic outcomes, others have proposed using a cardiac-focused scoring system. Patients at high risk for coronary artery disease, as defined by the Global Registry of Acute Coronary Events (GRACE) score >140, were shown to benefit from intervention in the absence of other EKG findings. There is no single guideline on how to determine which patients should go to immediate or early coronary intervention. Current recommendations are based on observational studies.

24.8 Post-Arrest Targeted Temperature Management

A revolution in post-arrest care came after the publication of several studies in the early 2000s. These studies described improved survival and neurologically intact survival in patients suffering out-of-hospital VF/VT arrest who were treated with a mild hypothermia protocol. This led many hospitals and EMSs to adopt hypothermia protocols designed to cool patients to a target temperature of 32–34°C as soon as possible after cardiac arrest.

The theory behind the improved survival and neurological outcomes was that the apoptotic cascade initiated by reperfusion of anoxic tissues could be mitigated by cooler temperatures. Subsequent studies were published showing an expanding role for therapeutic hypothermia in non-VF/VT patients and in in-hospital arrests.

All patients who present comatose post-cardiac arrest should be considered for post-arrest temperature management. Alternative sources of coma should be considered, but if there is the possibility that the patient has an altered mental status secondary to a cardiac arrest then the physician should err on the side of initiating management. This recommendation is based on the relatively benign side effect and complication profile found in the TTM study.

Conflicting evidence also started to emerge regarding worse outcomes in patients that reach target temperature early and in a single retrospective study of post-arrest patients treated with or without hypothermia. This set the stage for the largest prospective post-arrest trial to date, the Targeted Temperature Management trial (TTMT). This international trial with a large number of patients (939) compared cooling protocols that were identical with the exception of the target temperature of 33°C or 36°C. The 33°C target was not found to be superior to 36°C in either mortality or good neurological outcome.

For many in the post-arrest community the TTMT called into question the benefits of hypothermia in post-arrest patients. Some even looked at the totality of data and questioned the efficacy of TTM in general. The near normothermic temperature of 36°C is not thought to have an effect on the apoptotic cycle. Several additional research questions resulted from the TTMT: Is it merely the prevention of post-arrest fever that incurs the clinical benefit? Is it the protocol itself with the extra attention being given to the patients that provides the true benefit? The TTMT did not compare therapeutic hypothermia at 33°C to no active temperature management. Like many seminal studies, the TTMT created more questions than it answered.

The most contentious question and the one with the least data to guide the clinician is what is the target temperature? If 36°C is not inferior to 33°C with regard to key clinical outcomes, should that temperature be adopted as a new standard? The post-arrest community is divided between a target of 36°C and 33°C. There is a dearth of evidence in this area and further research is needed. Those who support 33°C cite that the early studies were based on 33°C and that while 36°C may not be inferior, the more robust data at the lower temperature makes them more comfortable using the 33°C standard. Those who favor 36°C argue that the near-normothermia attained in the 36°C group gives patients a better side effect and complication profile, though the data supporting these positions are based on post-hoc analysis of the original TTMT dataset. The original study, while showing a trend toward more complications in the 33°C group, did not reach clinical significance. Further, the TTMT was a noninferiority trial and by design is underpowered to show that 36°C is superior to 33°C. Current guidelines leave a wide range of target temperatures from which the clinician may choose (32°C to 36°C).

Clinical experience suggests that the sicker (older, more comorbidities, prolonged resuscitation) patients seem to tolerate 36°C better than 33°C. Younger, previously healthy patients with no concerns of bleeding, infection, or unstable bradycardia are typically easily cooled to 33°C. Other centers have adopted a one-size-fits-all approach at either 33°C or 36°C. This approach is reasonable as well, as there are not enough data at this time to strongly recommend a particular temperature for any group of post-arrest patients. Temperature variability while under TTM doesn't seem to affect outcome.

Once a choice of target temperature is made, the question remains as to what is the best mechanism to reach the goal. There are many methods of cooling a patient. There are complex devices that allow for minimal intervention and monitoring for the nursing staff, and there are simple cold fluids and ice packs, which are inexpensive but labor-intensive. All mechanisms can provide adequate temperature control, but have their own complications and cost–benefit profiles. A thorough, but likely prone to bias, meta-analysis found that certain device factors, such as invasive devices and those with temperature feedback control, tend to have slightly better neurological outcomes.

Cold saline (4°C) is effective at quickly lowering core temperature but is impractical for prolonged cooling. Ice packs and cooling blankets are relatively cheap but require the nurses to monitor the temperature and apply or remove materials as temperatures change. The temperature of the patient as well as the trend in temperature change over time must be considered; cooling a patient quickly to 33°C with multiple methods may have the patient overshoot and result in a temperature under 32°C, making the patient vulnerable to arrhythmia. Similarly, the patient also may get too warm if the target is 36°C and cooling is reapplied too late. Rewarming these patients is passive and less controlled than with commercial devices.

Cooling devices with smart technology and temperature feedback control allow the physician to set the target temperature and the rate of temperature change and are much easier for the nursing staff to use. The device can be programmed and will then control the temperature tightly throughout the cooling, rewarming, and fever-prevention stages. These are more costly, requiring both the investment in the permanent hardware and the disposable pads or catheters.

Commercial surface cooling devices are noninvasive, easy to apply, and can provide rapidly controlled cooling. These cover parts of the trunk and the thighs and can therefore restrict access to those areas; however, they are easy to peel back and to reapply. These cool from the surface of the skin; hence the skin where the cutaneous temperature sensors are applied is cooled first. The surface temperature must first be cooled and the body's response to cold (shivering and vasoconstriction) overcome before the core can be cooled. These mechanisms can be overcome with opiates, sedatives, and, if needed, paralytics. Many post-arrest patients have a blunted response to temperature that makes them easier to thermoregulate as well. In summary, commercially available surface cooling devices are noninvasive, easy to apply and manage, but may restrict access to the patient and may induce a more robust thermoregulatory response.

24.9 Timing of Cooling

There are limited data on the ideal duration of temperature control after cardiac arrest. The TTM for 48 vs 24 hours (TTH48) sought to answer this and found no significant difference between the two time lengths. This study was of modest size and the Influence of Cooling Duration on Efficacy in Cardiac Arrest Patients (ICECAP) trial hopes to answer this question more definitively. In the absence of clear evidence-based data, many centers continue to use 24 hours as a standard cooling time.

There is also a paucity of data describing the ideal time after arrest when temperature management should be initiated. A large prospective observational study found that there was no difference in outcome for patients when hypothermia was initiated 60 or 190 minutes post-arrest. Initiating hypothermia by rapid infusion of saline while a patient was still pulseless resulted in decreased likelihood of ROSC. However, these studies were done using the lower target temperatures of 32–34°C. This dichotomy of outcomes in combination with the lower target temperatures and the results of the large pre-hospital study makes it clear that there is no role for pre-hospital initiation of cooling in most patients. Examining the results of the Nielsen registry shows that the average temperature at presentation was already less than 36°C, meaning that more than half of the patients arrived already at target temperature regardless of when the hypothermia protocol was activated. Initiation of a pre-hospital cooling protocol does not seem to be helpful and many patients will reach the more modest temperature goal of 36°C on their own.

Observational data from a large Canadian registry found that a door to TTM time of less than 2 hours was associated with improved overall survival, but not favorable neurological outcome in all post-arrest patients. Patients with a Vfib/Vtach arrest were found to have modest improvements in both survival and favorable neurological outcome. This modest improvement in combination with a time frame sufficient for most facilities to initiate the procedure makes the 2-hour goal a reasonable one to include in a post-arrest protocol.

24.10 Seizures

The presence of seizures in the patient is an ominous sign. Up to 20% of post-arrest patients have seizures at some point in the post-arrest period. Seizures usually occur during the first 24 hours post-arrest and are associated with high short-term mortality. A review of EEG results with clinical outcomes shows that certain activities are associated with dismal outcomes. One series of 258 patients found that only 2 had final outcomes with a modified Rankin score of 2 or better (able to look after own affairs). There have also been case reports of individual patients surviving with good neurological outcomes despite electroencephalogram (EEG)-confirmed seizure activity. While seizure activity is not a 100% sign of death or poor outcome, seizure activity is still an ominous sign.

Myoclonic activity is common in post-arrest patients. The physical exam finding of myoclonic activity should be differentiated from myoclonic status epilepticus; myoclonic epileptiform activity can be further divided into multifocal and generalized. Fifteen percent of patients with myoclonus alone on physical exam were found to have a reasonable survival with good neurological outcome compared with those found to have myoclonus with seizure activity on EEG (2% with good neurological survival). Further research is needed to refine the diagnosis of myoclonic seizure activity to assess their utility in prognostication.

Different modalities of seizure monitoring have been incorporated into post-arrest protocols. Continuous EEG monitoring and episodic monitoring have been found to have similar results as far as neurological outcomes are concerned. This is encouraging in settings where continuous monitoring may not be available.

There is limited data on how to best treat post-arrest seizures and whether treatment is effective. The degree of anoxic injury incurred in order to induce seizures may be more damaging than the effect of the seizures themselves. Seizure prophylaxis has not been shown to be effective and is not recommended for post-arrest patients. Different modalities may be applied, such as standard antiseizure medications and sedative anesthetics such as propofol or benzodiazepines. There have been no quality studies comparing any one of these modalities to another with or without placebo.

24.11 When to Withdraw Care

Despite recommendations to delay neuroprognostication in post-arrest patients, a large number of patients are described as having a "poor" or "grave" prognosis early in the treatment course. Twenty percent of these patients went on to have good neurological outcomes. This finding was supported by a reanalysis of the ROC trial that found that one-third of subjects had withdrawal of care before the 72-hour mark due to an expected poor neurological outcome. When these patients were risk-stratified, 16% were expected to survive with good neurological outcome.

The combination of a lack of brainstem reflexes and somatosensory evoked potentials has been found to be the best data for an accurate diagnosis of a universally poor neurological outcome. The lack of corneal reflexes and pupillary reflexes in combination with the lack of evoked potentials more than 72 hours post-arrest is very specific for poor neurological outcomes (see Chapter 27).

The presence of myoclonus and myoclonic status can assist in prognostication. As discussed in the preceding section, one must be careful with how these terms are used and what the prognostic outcomes are in those categories. The presence of seizures or myoclonus alone should not prompt one to consider withdrawal of care.

Serum markers such as neuron-specific enolase and tau protein have been studied for their use in neuroprognostication with mixed results. These tests may have some value to the physician well versed in their use; however, the heterogeneity of cutoff values used and the weak levels of evidence would make their use in most post-arrest protocols extremely limited.

Pearls and Pitfalls

- Target temperature management of 36°C had similar results to 33°C.
- Supraglottic airways should be replaced as soon as possible to avoid obstructing cerebral blood flow.
- Seizure prophylaxis has not shown any benefit post-arrest.
- Avoid hypoxia in the early care of post-arrest patients, and when successful avoid hyperoxia to keep PO_2 at 94–100%.
- Consider catheterization lab activation in patients showing a new STEMI on post-arrest 12-lead EKG.

Bibliography

Bernard SA, Gray TW, Buist MD, et al. Treatment of comatose survivors of out-of-hospital cardiac arrest with induced hypothermia. *N Engl J Med* 2002;**346**(8):557–563.

Calabró L, Bougouin W, Cariou A, et al. Effect of different methods of cooling for targeted temperature management on outcome after cardiac arrest: a systematic review and meta-analysis. *Crit Care* 2019;**23**(1):285.

Callaway CW, Donnino MW, Fink EL, et al. Part 8: Post-Cardiac Arrest Care: 2015 American Heart Association Guidelines update for cardiopulmonary resuscitation and emergency cardiovascular care. *Circulation* 2015;**132**:S465–S482.

Callaway CW, Schmicker RH, Brown SP, et al. Early coronary angiography and induced hypothermia are associated with survival and functional recovery after out-of-hospital cardiac arrest. *Resuscitation* 2014;**85** (5):657–663.

Dragancea I, Horn J, Kuiper M, et al. Neurological prognostication after cardiac arrest and targeted temperature management 33°C versus 36°C: results from a randomised controlled clinical trial. *Resuscitation* 2015;**93**:164–170.

Dumas F, Grimaldi D, Zuber B, et al. Is hypothermia after cardiac arrest effective in both shockable and nonshockable patients? Insights from a large registry. *Circulation* 2011;**123**(8):877–886.

Faro J, Coppler PJ, Dezfulian C, et al. Differential association of subtypes of epileptiform activity with outcome after cardiac arrest. *Resuscitation* 2019;**136**:138–145.

Kalra R, Arora G, Patel N, et al. Targeted temperature management after cardiac arrest: systematic review and meta-analyses. *Anesth Analg* 2018;**126**(3):867–875.

Kilgannon JH, Jones AE, Shapiro NI, et al. Association between arterial hyperoxia following resuscitation from cardiac arrest and in-hospital mortality. *JAMA* 2010;**303** (21):2165–2171.

Knight WA, Hart KW, Adeoye OM, et al. The incidence of seizures in patients undergoing therapeutic hypothermia after resuscitation from cardiac arrest. *Epilepsy Res* 2013;**106** (3):396–402.

Lucas JM, Cocchi MN, Salciccioli J, et al. Neurologic recovery after therapeutic hypothermia in patients with post-cardiac arrest myoclonus. *Resuscitation* 2012;**83** (2):265–269.

Lupton JR, Schmicker RH, Stephens S, et al. Outcomes with the use of bag-valve-mask ventilation during out-of-hospital cardiac arrest in the pragmatic airway resuscitation trial. *Acad Emerg Med* 2020;**27**:5.

Lybeck A, Friberg H, Aneman A, et al. Prognostic significance of clinical seizures after cardiac arrest and target temperature management. *Resuscitation* 2017;**114**:146–151.

Nichol G, Huszti E, Kim F, et al. Does induction of hypothermia improve outcomes after in-hospital cardiac arrest? *Resuscitation* 2013;**84**(5):620–625.

Nielsen N, Wetterslev J, Cronberg T, Erlinge D, et al. Targeted temperature management at 33°C versus 36°C after cardiac arrest. *N Engl J Med* 2013;**369**(23):2197–2206.

Perman SM, Kirkpatrick JN, Reitsma AM, et al. Timing of neuroprognostication in postcardiac arrest therapeutic hypothermia. *Crit Care Med* 2012;**40**(3):719–724.

Rab T, Kern KB, Tamis-Holland JE, et al. Cardiac arrest: a treatment algorithm for emergent invasive cardiac procedures in the resuscitated comatose patient. *J Am Coll Cardiol* 2015;**66**(1):62–73.

Rittenberger JC, Weissman A, Baldwin M, et al. Preliminary experience with point-of-care EEG in post-cardiac arrest patients. *Resuscitation* 2019;**135**:98–102.

Roberts BW, Kilgannon JH, Chansky ME, et al. Association between postresuscitation partial pressure of arterial carbon dioxide and neurological outcome in patients with post-cardiac arrest syndrome. *Circulation* 2013;**127**(21):2107–2113.

Seder DB, Sunde K, Rubertsson S, et al. Neurologic outcomes and postresuscitation care of patients with myoclonus following cardiac arrest. *Crit Care Med* 2015;**43** (5):965–972.

Soar J, Berg KM, Andersen LW, et al. Adult Advanced Life Support: 2020 International Consensus on Cardiopulmonary Resuscitation and Emergency Cardiovascular Care Science with Treatment Recommendations. *Resuscitation* 2020;**156**: A80–A119.

Stanger D, Kawano T, Malhi N, et al. Door-to-Targeted temperature management initiation time and outcomes in out-of-hospital cardiac arrest: insights from the Continuous Chest Compressions Trial. *J Am Heart Assoc* 2019;**8**(9):e012001.

Szarpak L, Filipiak KJ, Mosteller L, et al. Survival, neurological and safety outcomes after out of hospital cardiac arrests treated by using prehospital therapeutic hypothermia: a systematic review and meta-analysis. *Am J Emerg Med* 2020;**20**:S0735-6757.

Testori C, Sterz F, Behringer W, et al. Mild therapeutic hypothermia is associated with favourable outcome in patients after cardiac arrest with non-shockable rhythms. *Resuscitation* 2011;**82** (9):1162–1167.

Yang MC, Meng-Jun W, Xiao-Yan X, et al. Coronary angiography or not after cardiac arrest without ST segment elevation: a systematic review and meta-analysis. *Medicine (Baltimore)* 2020;**99**(41):e22197.

Yoshida M, Yoshida T, Masui Y, et al. Association between therapeutic hypothermia and outcomes in patients with non-shockable out-of-hospital cardiac arrest developed after emergency medical service arrival (SOS-KANTO 2012 Analysis Report). *Neurocrit Care* 2019;**30**(2):429–439.

Chapter

25

Neurotoxicology

Matthew Stripp

25.1 Introduction

Emergency medicine patients may present with a variety of symptoms secondary to the effects of drugs and toxins on the nervous system. A clear understanding of the unique susceptibilities and mechanisms of toxicity can aid in diagnosis and management. Observed effects may be secondary to alterations in neurologic function at any point in signal transmission or development. The number of xenobiotics resulting in disruptions to neurologic function can seem overwhelming, but many characteristics can be examined to inform the care of acutely poisoned patients.

25.2 General Approach

As with any emergency medical condition with the potential for significant morbidity or mortality, excellent supportive care instituted immediately after the recognition of inadequacy of the airway, respiratory, or circulatory function is critical. Vital sign abnormalities on presentation/initial evaluation may inform the need for immediate intervention. Patients with impairment in consciousness should undergo quick evaluation for derangements in blood glucose with rapid beside testing. Alternative underlying medical conditions resulting in alterations of consciousness or neurologic effects should be considered in addition to causes secondary to the effects of xenobiotics.

Evidence of exposure to drugs, chemicals, and toxins upon initial presentation may be present, such as traces on the patient or their belongings. Care should always be taken to prevent the exposure of healthcare personnel to toxic agents, in the form of universal precautions or more aggressive protective measures as the situation dictates. Exposures may be reported by EMS, bystanders, or friends/family of the patient. A specific toxic exposure may not be reported. A large number of patients presenting with similar symptoms and/or signs within a defined time frame should prompt consideration of mass exposure or malicious intent.

If the patient or others are able to provide information, a detailed history is valuable. Careful attention should be given to the circumstances surrounding the exposure, such as timing, duration, quantity, intent, route, frequency, and concurrent exposures. Listing of prescription and nonprescription medications, supplements, herbal products, alternative therapies, infusions, prior treatments, vitamins, hobbies, nutrition/dietary habits, water sources, chemical, and occupational exposures can provide clues to the etiology of a toxic exposure. Patients may provide a history of alcohol or other substance use.

Physical examination can reveal findings that point to a specific toxin or a group of toxic agents. A thorough physical evaluation is paramount in cases with limited history.

Evidence of intentional drug use may include injection markings over areas of intravenous access or subcutaneous administration. Medication patches should not be overlooked. Neurologic examination may reveal the presence of inducible clonus or hyperreflexia. Groups of exam findings known as toxidromes can relate exposures to a specific class of xenobiotics.

The choice of diagnostic testing should be directed to specific agents that are suspected based on history and physical examination. Quantitative levels for acetaminophen and salicylates should be strongly considered in most cases to more rapidly institute critical therapies such as n-acetylcysteine for acetaminophen toxicity. The history of use may not be reported, and these common medications are widely available. Routine screening for a large number of drugs may have a low diagnostic yield. Specific drug levels can be helpful when available and a specific exposure is suspected. Drug levels can help guide management or indicate the degree of toxicity. Direct CSF analysis can evaluate for comorbid disease in addition to providing the opportunity to obtain drug levels and other indicators of CNS toxicity in select cases. Concentrations in the serum and blood may not accurately reflect levels in the CNS. Electroencephalograms (EEGs) may have a role in xenobiotic toxicity that is neuroexcitatory with concern for seizure. An autopsy may demonstrate anatomic changes concerning for xenobiotic-induced injury to the CNS.

25.3 General Toxicology Management Techniques

Specific therapies for decontamination and enhanced elimination can be considered to decrease toxic effects. Activated charcoal can be used to adsorb many pharmaceutical drugs. There are some notable exceptions where significant adsorption to charcoal would not be expected and therefore would not be recommended. No significant benefit is expected with ingestions of alcohols, most metals, and caustic agents. Toxic agents not significantly adsorbed by charcoal are listed in Table 25.1. The use of syrup of ipecac is no longer routinely recommended for the induction of emesis. Orogastric lavage is also no longer routinely recommended but can be considered in specific cases of recent ingestion and cases with the expectation of severe irreversible toxicity that may be refractory to conventional supportive measures such as large ingestion of colchicine. Whole bowel irrigation is also

Table 25.1 Substances not significantly adsorbed by activated charcoal

Borates
Iron
Lithium
Alcohols
Acid and alkali materials
Potassium
Magnesium
Sodium salts

reserved for specific cases when the benefits of use will outweigh the risks. The controversy regarding the use of decontamination measures, indications, and contraindications are further explored in publications by the American Academy of Clinical Toxicology (AACT) and European Association of Poison Centres and Clinical Toxicologists (EAPCCT). These measures should be taken into consideration on an individual basis.

Enhanced elimination methods can involve the use of hemodialysis, hemofiltration, hemoperfusion, exchange transfusion, plasmapheresis, metal chelation, multiple-dose activated charcoal, resins, cerebrospinal fluid replacement, and alteration of urinary pH. These measures should be considered in patients with inadequate response to supportive care, impaired elimination, significant medical comorbidities, or metabolic disturbance. Decisions to institute measures for enhanced elimination should include consideration of pharmacokinetic/toxicokinetic factors for the individual agent. Forced diuresis beyond the repletion of extracellular fluid volume has little expectation of benefit for most cases.

25.4 Xenobiotic-Induced Neurologic Effects

Evaluating the neurologic effects of xenobiotics requires attention to the specific factors related to the nervous system. The blood–brain barrier and blood–CSF barrier offer a degree of protection from many drugs and toxins. Transendothelial movement across the blood–brain barrier can occur via diffusion, transport proteins, or endocytosis. Lipophilic substances cross more readily through direct movement across the endothelial membranes. Endothelial cells may offer further protection through the metabolism of some substances. Transport proteins (which include p-glycoprotein) can efflux molecules back to the capillary lumen.

25.5 CNS Excitation: Excitotoxicity and Seizure

A link between excitation and neurotoxicity has been established. Multiple mechanisms by various xenobiotics can result in derangements leading to excess CNS activity either through direct toxicity or withdrawal of inhibitory effects. Stimulation of N-methyl-d-aspartate (NMDA) receptors has been implicated in the process of excitotoxicity. Other mechanisms may be due to decreased activity at GABA receptors or enhancements in excitatory neurotransmitter activity. Neuronal cell death can occur when more energy is expended than the cell can produce.

Xenobiotic-induced seizures can be triggered by many agents, but some are more closely associated with seizure induction. Bupropion is one prominent example and is commonly associated with a lower seizure threshold even at therapeutic doses. Severe toxicity can result in status epilepticus (as well as QRS widening and QTc prolongation with ventricular dysrhythmia). Tricyclic antidepressants (TCAs), tramadol, theophylline, and isoniazid are other agents that are commonly associated with the induction of seizures. Water hemlock contains a naturally occurring toxin, ciguatoxin, which induces seizures through antagonism at the $GABA_A$ receptor. Ingestion may occur after mistaken identity following foraging. Withdrawal-associated seizures can be seen with ethanol, benzodiazepines, baclofen, and gamma-hydroxybutyrate (GHB). Table 25.2 shows agents commonly associated with seizure.

Treatment of drug-induced seizures often consists of the administration of medications to enhance GABAergic tone. Liberal use of benzodiazepines is usually indicated as first-line therapy, with escalation to barbiturates for refractory seizures. Special consideration should be given to the

Table 25.2 Selected seizure inducers

Psychotropic medications

Citalopram/escitalopram

Bupropion

Venlafaxine/desvenlafaxine

Quetiapine

MAOIs (monoamine oxidase inhibitors)

Drugs of abuse

Synthetic cannabinoids

Cathinones ("bath salts")/amphetamines

Cocaine

Ethanol withdrawal

Sedative-hypnotic withdrawal

GHB withdrawal

Analgesics/musculoskeletal

Tramadol

Propoxyphene

Lidocaine

Mefenamic acid

Meperidine

Phenylbutazone (veterinary)

Baclofen (overdose or withdrawal)

Environmental

Domoic acid contaminated mussels

Other pharmaceutical

Isoniazid

Hypoglycemics

Antihistamines

Carbamazepine

Theophylline

Chloroquine

Plant-based

Thujone from wormwood (*Artemisia absinthium*)

Gyromitrin from *Gyromitra* spp. mushrooms

Nicotine (*Nicotiana tabacum*)

Japanese star anise (*Illicium anisatum*)

Table 25.2 (cont.)

4-methylpyridoxine in *Ginkgo biloba* seeds

Cicutoxin from water hemlock (*Cicuta maculata*)

N-methylcytisine from blue cohash (*Caulophyllum*)

Household

Caffeine

Camphor

War agents/pesticides/occupational

Organophosphorus compounds

Organic chlorines

Carbon monoxide

Ethylene oxide

Methyl bromide

Cyanide

Seizure mimics

Strychnine

Tetanus

Brucine

treatment of agents that deplete GABA and require therapy with pyridoxine (vitamin B6) as a cofactor for the synthesis of additional GABA (e.g., isoniazid- and gyromitrin-containing mushrooms). The use of phenytoin should be avoided in most cases of toxin-induced seizures because of lack of efficacy, and it may be harmful when used to treat seizures caused by lidocaine, theophylline, or TCAs. The efficacy and risks of newer agents, such as levetiracetam, for toxin-induced seizure is an area of active investigation.

Some agents can induce convulsions with preservation of consciousness through inhibition of glycine in the spinal column. Potential exposure to strychnine can occur from rodenticide or the tree *Strychnos nux-vomica* (postsynaptic glycine receptor inhibitor). Tetanus toxin (presynaptic glycine receptor inhibitor) may produce similar symptoms and is produced by the bacterium *Clostridium tetani*. Exposure to these agents should be considered in cases where seizure-like movements occur while the patient remains conscious.

25.6 Toxidromes

A toxidrome is a clinical syndrome that refers to the effects of a specific toxin or group of toxins. The presence of a toxidrome can help guide management when found by patient examination. Syndromes may appear partially/incompletely, and elements may vary over time. This may be especially important in cases of exposure to multiple agents. Toxidromes are the outcome of xenobiotic effects resulting in changes in neurotransmission at various receptor sites throughout the body.

25.6.1 Cholinergic

The cholinergic toxidrome is the result of increased stimulation of cholinergic receptors. Multiple mechanisms may lead to increased activity at these receptors either through decreased breakdown of acetylcholine or direct stimulation of the cholinergic receptors. Both nicotinic and muscarinic subtypes can be found throughout the central and peripheral nervous systems. Significant exposure can occur by the dermal, oral, and inhalation routes. Organophosphates (OPs) and carbamates are commonly used as pesticides, and the number of patients affected by acute poisoning from these agents is devastating on a global scale. The rapid onset and severe, incapacitating effects from a few drops are the reason that these xenobiotics have been used in warfare. Sarin (GB), Soman (GD), tabun, and VX are examples that are considered chemical weapons and are sometimes referred to as "nerve agents."

OPs and carbamates are well known for inhibiting acetylcholine esterase (AChE), the enzyme responsible for the breakdown of acetylcholine in the synapse. Inhibition of AChE can produce the cholinergic toxidrome. The mnemonic DUMBBELS (defecation, urination, miosis, bronchorrhea, bronchospasm, emesis, lacrimation, salivation) and SLUDGE (salivation, lacrimation, urination, defecation, gastric emptying) are helpful to remember these effects. In an acute presentation it is important to remember that nicotinic receptor stimulation may lead to adrenergic effects secondary to catecholamine release, which may produce confounding findings such as tachycardia. Sympathetic nervous system stimulation may be present. Nicotinic stimulatory effects at neuromuscular junctions include muscular weakness, paralysis, and fasciculations. Direct-acting muscarinic agonists such as pilocarpine and *Clitocybe* mushrooms can produce cholinergic effects without the sympathetic and somatic effects of nicotinic receptor stimulation.

Intubation with mechanical ventilation may be required for management of respiratory failure. Red blood cell cholinesterases and butyrylcholinesterase can be used for monitoring; however, they may have low clinical utility in the acute setting. Atropine is an antimuscarinic medication that reverses the effects of cholinergic toxicity through competitive blockade. Atropine should be administered to the end-point of reversal of excess airway secretions. Bronchorrhea is considered the most life-threatening manifestation.

An OP will undergo a process of aging in which the cholinesterase will become irreversibly inactivated. An oxime, such as pralidoxime (2-PAM), can be administered for reactivation of the cholinesterase that has been inactivated by an OP in an attempt to prevent aging. Pralidoxime will only be effective if administered prior to the enzyme becoming "aged." Individual OPs will have a different amount of time between initial exposure to the OP until aging occurs. Some OPs may undergo significant aging in minutes and others may take days. This makes the rapid administration of antidotal therapy critical in some cases. Carbamates do not undergo aging.

Decontamination is essential. Associated seizure activity should be treated with benzodiazepines. Consultation with a toxicologist should be considered for patients affected by cholinergic toxicity.

25.6.2 Anticholinergic

Xenobiotics that block acetylcholine effects at muscarinic cholinergic receptors are termed *anticholinergic*. A great number of medications have anticholinergic effects, and these effects may be much more pronounced in an overdose setting. Some examples include antihistamines, antipsychotics, antispasmodics, skeletal muscle relaxers, some plants/mushrooms, and TCAs. A classic toxidrome is associated with anticholinergic toxicity, which consists of increased sedation, confusion, disorientation, delirium, agitation, hallucinations, trailing/incomprehensible speech patterns, and characteristic "picking" behaviors. Peripheral effects include hyperthermia, flushed skin, anhidrosis (especially axillary), tachycardia, decreased gastrointestinal motility, mydriasis, and urinary retention.

Anticholinergic toxicity is treated with supportive care, including benzodiazepines for agitation/seizure and fluid hydration. Physostigmine is a reversible inhibitor of cholinesterases and is used to reverse anticholinergic toxicity. This medication is contraindicated for use with concomitant TCA toxicity. Other contraindications include use with patients with intraventricular conduction delay, atrioventricular block, and concurrent use of succinylcholine or choline esters. Physostigmine may be diagnostic if rapid reversal of symptomatology is achieved.

25.6.3 Sympathomimetic

Sympathomimetic toxicity is a broad categorization of effects secondary to stimulant toxicity. The list of common agents that can induce this syndrome is extensive and includes cocaine, amphetamines (and derivatives), caffeine, phenylephrine, theophylline, albuterol, epinephrine, and methylphenidate. These effects include agitation, tremor, seizures, tachycardia, hypertension, hyperthermia, tachypnea, diaphoresis, and mydriasis. Vital signs abnormalities alone may be insufficient to distinguish between anticholinergic and stimulant toxicity. ECG should be obtained to assess for myocardial ischemia or dysrhythmia.

Benzodiazepines should be used to control agitation and seizure. Escalation to barbiturates may be required. Caution should be used when considering sedation with agents that have anticholinergic side effects (e.g., antipsychotics, antihistamines). The use of ketamine for control of undifferentiated agitation is increasing, although ketamine has some sympathomimetic effects. Further research is needed to determine the role of ketamine for control of agitation in patients with sympathomimetic toxicity. The use of antipsychotics for symptomatic control has traditionally been avoided due to potential for seizure, QT interval prolongation, and issues with heat dissipation. While definitive evidence for harm from antipsychotics is lacking, there is little evidence to support the use over benzodiazepines or alternatives. If dexmedetomidine is used as an adjunct, close monitoring of vital signs for bradycardia and hypotension is recommended.

Core temperature monitoring with careful management of temperature elevation is critical. Rapid external cooling for hyperthermic patients should be a primary focus. Paralytics in conjunction with endotracheal intubation and mechanical intubation should be considered for refractory hyperthermia. Creatine kinase level should be sent. Affected patients should have intravenous fluid hydration with monitoring for rhabdomyolysis and myoglobinuric renal failure (when feasible to implement safely in the setting of severe agitation). Hypertension typically responds to benzodiazepines or barbiturates. Short-acting agents should be considered if refractory hypertension occurs.

25.6.4 Sedative-Hypnotic

A reduction in excitability or the induction of sleep is the result of exposure to this class of xenobiotic, as may be expected from the terminology *sedative-hypnotic*. A sedative-hypnotic toxidrome will typically present with depressed mental status in association with bradycardia, hypotension, bradypnea, hypoactive bowel sounds, hyporeflexia, and ataxia/decreased coordination. Different xenobiotics in this class can have varying degrees of manifestations such as respiratory depression. An isolated oral overdose of benzodiazepines or sleep aids such as zolpidem does not typically produce life-threatening respiratory depression. Other agents in this class (e.g., chloral hydrate, which can cause lethal ventricular dysrhythmias) may have unique effects that should be taken into consideration on an individual basis. Tolerance may develop and increasing doses over time may be required to produce the same effects.

Routine drug screening will often have low clinical utility in the setting of acute toxicity and can be misleading. Many urine drug screens for benzodiazepines are designed to detect metabolites that are not universal to all agents in this drug class, and this may lead to false negative results. Relatively common benzodiazepines such as alprazolam and clonazepam can go undetected despite overdose involving these xenobiotics. Obtaining specific drug levels may confirm exposure but availability and laboratory turnaround times may limit clinical utility.

25.6.5 Opioid

Opioid use has become widespread, and the concern for addiction and toxicity is increasing. This epidemic has been compounded by the development of opioids with high potency and greater potential for adverse outcomes. Fentanyl exemplifies these concerns and significant toxicity can be realized from small doses. Effects secondary to opioid receptor stimulation produce a syndrome consisting of hypoventilation, hypoperistalsis, mental status depression, and miosis. Other effects may include seizure, bradycardia, pruritis, analgesia, euphoria, and endocrine effects. Hypotension may be present, although this effect can vary among different opioids due to the degree of associated histamine release. QT interval lengthening can occur with toxicity of some opioids such as methadone.

Naloxone, an opioid antagonist, is considered the antidote to opioid toxicity and will reverse the effects rapidly by competing for receptor sites. Appropriate dosing is essential to avoid precipitation of withdrawal effects. Patients should be monitored very closely for recurrence of respiratory depression after administration of naloxone. The effects of opioid toxicity can last longer than the effects of naloxone. Please refer to Table 25.3 for an approach to the use of naloxone in patients with opioid intoxication.

The risks of secondary exposure to pre-hospital and hospital personnel are expected to be minimal with the use of standard precautions. For further discussion of this topic, refer to the ACMT/AACT Position Statement on preventing occupational fentanyl and fentanyl analog exposure to emergency responders.

25.7 Withdrawal Syndromes

Withdrawal is a constellation of symptoms that can occur following the abrupt discontinuation (or decrease) of a continuously present xenobiotic. Withdrawal effects are due to physiological changes that have taken place in response to continued exposure to the drug or toxin. Physiologic changes can result from a combination of alterations in the number or conformation of the receptors, increased counter-regulatory signaling, and decreased endogenous activity of similar mechanisms.

Ethanol withdrawal is commonly encountered and a prominent example. Symptoms are diverse and overlap with other $GABA_A$ modulating agents such as benzodiazepines, barbiturates, and some volatile solvents. $GABA_B$-active agents, which include baclofen and gamma-hydroxybutyrate (GHB), also produce similar and significant withdrawal

Table 25.3 Naloxone use

Naloxone nasal spray 4 mg is often used by the public and pre-hospital personnel. One full dose is insufflated into the nostril of the patient and may be repeated within 2–3 minutes. Patients should be evaluated by medical personnel if successful.

1. If IV access is available, bolus (start with 0.04 mg IV and titrate up to reverse respiratory depression) and when successful, administer two-thirds of the effective bolus dose per hour by IV infusion.

2. If respiratory depression is not reversed, administer up to 10 mg of naloxone as an IV bolus and if not successful intubate the patient and evaluate for other causes.

3. If respiratory depression recurs, administer half of the initial bolus dose and begin an IV infusion at two-thirds of the new bolus dose per hour.

4. If the patient develops withdrawal signs or symptoms during infusion, stop the infusion until the symptoms abate and restart the infusion at half of the initial rate.

5. If the patient develops respiratory depression during the infusion, readminister half of the initial bolus dose and repeat until reversal and increase the infusion rate an additional 50%. Careful reassessment is required to exclude other causes, such as re-administration of opioids, delayed absorption, or other medical causes of respiratory depression.

effects. Treatment is supportive and therapeutic agents are often directed at rebalancing the receptor activity in a tapering fashion. Long-acting benzodiazepines are useful for alcohol withdrawal to agonize $GABA_A$ receptors after ethanol use cessation. Occasionally, the same agents, or agents from the same class, are necessary to control the withdrawal effects. This is often the case in benzodiazepine withdrawal. Withdrawal symptoms can occur while the patient still has detectable levels of the inciting xenobiotic.

25.8 Use of Antidotal Therapy

When a diagnosis of a specific toxicity is strongly suspected or reported, the use of an antidote may be considered when available. Sufficient knowledge regarding the indications, contraindications, and method of proper administration is critical when administering antidotal therapy. Appropriate antidote usage can be potentially lifesaving, whereas inappropriate use can result in negative effects. For example, flumazenil, a competitive inhibitor of the $GABA_A$ benzodiazepine receptor complex, can reverse the effects of benzodiazepine toxicity but may precipitate seizures in individuals who are chronically exposed to this drug class. Another common example includes the use of physostigmine, a reversible anticholinesterase that increases the concentration of acetylcholine at receptor sites, for the treatment of anticholinergic toxicity. Physostigmine should be avoided in patients with exposures to TCAs. Prior to administration of an uncommonly used antidote, members of the care team should have a complete understanding of the proper use of the therapeutic agent. Consultation with a local poison control center in conjunction with a clinical toxicologist is strongly recommended, especially in cases where the diagnosis is unclear, the situation involves significant potential morbidity or mortality, or antidotal therapy is being considered.

25.9 Serotonin Toxicity

When excess stimulation occurs at serotonin receptors, a spectrum of toxicity occurs consisting of tremor, altered mental status, hyperthermia, tachycardia, diaphoresis, myoclonus, agitation, hyperreflexia, and hyperactive bowel sounds/diarrhea. The severity of the clinical manifestations can range from mild to life-threatening. Serotonin toxicity can occur when a new serotonergic medication is added or a dose is increased. It is important to recognize this syndrome and discontinue serotonergic medications. A significant number of drugs are not commonly known to be serotonergic, including antibiotics (linezolid) and antimigraine (sumatriptan). Care should be taken to eliminate exposure to serotonergic medications when possible and especially in cases of life-threatening toxicity. A detailed medication history is essential in cases where serotonin toxicity is suspected. There is no specific laboratory derangement that implicates serotonin toxicity. Clonus is considered to be the most important diagnostic finding for establishing this diagnosis. Lower extremity findings are usually more prominent than upper extremity exam findings. Various diagnostic criteria have been set forth with differing degrees of sensitivity and specificity. One method is outlined in Figure 25.1. For optimal patient management it is imperative to differentiate serotonin syndrome from other drug toxicity syndromes with similar features, such as neuroleptic malignant syndrome, anticholinergic poisoning, and malignant hyperthermia. The duration may be prolonged if the involved agents have long elimination half-lives and active metabolites.

Management should consist of benzodiazepines for agitation and hyperadrenergic effects. Rapid external cooling should be initiated in cases of hyperthermia. Cyproheptadine is a serotonin receptor antagonist that may be beneficial in serotonin toxicity. The therapeutic efficacy and optimal dose are not well established.

25.10 Neuroleptic Malignant Syndrome

The development of neuroleptic malignant syndrome (NMS) secondary to xenobiotic-induced changes in the neurotransmission of dopamine can be challenging diagnostically. The specific mechanism of NMS is not clear and is associated with a decrease in dopaminergic neurotransmission. This may lead to alterations in thermoregulation/hyperthermia, muscular rigidity ("lead pipe"), confusion, tremor, and autonomic dysfunction. NMS is typically associated with dopamine receptor antagonists; however, similar effects may occur with dopamine agonist withdrawal. More cases occur with therapeutic doses of antipsychotics compared to the overdose setting. These effects will often occur within 2 weeks of a medication addition, dosage change, or with coinciding disease. Patients should be monitored for rhabdomyolysis. Supportive treatment with rapid temperature control should be started. Drugs with dopamine blockade should be discontinued and dopamine agonists should be resumed rapidly. Respiratory failure may require aggressive management in an intensive care setting. IV fluid resuscitation should be administered for hypotension, with escalation to vasopressors if required. Benzodiazepines can be used for treatment since other therapies remain more controversial. Dantrolene has been used in the past, especially in patients who have significant muscular rigidity, but this medication has also been associated with a higher mortality and prolonged recovery. Dopaminergic agonists such as bromocriptine can be considered as antidotal therapy.

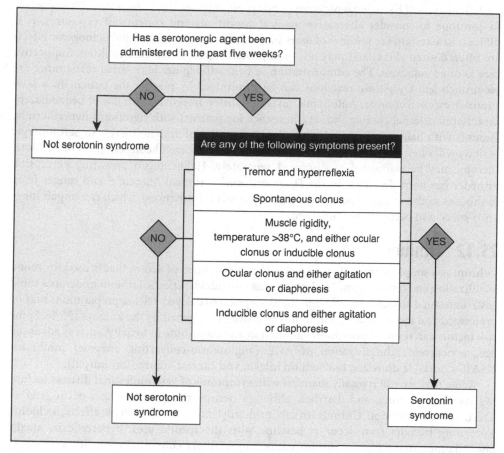

Figure 25.1 Evaluation of serotonin syndrome: algorithm for diagnosis. The neuromuscular features of clonus and hyperreflexia are highly diagnostic for serotonin syndrome, and their occurrence in the setting of serotonergic drug use establishes the diagnosis. Clinicians should be aware that muscle rigidity can overwhelm other neuromuscular findings and mask the diagnosis. Reproduced with permission from Boyer EW, Shannon M. The serotonin syndrome. *N Engl J Med* 2005;352(11):1112–1120. doi:10.1056/NEJMra041867. Criteria adapted from Dunkley EJ, Isbister GK, Sibbritt D, Dawson AH, Whyte IM. The Hunter Serotonin Toxicity Criteria: simple and accurate diagnostic decision rules for serotonin toxicity. *QJM* 2003;96(9):635–642. doi:10.1093/qjmed/hcg109

25.11 Hallucinogenic Agents

Compounds that produce disturbances in perception that do not have a basis in the external environment are termed hallucinogens. Classes are often differentiated based on chemical structure. Lysergamides, tryptamines, hallucinogenic amphetamines such as phenylethylamines, MAOIs, and anticholinergic compounds are some examples. Some other agents include salvinorin A (a compound derived from the plant *Salvia divinorum*), psychoactive components found in *Myristica fragrans* (nutmeg), and psilocybin, which is a naturally occurring prodrug found in some hallucinogenic mushrooms. Many hallucinogenic effects are the result of action at serotonin receptors. Lysergic acid diethylamide (LSD) exerts its effects primarily through its action at the 5-HT2 family of serotonin receptors. Salvinorin A is a notable exception that acts on kappa opioid receptors.

When users of hallucinogenic compounds present to healthcare facilities, it is important to continue to consider alternative medical conditions and concurrent exposures. It is difficult to ascertain the number of users in the general population as hallucinogenic effects are often desired effects and may not prompt visits to the healthcare facilities. Supportive care is often sufficient. The administration of benzodiazepines and verbal reassurance are recommended. Dysphoric reactions can be minimized by placing the patient in a low-stimulatory environment. Autonomic instability often improves with use of benzodiazepines. Rapid external cooling should commence for patients with significant hyperthermia. Patients with hallucinations and other signs suggestive of anticholinergic or serotonergic toxicity will often respond to benzodiazepines; however, careful consideration of antidotal therapy may be warranted as discussed separately. Hallucinogen persisting perception disorder has been described in the *Diagnostic and Statistical Manual 5* and ranges from flashbacks to alterations in perception (usually visual disturbances), which can impair long-term social and occupational function.

25.12 Lithium

Lithium is a simple xenobiotic with a complex mechanism of action that is used for mood stabilization and bipolar disorder. Lithium has antisuicidal effects. Lithium undergoes rapid gastrointestinal absorption, although the absorption of delayed-release preparations may be prolonged and more variable. Lithium is primarily eliminated by the kidneys (95%). Some risk factors can result in prolonged elimination and contribute to toxicity, such as advanced age, concurrent administration of ACE (angiotensin-converting enzyme) inhibitors, NSAIDs, thiazide diuretics, low sodium intake, and cardiac failure (low output).

Acute toxicity will typically manifest with symptoms of gastrointestinal distress including nausea, vomiting, and diarrhea, although neurologic symptoms can occur later as a result of redistribution. Chronic toxicity primarily consists of neurologic effects, including worsening tremors (can occur at baseline with therapeutic use), hyperreflexia, ataxia, fasciculations, nystagmus, confusion, coma, and seizure. Acute-on-chronic lithium toxicity may have features of both types. The syndrome of irreversible lithium-effectuated neurotoxicity (SILENT) refers to the neurologic effects that have been described after lithium toxicity. This dysfunction persists for at least two months after discontinuation of lithium, is not explained by pre-existing neurologic disease, and is primarily cerebellar. The mechanism of this permanent CNS injury is unknown but has been suggested to involve the process of demyelination and cell death.

Evaluation should include serum lithium levels. Care should be taken to measure lithium using an appropriate blood tube that does not contain lithium-heparin as this may lead to falsely elevated measurements. ECG may reveal T-wave inversion/flattening and QT prolongation. Electrolytes/renal function may have implications for treatment. Hypernatremia may suggest the development of nephrogenic diabetes insipidus secondary to lithium. Thyroid function studies could be considered as lithium can cause hyper- or hypothyroidism.

Whole bowel irrigation may be indicated in select cases involving ingested sustained-release preparations. Intravascular volume should be maintained as tolerated (1.5–2 times maintenance rate with normal saline). Consensus recommendations regarding hemodialysis are available through the Extracorporeal Treatments in Poisoning (EXTRIP) Workgroup.

25.13 Carbon Monoxide

Carbon monoxide (CO) is a colorless, odorless gas that can lead to severe neurologic toxicity and is formed as a product of combustion of carbon-based material. Diagnosis may be challenging, especially where cases of exposure are not reported. Common sources of CO exposure are listed in Table 25.4. Self-injury attempts with CO should not be overlooked.

CO prevents oxygen delivery to the tissue by binding to hemoglobin as well as causing a leftward shift of the oxyhemoglobin dissociation curve. CO has additional adverse effects beyond tissue hypoxia. The binding of hemoglobin and CO does not predict neurologic injury; this injury is more likely related to effects on cellular respiration. CO interferes with the electron transport chain by binding to mitochondrial enzymes, leading to a series of downstream effects that may better account for the resultant neurologic injury and cellular loss. Hypotension may potentiate these pathologic effects.

Neurologic sequelae of acute CO exposure can take many forms. Dementia, psychosis, amnesia, parkinsonism, paralysis, chorea, agnosia, and neuropathy are some effects that have been described. Delay in onset may be up to 40 days post-exposure. The loss of consciousness with CO exposure is associated with the development of delayed neurologic sequelae.

Initial reported effects in an acute exposure may be nonspecific. A dull, continuous headache is the most common complaint. Children are usually more severely affected. Other effects can include dysrhythmia, chest pain/myocardial ischemia, syncope, visual changes, vomiting, ataxia, weakness, confusion, dizziness, and dyspnea/tachypnea. Exposures to higher levels of CO for longer durations will usually produce more severe neurologic manifestations. Signs of cerebrovascular infarction may be evident on exam.

Carboxyhemoglobin (COHB) levels should be obtained for cases of suspected acute exposure. Fetal hemoglobin may interfere with interpretation in neonates producing a falsely elevated level. Smokers may have levels up to 10% at baseline. Pulse co-oximeters are becoming more widely available for screening, but should not be used to direct patient care.

Table 25.4 Common sources of carbon monoxide

Anesthesia circuits (from carbon dioxide absorbents)
Banked blood
Gasoline powered vehicles and equipment, which includes but is not limited to:
Ice resurfacing equipment (Ice rinks)
Boats
propane-powered forklifts
Generators
Campfire stoves
Combustion furnaces
Building fire
Mines (especially with explosions)
Metabolized to CO:
methylene chloride (paint stripper)

Interpretation of the values obtained by these rapid noninvasive instruments should be approached with caution as inaccurate readings are frequent. An ECG should be obtained due to the potential for myocardial ischemia or dysrhythmia. Lactate elevation should prompt consideration of concurrent cyanide poisoning in the appropriate clinical setting. EEG may show diffuse frontal slow-wave activity. CT/MRI imaging may show decreased density of the globus pallidus and central white matter when obtained within hours to days of a severe exposure to CO. Neuropsychiatric testing can be considered to assess neurologic sequelae.

Delivery of 100% oxygen either through a facemask or another advanced airway intervention is critical. The half-life of COHB can be reduced with 100% oxygen therapy. Patients may require advanced supportive measures, including intravenous fluid resuscitation, vasopressors, glucose supplementation, and correction of acid–base disturbances. Hyperbaric therapy should be considered early for cases with significant exposure (confusion, loss of consciousness, seizure, chest pain, ataxia/cerebellar dysfunction) or in some cases with more mild exposure, such as with pregnancy. Early discussion with a toxicology or hyperbaric specialist with CO poisoning experience can assist in identifying patients who will benefit from hyperbaric therapy (prevention of neurologic sequelae). A careful neurologic examination is essential in the assessment of these patients and decision-making for hyperbaric therapy.

25.14 Drug-Induced Aseptic Meningitis

Headache, fever, nuchal rigidity, nausea, vomiting, and malaise are commonly reported in cases of drug-induced aseptic meningitis (DIAM). This condition is diagnostically challenging. Commonly implicated drugs are listed in Table 25.5. Systemic lupus erythematosus has been associated with this condition. DIAM cannot be distinguished from infectious meningitis based on clinical features alone, and concurrent testing with CSF cultures should be obtained. Treatment should focus on recognition and discontinuation of the offending agent. Re-challenging with the suspected provoking agent could be diagnostic, but may also carry significant risk. This approach is not routinely recommended.

25.15 Synthetic Drugs of Abuse

Recent advances in chemical synthesis have generated new compounds that may be structurally related to more classic drugs of abuse or they may represent new agents entirely. Many have psychoactive effects that may be similar or dissimilar to more well-described drugs. Drugs in the classes of designer benzodiazepines, synthetic cannabinoids, synthetic cathinones ("bath salts"), and amphetamines are rapidly expanding in number. The pharmacokinetic and pharmacodynamic properties of these new drugs may be unknown. Differing effects from these drugs could be secondary to changes in receptor binding affinity, binding to different receptors, drug distribution, or metabolism to different compounds.

Synthetic cannabinoids go by many street names, and these "brands" are constantly evolving. Some examples include "spice," "spike," or "legal marijuana." These compounds may have CNS effects that are profound and unpredictable. A wide variety of symptoms have been described, including nausea, vomiting, confusion, agitation, short-term memory loss, cognitive impairment, psychosis, seizure, arrhythmia, stroke, myocardial infarction, and death. The diagnostic testing for synthetic cannabinoids is often clinical as

Table 25.5 Selected drugs associated with DIAM

NSAIDs

Ibuprofen

Naproxen

Diclofenac

ASA (at high dose)

Antimicrobial

Sulfamethizole

TMP-SMX

Isoniazid

Ciprofloxacin

Penicillin

Metronidazole

Cephalosporins

Pyrazinamide

Sulfisoxazole

Indianivir

Valcyclovir

Immune-related

IVIg

OKT3 monoclonal ab

Infliximab

Azathioprine

Sulfasalazine

Other

Carbamazepine

Allopurinol

Chemotherapeutics

Corticosteroids

Levamisole

confirmatory testing is not readily available and may take several days. Urine drug screening for THC (tetrahydrocannabinol) will be negative for exposures to synthetic cannabinoids alone. Reasonable initial tests include an ECG, electrolytes/renal function, and symptom-directed testing (e.g., cardiac enzymes for patients presenting with chest pain). Supportive care is the mainstay of management for toxicity from these compounds. Management should also be directed primarily at symptoms due to the less frequently reported but potentially severe effects.

25.16 Brain Death Mimicry

When a patient is undergoing an evaluation for the establishment of brain death, it is critical to ensure that no xenobiotics might account for the clinical effects or EEG findings. Some drugs and toxins such as sedative-hypnotic agents have been found to mimic brain death. Drug elimination half-life may be prolonged in the setting of overdose and severe critical illness. Pharmacokinetic calculations/estimations may be unreliable. Observation periods beyond five drug half-lives may be appropriate in select cases. Serum/blood levels may not represent the amount of drug present at the site of action. The specific duration of observation is not standardized and should be tailored to each clinical circumstance with consideration of the suspected exposures and anticipated duration effect. Drug screens may not detect agents that could account for significant CNS depression and testing should focus on the specific suspected agents involved in the overdose based on clinical findings. Consultation with a toxicologist is recommended for cases when the management is complex or unclear. Further discussion of this topic can be explored with the American College of Medical Toxicology (ACMT) Position Statement on the determination of brain death in patients after a suspected drug overdose.

Pearls and Pitfalls

- Co-ingestion of substances occurs regularly, and specific attention should be paid to possible acetaminophen and salicylate exposure.
- Toxidromes are syndromes that can be used to identify toxins or groups of toxins in the management of undifferentiated poisoned patients.
- The potential for unknown and undescribed effects secondary to designer/synthetic drug toxicity is increasing.
- An ample period of observation should take place in cases of brain death evaluation where suspicion of exposure to CNS-depressing medications is suspected.

Bibliography

Boyer EW, Shannon M. The serotonin syndrome. *N Engl J Med* 2005;**352** (11):1112–1120.

Connors NJ, Alsakha A, Larocque A, et al. Antipsychotics for the treatment of sympathomimetic toxicity: a systematic review. *Am J Emerg Med* 2019;**37**(10):1880–1890.

Decker BS, Goldfarb DS, Dargan PI, et al. Extracorporeal treatment for lithium poisoning: systematic review and recommendations from the EXTRIP Workgroup. *Clin J Am Soc Nephrol* 2015;**10** (5):875–887.

Gurney SM, Scott KS, Kacinko SL, Presley BC, Logan BK. Pharmacology, toxicology, and

adverse effects of synthetic cannabinoid drugs. *Forensic Sci Rev* 2014;**26**(1):53–78.

Hoffman RS, Howland MA, Lewin NA, Nelson LS, Goldfrank LR (eds.) *Goldfrank's Toxicologic Emergencies*, 10th ed. McGraw-Hill, 2015.

Hopper A, Vilke G, Castillo EM, et al. Ketamine use for acute agitation in the emergency department. *J Emerg Med* 2015;**48**(6):712–719.

Marinac JS. Drug- and chemical-induced aseptic meningitis: a review of the literature. *Ann Pharmacother* 1992;**26**(6):813–822.

Moris G, Garcia-Monco JC. The challenge of drug-induced aseptic meningitis. *Arch Intern Med* 1999;**159**(11):1185–1194.

Neavyn MJ, Stolbach A, Greer DM, et al. ACMT Position Statement: determining brain death in adults after drug overdose. *J Med Toxicol* 2017;**13**(3):271–273.

Olson KR, Anderson IB, California Poison Control System. *Poisoning & Drug Overdose*, 7th ed. Lange Medical Books and McGraw-Hill, 2018.

Sud P, Gordon M, Tortora L, et al. Retrospective chart review of synthetic cannabinoid intoxication with toxicologic analysis. *West J Emerg Med* 2018;**19**(3):567–572.

Sullivan R, Hodgman MJ, Kao L, Tormoehlen LM. Baclofen overdose mimicking brain death. *Clin Toxicol (Phila)* 2012;**50**(2):141–144.

Weaver LK, Churchill SK, Deru K, Cooney D. False positive rate of carbon monoxide saturation by pulse oximetry of emergency department patients. *Respir Care* 2013;**58**(2):232–240.

Neurologic Emergencies of Pregnancy

Ronald L. Thomas, Andrea Synowiec, Roseann Covatto, and Thomas P. Campbell

26.1 Introduction

The spectrum of neurologic emergencies in pregnancy extends from life-threatening eclamptic seizures to self-limiting paresthesias. Pregnancy markedly modifies human physiology, creating a unique and challenging physical and laboratory evaluation. In addition, pregnant patients may present with gestational and peripartum conditions resulting directly from pregnancy, but also a portent of future disease as well as exacerbation of pre-existing conditions changed by the patient's gravid state. All of these issues can be complicated by the "second patient" (the fetus), which requires careful consideration.

26.2 Eclampsia

Eclampsia is the presence of new-onset grand mal seizures in a pregnant patient diagnosed with preeclampsia. Eclampsia may occur before, during, or after labor:

1. 45% occur before labor
2. 5% occur during labor
3. 55% occur in the postpartum period (10% of eclamptic patients do not develop seizure until after 48 hours)

The peak incidence occurs in adolescence and in the early twenties but is also seen in women over 35 years of age. Other risk factors include nonwhite, nulliparous, and females from lower socioeconomic backgrounds, and molar and multifetal pregnancies. The precise cause of seizure in the preeclamptic patient is not clear.

Preeclampsia is a syndrome that includes the development of new-onset hypertension (BP 140/90) and new-onset proteinuria (≥300 mg protein in 23 hours). Preeclampsia can be diagnosed in the absence of proteinuria with new-onset thrombocytopenia, renal insufficiency, impaired liver function, pulmonary edema, or cerebral or visual symptoms (Table 26.1).

26.2.1 Evaluation and Differential Diagnosis

When convulsions and altered sensorium occur in the pregnant patient past 20 weeks' gestation or in the first 2 weeks postpartum, eclampsia is the working diagnosis. Most patients will have premonitory signs or symptoms in the hours before the initial seizure. The most common of these are:

- hypertension – 75%
- headache that can either be persistent frontal or occipital, or thunderclap – 66%

Table 26.1 Preeclampsia Criteria Task Force on Hypertension in Pregnancy – ACOG

Blood pressure	• ≥140 mm Hg systolic or ≥90 mm Hg diastolic on two occasions at least 4 hours apart after 20 weeks of gestation in a patient without a history of hypertension • ≥160 mm Hg systolic or ≥105 mm Hg diastolic on two occasions that can be within minutes of each other to facilitate diagnosis of hypertensive emergency
AND	
Proteinuria	• ≥300 mg/24-hour urine collection (or extracted from a 12-hour urine collection) • Protein/creatinine ratio ≥0.3 (also known as a urine spot test and both values are measured in mg/dL)
OR IN THE ABSENCE OF PROTEINURIA, NEW-ONSET HYPERTENSION AND ANY OF THE FOLLOWING	
Thrombocytopenia	• Platelet count <100,000/µL
Renal insufficiency	• Serum creatinine greater than 1.1 mg/dL or a doubling of the serum creatinine concentration in the absence of other renal disease
Impaired liver function	• Elevated liver transaminases (AST, ALT) to twice the normal lab value
Pulmonary edema	
Cerebral or visual symptoms	

- visual disturbances such as scotoma, loss of vision, blurred vision, diplopia, visual field defects – 27%
- right upper quadrant or epigastric pain – 25%
- asymptomatic – 25%

The laboratory work-up for eclampsia should include a complete blood count, electrolytes, glucose level, uric acid, BUN, creatinine, and liver function panel. Urine should be sent for a protein/creatinine ratio and a drug screen. Although the lab findings in eclampsia can be inconsistent and none is pathognomonic, Table 26.2 can be helpful in establishing a diagnosis and distinguishing eclampsia from nonpregnancy-related causes.

26.2.2 Management of Eclamptic Seizures

Systematic reviews of magnesium sulfate for the treatment of eclampsia have documented its superiority to phenytoin and diazepam. Women who have had an eclamptic seizure should have magnesium sulfate continued 24 hours after delivery, or if already delivered,

Table 26.2 Eclampsia lab findings

	Eclampsia	New-onset nonpregnancy-related seizure	Established seizure disorder
Hemoglobin and hematocrit	Hemoconcentration suggests eclampsia	WNL	WNL
Platelet count	<100,000 suggests eclampsia	WNL	WNL
Electrolytes	WNL	+/− abnormal	WNL
Serum glucose	WNL	+/− abnormal	WNL
Serum uric acid	increased	WNL	WNL
Serum creatinine	+/− increased	WNL	WNL
AST	Elevated	WNL	WNL
ALT	Elevated	WNL	WNL
LDH	Elevated	WNL	WNL
Spot urine protein to creatinine ratio ×1000	>300	<300	<300
Urine drug screen/serum alcohol level	Negative	+/− abnormal	WNL
Antiseizure medication serum level	N/A	N/A	decreased

WNL, within normal limits.

24 hours after the seizure (Table 26.3). Diuretics and hyperosmotic agents are avoided and intravenous fluids are limited unless fluid loss is excessive. If the patient is undelivered, prompt delivery of the fetus is necessary.

Early symptoms of magnesium toxicity include nausea, a sensation of warmth and flushing, somnolence, diplopia, dysarthria, and weakness (Table 26.4).

At the first sign of magnesium toxicity, 1 g of calcium gluconate should be given intravenously and the magnesium infusion should be discontinued. Magnesium sulfate is contraindicated in patients with myasthenia gravis.

A second loading dose of magnesium can be given following seizure recurrence. If unsuccessful, other agents that can be used as adjunctive agents for acute seizures include benzodiazepines, such as midazolam, diazepam, and lorazepam, and phenytoin. Diazepam and lorazepam can be given rapidly but should be used with caution as large doses are known to suppress fetal activity and cause maternal hypoventilation. Phenytoin can be used to control seizures and has little effect on respiratory drive, gastric emptying, or the level of consciousness. Phenytoin is free of tocolytic activity and neonatal effects. Contraindications to the use of this medication include allergy to phenytoin, marked bradycardia, especially if associated with atrial flutter or fibrillation, and patient monitoring for prolongation of QT interval is needed.

Table 26.3 Magnesium sulfate dosage

Loading dose – IV

1. Give 4–6 g magnesium sulfate diluted in 100 mL IV fluid over 15–20 minutes

Loading dose – IM

1. Give 5 g magnesium sulfate IM into each buttock for a total of 10 grams (therapeutic onset is slower than IV administration and the injection is painful for the patient)

Maintenance dose

1. Begin 2 g/h magnesium sulfate in 100 mL IV of IV maintenance solution

2. Monitor for magnesium toxicity (see Table 26.4)

3. Assess deep tendon reflexes periodically (~q 2 h)

4. Measure serum magnesium periodically if absent reflexes or creatinine ≥1.0 mg/dL. Levels should be between 4–6 mEq/L or 4.8–8.4 mg/dL

5. Magnesium sulfate is discontinued 24 h after delivery

Table 26.4 Magnesium toxicity levels

4–8 mg/dL	Target dose that typically controls seizures
9–12 mg/dL	Feelings of warmth and flushing and loss of patellar reflexes
10–12 mg/dL	Somnolence and slurred speech
15–17 mg/dL	Respiratory compromise, muscular paralysis
30–35 mg/dL	Cardiopulmonary arrest

26.2.3 Management of Hypertension

Adequate control of hypertension is essential for prevention of CNS complications. Acute-onset, severe systolic (≥160 mm Hg) and/or severe diastolic (≥110 mm Hg) hypertension that is persistent for 15 minutes or more is considered a hypertensive emergency. These severe elevations in blood pressure can cause CNS injury, including hemorrhagic stroke and infarction. The goal of antihypertensive therapy in these cases is not to normalize the patient's blood pressure but to achieve the range of 140–150/90–100 mm Hg.

The medications that have been traditionally used as first-line therapy for the management of acute-onset severe hypertension in pregnant women and women in the postpartum period are intravenous labetalol and hydralazine. The more current evidence available suggests that oral nifedipine may also be considered first-line therapy. Some studies have shown that women who received oral nifedipine had their blood pressure lowered more quickly than with either IV labetalol or hydralazine and had a significant increase in urine output. With the concurrent use of nifedipine and magnesium sulfate there is concern for neuromuscular blockade and severe hypotension (Figure 26.1).

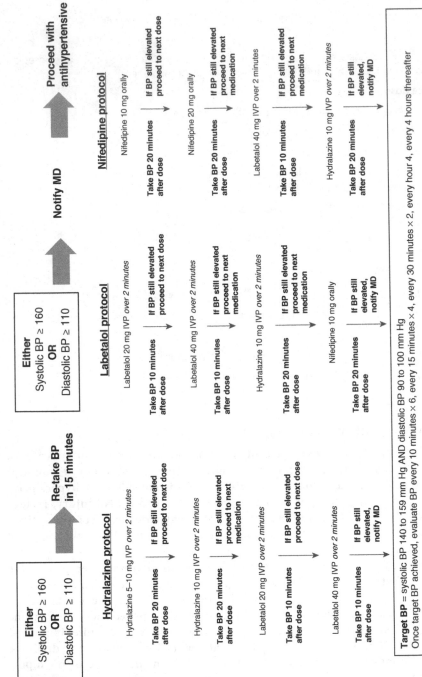

Figure 26.1 Blood pressure management.

26.2.4 Disposition

All patients that are suspected of having preeclampsia or eclampsia need to be evaluated by an obstetrician, preferably in the labor and delivery suite.

26.3 Noneclamptic Seizures in Pregnancy

Seizures are one of the most frequent neurological disorders encountered in pregnancy and carry an increased risk to the fetus from trauma, hypoxia, and metabolic acidosis. Rarely, seizures have been reported to cause intracranial hemorrhage and stillbirth. Even a single brief convulsive seizure has been shown to cause depression of the fetal heart rate for greater than 20 minutes. Status epilepticus is especially risky, with a high maternal and fetal mortality rate.

Immediate ED management of the noneclamptic convulsing pregnant patient is similar to that of the nonpregnant patient. All pregnant and peripartum patients should be treated for eclampsia until proven to be noneclamptic. Benzodiazepines can be used initially to abort a cluster of noneclamptic seizures or status epilepticus. Fetal monitoring is suggested in the viable fetus because of the prolonged effects of a brief seizure on the fetal heart rate. Use of a longer-acting antiseizure drug is often indicated in addition to initial benzodiazepines. Basic knowledge of the risk of long-acting antiseizure medication (ASM) use during pregnancy should be considered and eventually discussed with the patient and/or family members (Table 26.5).

Table 26.5 Treatment of acute seizure

1. Avoid maternal injury:
   a. Insert padded tongue blade
   b. Avoid inducing gag reflex
   c. Elevate padded bedside rails
   d. Physical restraints as needed
2. Maintain oxygenation to mother and fetus
   a. Apply face mask with 8–10 L of oxygen
   b. Monitor metabolic and oxygenation status – pulse oximetry or arterial blood gas
   c. Correct metabolic or oxygen status before administration of anesthetics that may depress myocardial function
   d. Fetal bradycardia lasting 3–5 minutes during and immediately after an eclamptic seizure is a common finding; this does not require emergent delivery.
3. Minimize aspiration
   a. Left lateral decubitus position
   b. Suction oral secretions and vomitus
   c. Consider chest x-ray after seizure resolution to rule-out aspiration
4. Treat/prevent seizure until definitive diagnosis is made. The ASM of choice is magnesium sulfate. This should be started immediately after the initial seizure to prevent further seizures. Loading dose:
   - IV – 4–6 g magnesium sulfate in 100 mL IV fluid over 15–20 minutes
   - IM – 5 g magnesium sulfate

Hyperemesis gravidarum, medical noncompliance, and pregnancy itself can lower ASM serum levels and precipitate seizures. Sleep deprivation, which is a common complaint in pregnancy, can lower the seizure threshold, causing an increase in seizures in these patients.

26.4 Headache

Quite common during pregnancy, headache is generally benign, but it can occasionally herald serious pathology. Headache with new onset in the pregnant patient should alert the emergency physician to serious disorders such as preeclampsia, eclampsia, uncontrolled hypertension, pheochromocytoma, vasculitis, arteriovenous malformation, stroke, subarachnoid hemorrhage, cerebral venous thrombosis, pituitary tumor, choriocarcinoma, pseudotumor cerebri, a rapidly expanding tumor, and infectious etiologies such as encephalitis and meningitis (Tables 26.6–26.8).

Table 26.6 Headaches in pregnancy differential diagnosis

1. Pre-pregnancy established headache disorder – primary headaches
   a. Migraine headache
   b. Tension headache
   c. Cluster headache
2. New-onset nonpregnancy-related headache
   a. Primary headaches – approximately 10% initially present or are first diagnosed in pregnancy
   b. Pregnant women with onset of new or atypical headaches:
      i. One-third – migraine
      ii. One-third – other causes
3. Pregnancy-related headache – preeclampsia/eclampsia

Table 26.7 Initial evaluation of headache in pregnancy

1. Vital signs
2. Fetal heart tones/nonstress test if patient still pregnant
3. Labs:
   a. CBC with differential
   b. Electrolyte panel
   c. Serum glucose
   d. Serum uric acid
   e. Serum creatinine
   f. AST
   g. ALT
   h. LDH
   i. Urine spot – random urine protein and creatinine
   j. ASM serum level if known diagnosis of epilepsy
   k. Urine drug screen/blood alcohol level

Table 26.8 Physical and laboratory findings suggestive of preeclampsia

Systolic blood pressure ≥160 mm Hg
Diastolic blood pressure ≥110 mm Hg
New diagnosis of proteinuria, especially if 2.0 g or more in 24 h. A qualitative result of 2+ or 3+ is also suggestive.
Serum creatinine greater than 1.2 mg/dL (106 mmol/L)
Platelet count less than 100,000 cells/mm³
Evidence of microangiopathic hemolytic anemia (e.g., elevated lactic acid dehydrogenase)
Elevated liver enzymes (e.g., alanine aminotransferase or aspartate aminotransferase)
Persistent headache or other cerebral or visual disturbances
Persistent epigastric pain

If the patient is suspected to have preeclampsia, then consult Obstetrics. If the patient does not have preeclampsia then see Figures 26.2 and 26.3.

Indications for neuroimaging and lumbar puncture are the same as in the nonpregnant patient. Choose the modality that is most appropriate for the suspected diagnosis.

1. MRI. Most consider this modality safe in pregnancy without the gadolinium contrast (limited experience in pregnancy). It is considered the modality of choice over CT for evaluation of nontraumatic and nonhemorrhagic lesions such as edema, infection, tumor, or vascular disease.

   a. MRA can be done without gadolinium to evaluate for arterial lesions.
   b. MRV can be done without gadolinium to evaluate for venous thrombosis.

2. CT. The fetus has the potential of being exposed to ionizing radiation, although this is thought to be minimal. Iodinated contrast does cross the placenta and can affect the fetal thyroid gland. Limited data have shown this exposure risk to be minimal.

3. Lumbar puncture. This should be performed when either increased intracranial pressure (ICP) or infection is suspected.

26.4.1 Treatment of Acute Headaches

1. **Preeclampsia** – start magnesium sulfate and transfer the patient to an obstetrical unit.

2. **Acute migraine** – initial treatment should be acetaminophen 1,000 mg. This can be an effective treatment and there is extensive evidence that it does not increase the risk to the developing fetus. If the migraine does not respond to acetaminophen alone, then acetaminophen in combination with metoclopramide (10 mg), acetaminophen–codeine, or acetaminophen–caffeine–butalbital can be used. Treatment with butalbital should be limited to four or five days/month and codeine to nine days/month. Nonsteroidal anti-inflammatory drugs (NSAIDs) such as ibuprofen or naproxen are second-line options. These are safest when used in the second trimester. NSAIDs use in the first trimester has been associated with an increased risk of miscarriage and some birth defects such as gastroschisis and ventricular septal defects. Use in the third trimester raises concerns of premature closure of the ductus arteriosus, therefore use of these medications should be

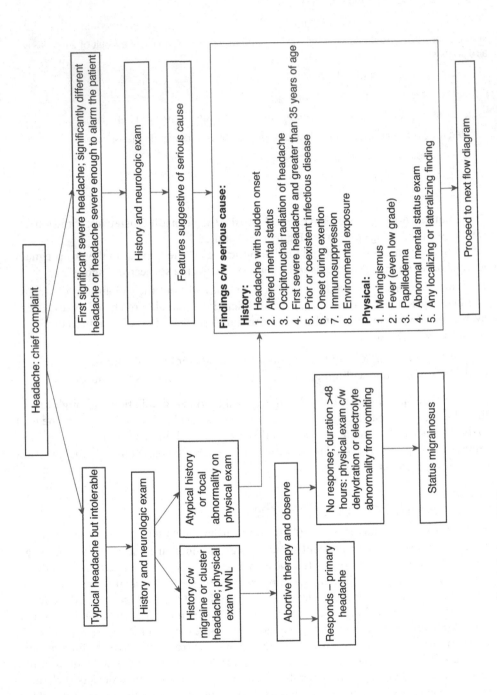

Figure 26.2 Evaluation of headache in pregnancy.

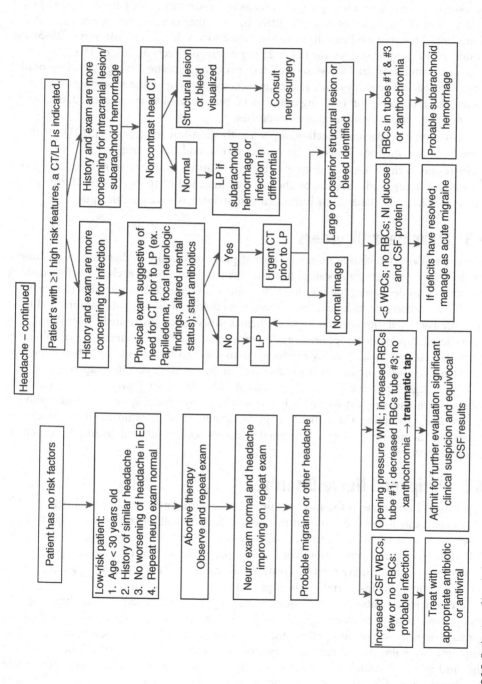

Figure 26.3 Evaluation of headache in pregnancy continued.

limited to 48 hours. Sumatriptan may be indicated for severe attacks during pregnancy that do not respond to the above medications. Human experience with sumatriptan exposure in several hundred pregnancies has been reassuring. In patients experiencing nausea and vomiting, opioids are an option because they can be given by rectal, IV, or IM injection. Preferred medications to reduce nausea include diphenhydramine (25–50 mg orally or IV) and promethazine (12.5–25 mg orally, per rectum, IM, or IV). Metoclopramide 10 mg IV, IM, or orally) or prochlorperazine (10 mg IV, IM, or orally) can be used, but acute dystonic reactions sometimes occur in the mother. As an alternative, ondansetron (4–8 mg orally or IV may be used to treat severe nausea and vomiting associated with migraine headaches.

3. **Tension-type headaches** – acetaminophen is the first-line treatment. NSAIDs, with restrictions as mentioned above, are considered second-line therapy.

4. **Cluster headaches** – First- and second-line therapies are similar to those in nonpregnant women. Cluster headaches can be aborted by inhalation of 100% oxygen. If this is unsuccessful, subcutaneous or intranasal sumatriptan is a reasonable option.

26.5 Movement Disorders

Chorea gravidarum is chorea occurring during pregnancy and is a diagnosis of exclusion. Inherited and other identifiable causes of choreiform movements are excluded before making the diagnosis. In developing nations, the vast majority of these cases are related to rheumatic heart disease, whereas in industrialized nations the etiology is usually autoimmune and most frequently associated with systemic lupus erythematosus; medication-related causes should also be considered. Psychiatric symptoms are often related and can range from emotional liability to psychosis. Chorea gravidarum may resolve spontaneously in several months when associated with rheumatic disease, or after parturition. Medications are discussed in Chapter 21.

Restless legs syndrome has an incidence of 11–19% during pregnancy and can be confused with chorea gravidarum. It is characterized by crawling dysesthesias involving the legs and prompting the patient to move about, most commonly at night during relaxation. The neurologic exam is normal and this resolves after delivery. Treatment is usually supportive.

26.6 Peripheral Nerve Disorders

Carpal tunnel syndrome is the most common nerve entrapment syndrome associated with pregnancy. It usually resolves postpartum. Supportive care with nocturnal wrist splints until delivery is most common, but severe cases may require consult from a hand surgeon for repair.

Bell's palsy is three times more common in pregnant women than nonpregnant, with 85% occurring in the third trimester. Treatment is the same as that for nonpregnant patients and protection of the ipsilateral eye is important.

Lateral femoral cutaneous neuropathy (meralgia paresthetica) is a self-limiting sensory syndrome caused by trapping of the lateral femoral cutaneous nerve under the inguinal ligament or retroperitoneally where the nerve angulates over the sacroiliac joint. The symptoms are pain, paresthesias, or dysesthesias in the middle one-third of the lateral thigh and may be bilateral. The onset is usually later in pregnancy with larger uterine size and exaggeration of lumbar lordosis. Management is symptomatic and usually relieved at rest and resolves with delivery.

26.7 Cerebrovascular Diseases in Pregnancy

26.7.1 Idiopathic Intracranial Hypertension (Pseudotumor Cerebri)

Idiopathic intracranial hypertension (IIH), formerly referred to as pseudotumor cerebri, is a disease/syndrome entity first described over a century ago by Quincke. The current definition is a modification of the original by Dandy and Smith. IIH is defined by signs and symptoms that can be explained by either increased ICP or papilledema that have no other explanation. Signs include papilledema, visual field defects, and sixth nerve palsy. Symptoms include headache and visual changes. Following headache, transient visual loss is the most common presenting symptom.

26.7.1.1 Modified Dandy Criteria for Diagnosis

1. Signs and symptoms of an increased ICP
2. No localizing neurologic findings (with the exception of sixth nerve palsy)
3. Increased CSF opening pressure noted with lumbar puncture (performed in lateral decubitus position with legs extended).
4. CT and/or MRI do not demonstrate enlargement of the ventricles or any structural explanation for an elevated ICP.
5. There are no other identifiable causes (intracranial or systemic) for an elevated ICP.

Obstetricians must have an awareness of this diagnosis, as must emergency physicians seeing obstetric patients. Although seen in other populations, IIH is frequently seen in overweight females of reproductive age. IIH is increased 10-fold in women, and obesity increases the risk 20-fold. The incidence in the general population is reported as 1–5 per 100,000.

26.7.1.2 Evaluation

The differential diagnosis includes other etiologies of headache that are seen most commonly in association with pregnancy, including eclampsia/preeclampsia (PET), cerebral venous sinus thrombosis (CVT), posterior reversible encephalopathy syndrome (PRES), and reversible cerebral vasoconstriction syndrome (RCVS). Of these, CVT is the only common (although still rare) additional consideration with a typical presentation with IIH. The evaluation of headache with papilledema should trigger imaging investigations that would provide a more precise diagnosis. Noncontrast CT scans may not be definitive (30% showing clot or infarction). MRI (venography) is typically diagnostic.

Imaging concerns are typically directed at fetal safety issues for contrast agents. Iodinated contrast is classified by the FDA as class B. Gadolinium is a class C. There should be little hesitation in performing CT scans; a noncontrast CT scan provides very limited fetal radiation exposure. As with any medication, avoidance is best but risk vs benefit considerations must be weighed. Informed consent is suggested for using contrast agents. Both contrast agents are considered safe for breastfeeding.

26.7.1.3 Treatment

Once the diagnosis is established (see the modified Dandy criteria above), treatment options include medical and surgical treatments. The goals are headache resolution and vision preservation. Medically, the long-term advice is weight loss for those patients with obesity. Modest weight loss (5–10%) may be effective for resolving signs and symptoms of IIH. In the short term, the mainstay of treatment is acetazolamide (Diamox), a carbonic anhydrase inhibitor, and to a lesser extent furosemide (Lasix). Both presumably decrease the production of CSF and thus reduce the ICP. Although no standardized dose of acetazolamide exists, a "reasonable dose" from one current review is 500 mg twice daily, titrated upward to a maximum dose of 2000 mg twice daily. Use of furosemide, a diuretic, and to a lesser extent topiramate, a weak carbonic anhydrase inhibitor, is a secondary option. Furosemide is commonly used at a dose of 20–40 mg once or twice daily. Topiramate also has no standard dose but may be started at a dose of 25 mg once daily, with titration up to 100 mg twice daily. Because of the patient population involved, the "pregnancy category" of drugs used in intervention is always a question. Acetazolamide is a category C drug; this implies limited data but no obvious negative fetal effect. There are two specific studies of acetazolamide in the second and third trimesters that suggest relative safety. Furosemide is also a category C drug. Topiramate is a category D drug.

Surgical options include lumbar puncture (also part of the diagnostic investigation) and CSF shunting. An elevated opening pressure in IIH is 250–400 mmH$_2$O (normal: 100–200 mmH$_2$O). This diagnostic test may be "curative" in reducing ICP with the associated headache and visual compromise. It has been suggested that pregnancy is one circumstance where serial lumbar punctures are the preferred treatment. Serial lumbar punctures are not risk-free. Particularly, after the first trimester, medical options are commonly considered. In obese patients fluoroscopic guidance may be required. Newer options also include ultrasound guidance being increasingly used in labor and delivery units in the United States for regional anesthesia in obese gravid patients requesting epidurals during labor or requiring regional anesthetics for surgical delivery. Large volumes, up to 30 mL, are removed during the procedure and approximately 25% of patients will fail medical management; headaches and visual compromise will continue. These patients are candidates for CSF diversions. Shunts may be ventriculoperitoneal (VPS) or lumbarperitoneal (LPS). Both procedures have limitations: infection rate (VPS) of 7–15%; high failure rate (50% for 2 years – LPS; 20% for 2 years – VPS). For the ED, patients may be seen anywhere along the continuum of their IIH disease process and considerations must be given to possible new-onset (in pregnancy) and complications in patients with "well established" IIH.

26.7.2 Stroke (Ischemic and Hemorrhagic)

Stroke in pregnancy and the puerperium is uncommon. Historically, "stroke" appears at the ends of the life span – at the beginning, in the guise of cerebral palsy, and in the aged as either ischemic or hemorrhagic strokes depending on pre-existing risk factors. In the pregnant patient there are diametric poles of risk; patients are physiologically hypercoagulable and, secondary to underlying hypertensive issues that may uniquely develop in pregnancy, they are at risk for intracranial hemorrhage.

The incidence of stroke from population-based studies ranges from 4 to 11 per 100,000. The US Nationwide Inpatient Sample (2000–2001) reported 2,850 pregnancies complicated by stroke, a population rate of 34.2 per 100,000 deliveries with a mortality rate of 1.4 per 100,000 (with a mortality rate of 10–13% for those experiencing strokes). What is epidemiologically striking is the noted increase in stroke events in past decades (mid-1990s to mid-

2000s). Stroke incidence has increased 47% in antenatal hospitalizations and 83% in postpartum hospitalizations. Of the periods of risk, the puerperium is especially dangerous for cardiovascular events (thromboembolic and ischemic), with a risk factor of 7–12 per 100,000.

26.7.2.1 Evaluation

Ischemic stroke has clearly identified risk factors, including a history of migraines (OR 15.05) and peripartum cardiomyopathy (RR 107.1). Also, it must be remembered that the increased thromboembolic risk in this younger population (i.e., reproductive age women) is set on a background risk of patent foramen ovale – 27% in adults – a common cause of stroke in this age group. Certain entities unique to pregnancy may be associated with both ischemic and hemorrhagic stroke. In this light, preeclampsia and eclampsia should always be in the differential list for pregnant women presenting with neurologic findings. As a single risk entity, preeclampsia exists as a diagnosis in 25–45% of cases of pregnancy-associated stroke with a relative risk of 3–12-fold. For ischemic stroke specifically, preeclampsia/eclampsia is identified as an etiologic association in 6–47% of cases. As medicine evolves, there is also a new recognition that a diagnosis of preeclampsia identifies a patient for increased cardiovascular risks in the future (i.e., women with a history of preeclampsia have a 60% greater likelihood of having a nonpregnancy ischemic stroke in the future).

26.7.2.2 Treatment

Diagnosis is based on suspicion and urgent imaging. A CT scan introduces ionizing radiation but, as noted above, clearly satisfies risk vs benefit considerations and exposes the fetus, if the patient is still pregnant, to minimal direct radiation effect. Once identified, considerations include thrombolysis; there is some supportive evidence available from case reports and series in pregnant patients.

Prevention serves as a primary consideration for both ischemic and hemorrhagic stroke. There are excellent guidelines available relative to thromboembolic prophylaxis. Under special circumstances, thrombophilias may be part of the decision-making process, but clinical history is nearly always superior to a laboratory evaluation performed without strong indications. Ideally, input from a local or regional stroke center is a necessity in these complex cases.

Fortunately, with aggressive care, patients survive both ischemic and hemorrhagic strokes and go on with their lives. On occasion they present for preconceptual counseling regarding pregnancy. A recent review suggested a recurrence risk of 1.8–2.7%. Of particular note in prevention strategies, most reviews suggest low-dose aspirin in subsequent pregnancies with some consideration for prophylactic low molecular weight heparin in certain circumstances of prior thromboembolic disease. In particular, as there are multiple connections to preeclampsia/eclampsia, preventive measures should be taken to decrease the incidence of preeclampsia. Such a preventive measure includes the use of low-dose aspirin (81 mg) taken on a daily basis in pregnancies at risk.

Other special, rare subcategories of stroke and stroke-like syndromes must also be considered in the clinical circumstances of pregnancy. These include PRES, RCVS, and CVT. Each of these can be compared and contrasted with eclampsia (Table 26.9).

Ultimately, the diagnoses of IIH and stroke (and the various subsets and subtypes) are diagnosed and managed for the most part as they are in the nonpregnant patient, i.e., assess

Table 26.9 Exam, lab, and imaging of pregnancy-related cerebrovascular diseases

	PRES	RCVS	CVT	Eclampsia
Mode of onset	Rapid (hours), usually postpartum	Abrupt, usually postpartum	Third trimester or postpartum, symptoms often progress over days	Antepartum, intrapartum, or postpartum (10–50%)
Key findings	Early prominent seizures, other symptoms (e.g., stupor, visual loss, and visual hallucinations) usually accompany seizures; headache dull and throbbing, not thunderclap	Thunderclap headache, multiple episodes; seizures occur but are less common than in PRES; transient focal deficits (could become permanent in cases with intracerebral hemorrhage or infarction)	Headache nearly universal at onset, generally progressive and diffuse, thunderclap in small minority; seizures occur in roughly 40% of patients; focal signs might develop later	Seizures, frequent visual symptoms, abdominal pain, hyperreflexia, hypertension, and proteinuria
Evolution over time	If blood pressure is controlled, symptoms resolve within days to weeks	Dynamic process over time; generally, headaches common during first week, intracerebral hemorrhage during second week, and ischemic complications during third week	Evolves over several days, nonarterial territorial infarcts and hemorrhages might develop	Can evolve (from preeclampsia) gradually or abruptly
CSF findings	Usually normal, might have slightly raised protein	Often normal (unless complicated by subarachnoid hemorrhage), but 50% of patients have slight pleocytosis and protein increases	Opening pressure raised in about 80% of patients; roughly 35–50% will have slightly raised protein or cell counts	Usually normal unless complicated by hemorrhage

Table 26.9 (cont.)

	PRES	RCVS	CVT	Eclampsia
Imaging aspects	CT positive in about 50% of patients; MRI shows prominent T2-weighted and FLAIR abnormalities nearly always in parieto-occipital lobes, but can involve other brain regions; intracerebral hemorrhage in about 15% of patients	CT usually normal (if no subarachnoid hemorrhage); 20% show localized convexal subarachnoid hemorrhage on MRI; CT angiogram and magnetic resonance angiogram usually show typical string-of-beads constriction of cerebral arteries; digital subtraction angiogram is more sensitive; might have associated cervical arterial dissection; initial arteriogram might be negative	CT often negative; MRI might show nonarterial territorial infarcts; hemorrhage common; MRV shows intraluminal clot flow voids; although MRV is preferred, CT venogram is also sensitive	Same as for PRES, some patients have coincident acute ischemic stroke or intracerebral hemorrhage

CVT, cerebral sinus thrombosis; FLAIR, fluid-attenuated inversion recovery; MRV, magnetic resonance venogram; PRES, posterior reversible encephalopathy syndrome; RCVS, reversible cerebral vasoconstriction syndrome.

blood pressure, assess blood sugar and electrolytes, and involve neurosurgical consultation as needed. Appropriate imaging should be obtained. Determine gestational age – if the fetus is viable (generally considered 24 weeks' gestation) establish the status of this second patient (fetal monitoring) with obstetrical interventions as indicated.

It is important to recognize potential devastating diagnoses in this otherwise young, healthy population. It is also important to realize that the unique diagnosis of preeclampsia/eclampsia markedly alters normal endothelial and vascular physiology. This can create opportunities for both ischemia and hemorrhage. Prevention of preeclampsia and early recognition and treatment can potentially prevent dire consequences.

Pearls and Pitfalls

- Magnesium sulfate is contraindicated in patients with myasthenia gravis.
- 10% of eclamptic patients do not develop seizures until 48 hours postpartum.
- Restless leg syndrome develops in 10–20% of pregnancies and resolves with delivery.
- Bell's palsy is three times more common in pregnant women and usually in the third trimester. Treatment is the same.
- When a pregnant patient presents with headache and visual changes, consider idiopathic intracranial hypertension.

Bibliography

ACOG Committee. ACOG Committee Opinion No 767, Emergent therapy for acute-onset severe hypertension during pregnancy and post-partum period, 2019.

ACOG Committee. ACOG Practice bulletin No. 222, Gestational hypertension and pre-eclampsia, 2020.

ACOG Committee on Obstetric Practice. Guidelines for diagnostic imaging during pregnancy. *Obstetr Gynecol* 2004;**104**:647–651.

Brown DW, Dueker N, Jamieson DJ, et al. Preeclampsia and the risk of ischemic stroke among young women: results from the Stroke Prevention in Young Women Study. *Stroke* 2006;**37**(4):1055–1059.

Bushnell CD, Jamison M, James AH. Migraines during pregnancy linked to stroke and vascular diseases: US population based case-control study. *BMJ* 2009;**10**(338):b664.

Cunningham F, Leveno KJ, Bloom SL, et al. (eds.) *Williams Obstetrics*, 25th ed. McGraw-Hill, 2018.

Del Zotto E, Giossi A, Volonghi I, et al. Ischemic stroke during pregnancy and puerperium. *Stroke Res Treat* 2011;**27**(2011):606780.

Demchuk AM. Yes, intravenous thrombolysis should be administered in pregnancy when other clinical and imaging factors are favorable. *Stroke* 2013;**44**(3):864–865.

Edlow JA, Caplan LR, O'Brien K, Tibbles CD. Diagnosis of acute neurological emergencies in pregnant and post-partum women. *Lancet Neurol* 2013;**12**(2):175–185.

Falardeau J, Lobb BM, Golden S, Maxfield SD, Tanne E. The use of acetazolamide during pregnancy in intracranial hypertension patients. *J Neuroophthalmol* 2013;**33**(1):9–12.

James AH, Bushnell CD, Jamison MG, Myers ER. Incidence and risk factors for stroke in pregnancy and the puerperium. *Obstet Gynecol* 2005;**106**(3):509–516.

Klein JP, Hsu L. Neuroimaging during pregnancy. *Semin Neurol* 2011;**31**(4):361–373.

Kuklina EV, Tong X, Bansil P, George MG, Callaghan WM. Trends in pregnancy hospitalizations that included a stroke in the United States from 1994 to 2007: reasons for concern? *Stroke* 2011;**42**(9):2564–2570.

Moatti Z, Gupta M, Yadava R, Thamban S. A review of stroke and pregnancy: incidence, management and prevention. *Eur J Obstet Gynecol Reprod Biol* 2014;**181**:20–27.

Quincke H. Meningitis serosa. Inn Med 1893;23:655. Cited by: Johnston I. The historical development of the pseudotumor concept. *Neurosurg FOCUS* 2001;**11**(2):1–9.

Saposnik G, Barinagarrementeria F, Brown RD Jr, et al. Diagnosis and management of cerebral venous thrombosis: a statement for healthcare professionals from the American Heart Association/American Stroke Association. *Stroke* 2011;**42**(4):1158–1192.

Shah AK, Rajamani K, Whitty JE. Eclampsia: a neurological perspective. *J Neurol Sci* 2008;**271**(1–2):158–167.

Tassi R, Acampa M, Marotta G, et al. Systemic thrombolysis for stroke in pregnancy. *Am J Emerg Med* 2013;**31**(2):448.e1–3.

Thurtell MJ, Wall M. Idiopathic intracranial hypertension (pseudotumor cerebri): recognition, treatment, and ongoing management. *Curr Treat Options Neurol* 2013;**15**(1):1–12.

Treadwell SD, Thanvi B, Robinson TG. Stroke in pregnancy and the puerperium. *Postgrad Med J* 2008;**84**(991): 238–245.

Worrell J, Lane S. Impact of pseudotumor cerebri (idiopathic intracranial hypertension) in pregnancy: a case report. *AANA J* 2007;**75**(3):199–204.

Brain Death

Rade Vukmir, James P. Valeriano, and Austin Oblack

The term "brain death" implies permanent absence of cerebral **and** brainstem functions. US law equates brain death with cardiopulmonary death, but specific criteria need to be met for a diagnosis of brain death or death by neurologic criteria (DBNC). There are established prerequisite criteria to consider a patient for brain death that include: (1) a cause of CNS catastrophe deemed irreversible; (2) no confounding metabolic abnormality; (3) no drug intoxication or CNS depressants; (4) a normothermic state; and (5) a normotensive state. If these criteria are met, then the patient can be formally considered for DBNC.

The process of determining brain death must allow decision-making to occur in the proper time frame, typically to include at least 24 hours of observation to ensure that the patient is in the proper homeostatic state (i.e., the parameters indicated above). This is because an abnormality of any of these parameters may mimic the appearance of brain death despite the patient not truly meeting the brain death criteria. It is important to note that the guidelines and criteria for establishing brain death vary from state to state and even from institution to institution within the same state.

The brain death criteria today are based on the 1995 American Academy of Neurology practice parameters, utilizing a four-step protocol (Table 27.1). First, the patient must meet all prerequisite criteria listed above. Again, be sure to verify your institution's specific values for blood pressure and body temperature before clearing the patient for a brain death examination. Second, a clinical evaluation needs to be performed and consistent with the designation of brain death; the clinical evaluation is broken down into a physical examination that assesses a patient's responsiveness and the integrity of brainstem reflexes (Table 27.2). This is followed by a formal 3-minute apnea test. Third, if the apnea test cannot be completed, then ancillary testing would be performed to gather evidence that would help support the diagnosis of brain death. Fourth, if all preceding steps are consistent with the designation of brain death, then formal documentation designating a time of death is required.

Ancillary tests can include any single or combination of the following: EEG, CTA, MRI/MRA, transcranial Doppler (TCD), nuclear scan, or cerebral angiography. If the apnea test can be completed, the time of ABG collection is the time documented for the time of death. Also note that pronouncement is a medical act and thus by law does not require family consent.

Brain death certification criteria are more stringent for pediatric patients, requiring two attending examiners with an interposed observation period of 12 hours for infants (>30 days) and children, and 24 hours for term newborns (37 weeks to 30 days).

Ancillary testing is required in the following circumstances: (1) the apnea test cannot be completed; (2) cranial nerves cannot be adequately assessed; (3) paralysis is present; or (4) to

Table 27.1 Brain death certification

1. Clinical prerequisites
    a. Irreversible and proximate cause of coma
    b. Normal core temperature
    c. Normal systolic blood pressure
2. Clinical evaluation consistent with brain death
    a. Lack of All Evidence of Responsiveness
    b. Absence of brainstem reflexes
    c. Presence of apnea, absence of urge to breathe
3. Use of ancillary tests (if needed)
    EEG, CTA, MRA, TCD
4. Documentation
    Time of death (time of ABG collection from apnea test if the latter is performed)

Table 27.2 Brainstem reflex testing consistent with brain death

1. No evidence of arousal, or awareness to maximal external stimulation, including noxious visual, auditory, and tactile stimulation.
2. Pupils are fixed and nonreactive to light in a midsized or dilated position.
3. The corneal, oculocephalic, and oculovestibular reflexes are absent.
4. Absence of facial movement to noxious stimulation.
5. Absent gag reflex to bilateral oropharyngeal stimulation.
6. Absent cough reflex to deep tracheal suctioning.
7. Absence of brain-mediated motor response to noxious stimulation of the limbs.
8. Absence of spontaneous respiration during apnea test targeting pH <7.30 and pCO_2 >60 mm Hg.

shorten an observation period. Ancillary testing is also required for infants less than 1 year old; at least two ancillary tests must be completed and consistent with the diagnosis of brain death in the assessment of an infant less than 2 months old.

Lastly, individual patient consideration is required, factoring in religious, societal, and cultural perspectives, legal requirements, and resource availability or scarcity.

In summary, brain death determination can be a difficult process and is rarely performed in an emergency department setting. Regional and local guidelines should be studied and followed. It is essential to coordinate with local organ procurement agencies to ensure that opportunity is provided for use of precious tissue and organs for life-sustaining purposes.

Pearls and Pitfalls
• Brain death determination is a very difficult decision-making process and must not be rushed.
• Eliminate all confounding variables as soon as feasible.
• Utilize two qualified examiners in pediatric and difficult adult cases.
• Perform a definitive apnea test as required.
• Utilize objective ancillary testing as needed.
• Consider organ donation referral early in the process if the condition warrants.
• Never forget the humanity of this event.

Bibliography

A definition of irreversible coma. Report of the Ad Hoc Committee of the Harvard Medical School to examine the definition of brain death. *JAMA* 1968;206:337–340.

Beresford HR. Brain death. *Neurologic Clin* 1999;17(2):295.

Greer DM, Shernie SD, Lewis A, et al. Determination of brain death/death by neurologic criteria: the World Brain Death Project. *JAMA* 2020;324 (11):1078–1097.

Landmark article August 5, 1968: A definition of irreversible coma. Report of the Ad Hoc Committee of the Harvard Medical School to examine the definition of brain death. *JAMA* 1984;252(5):677–679.

Nakagawa TA, Ashwal S, Mathur M, Mysore M, Society of Critical Care Medicine-Section on Critical Care, American Society of Pediatrics-Section on Neurology and the Child Neurology Society. Guidelines for the determination of brain death in infants and children: an update of the 1987 Task Force Recommendation. *Pediatrics* 2011;128(3): e720–740.

Quality Standards Subcommittee on the American Academy of Neurology. Practice parameter for determining brain death and adults (summary statement). 2015.

Wijdicks EFM, Varelas PN, Gronseth GS, Greer DM. Evidence-based guideline update: determining brain death in adults. Report of the Quality Standards Subcommittee of the American Academy of Neurology. *Neurology* 2010;74:1911–1918.

Winkfield v. Children's Hospital of Oakland, Temporary Restraining Order, No. RG13-707598, Super Ct Cal., December 23, 2013

Chapter 28

Hysteria

Arvind Venkat and Jon S. Brillman

28.1 Introduction

One of the most vexing issues in a busy emergency department (ED) is patients with neurologic psychogenic conversion disorders, also known as functional neurologic symptoms or hysteria. To understand and treat these patients requires patience, understanding, composure, knowledge of neuroanatomy and physiology, and a comprehension of human nature. Long experience evaluating patients with neurologic disorders may be the most important factor, and younger emergency physicians may not have this ability fully developed.

Even the term hysteria, which comes from the ancient Greek for "wandering womb," is highly controversial and implies an ulterior motive in the patient for his or her presentation. It is now clear that conversion disorder is a complex convergence of psychiatric etiologies of physical symptoms. Unlike malingering, where symptoms are clearly under the voluntary control of the patient, neurologic conversion disorders are not volitional. Functional MRI studies show that different parts of the brain are activated during neurologic conversion disorders, primarily the amygdala, in comparison to healthy control subjects. As such, the lack of an organic etiology of symptoms should not lead treating physicians to simply dismiss patients. Instead, differing methods of evaluation and treatment are required, and for emergency physicians establishment of a functional diagnosis should lead to a referral for appropriate psychiatric treatment in a sensitive manner.

In this chapter we review the common neurologic conversion or hysterical disorders that mimic, or sometimes accompany, organic disorders and how to differentiate between the two. We will emphasize that while laboratory and imaging studies can be helpful adjuncts, careful history and physical examination are critical for emergency physicians to diagnose accurately neurologic conversion disorders.

28.2 Epidemiology and Pitfalls of Diagnosis

One of the difficulties in evaluating the prevalence of neurologic conversion disorders is that there is a reluctance by physicians to apply this diagnosis. Instead, a negative statement is used. For example, a treating neurologist may state that there is an absence of a neurologic condition rather than diagnosing a functional disorder. In addition, concerns of misdiagnosis and resultant medicolegal liability may also lead to a vague lack of attribution of symptoms or signs to a conversion etiology.

With these limitations, studies suggest that the burden of neurologic conversion disorders is quite high. An estimated 15–30% of patients in a typical neurologic practice are found to have a functional disorder as the etiology of their presenting symptoms. These patients commonly receive extensive laboratory and imaging studies prior to a conclusion that signs do not have an

Table 28.1 Myths and cognitive errors leading to misdiagnosis of organic neurologic conditions as functional

1. Inconsistent or anatomically "nonsensical" presentations suggest a functional diagnosis. While such symptom manifestations can be functional, it is well recognized that both incomplete anatomical knowledge and the effect of provider or family encouragement can lead to a misattribution of inconsistent symptoms to a functional etiology.

2. Lack of familiarity with more obscure diagnoses. Given the broad spectrum of disease seen in the ED, it is easily foreseeable that patients with obscure disease processes may be misdiagnosed as having a neurologic conversion disorder due to ignorance of esoteric or unexpected acute presentations.

3. Flattened patient mood and affect (*la belle indifference*) in the face of significant neurologic impairment confirms a functional or hysterical diagnosis. Previous studies have suggested that individuals vary in their attitudes and outlook in the face of serious disease and that organic neurologic pathology can cause changes in mood and affect. As such, the use of perceived discordance between patient signs and symptoms and the seriousness of impairment as a confirmation of a neurologic conversion disorder is inappropriate.

4. Bias against pre-existing psychiatric illness or substance use disorders. It is well established that a significant source of misdiagnosis is the presumption that patients with psychiatric disease or substance use disorders may be presenting with symptoms that are factitious or functional in nature.

organic cause. At this point, patients may be transferred from the care of the neurologist, but without an appropriate referral, patients may feel abandoned. Alternatively, a reluctance to be forthright with patients about the nature of their symptoms as functional may lead to an overuse of healthcare resources as patients continue to present with acute symptoms and presume that medical treatment by itself will be effective.

The literature is replete with examples of misattribution of significant neurologic disease to conversion disorders. Some of the conditions diagnosed after an initial diagnosis of a functional disorder include stroke, transverse myelitis, and epidural abscess, among others. While the overall incidence of misdiagnosis of conversion disorder has declined over time, possibly due to improvements in diagnostic modalities, there are important pitfalls of which emergency physicians should be aware in presuming that odd or unexpected presentations may be attributable to a functional or hysterical cause (Table 28.1).

28.3 Presenting Signs and Symptoms of Neurologic Conversion Disorders

With this background, both common and rare presentations of neurologic conversion disorders using a signs-and-symptoms framework are discussed. We present history and physical examination findings that are suggestive of a functional cause, understanding the limitations discussed above.

28.4 Headache

Headache is unique in the assessment of functional or hysterical neurologic conditions. Unlike other neurologic conversion disorders, headaches do not classically have specific or reproducible neurologic signs or symptoms that can be tested. You cannot see a headache, only the patient can feel it. As such, in the spectrum of neurologic conversion disorders, headache holds a unique position.

Patients that come to the ED with headache generally fall into two categories: long-standing headache with exacerbation (often migrainous) and acute, new-onset headaches.

The former, when presenting to the ED, often have headaches that have not responded to their prescribed medications, may be drug-seeking, or have psychogenic headaches. For emergency physicians, the danger in presuming the latter with recurrent presentations is that more acute and serious pathology may be overlooked.

How can emergency physicians avoid falsely attributing a patient's headache to a psychogenic cause? Take a careful history and ask about the headache history and family history of headache. Important features are frequency, intensity, and accompanying autonomic symptoms (nausea, vomiting), visual disturbances, or focal neurological symptoms. Generally, headaches that occur all day every day, year in and year out are emotion-based. All patients with chronic or acute headache require imaging, at least a CT scan of the head at some point in their initial headache evaluation, though not subsequently with no change in symptoms. If there is a fever, a lumbar puncture should be considered.

Any number of medications, detailed elsewhere in this book, can be used for headache, but in general narcotics are avoided. The key is to not be dismissive of these patients, even "frequent flyers."

Once imaging is performed and a lumbar puncture is done (if subarachnoid hemorrhage or meningitis is suspected), the emergency physician's responsibility is largely completed and neurological and/or psychological referral may prove helpful.

28.5 Coma

Patients with psychogenic coma are rare but usually have severe emotional issues. Compounding the difficulty is that misattributing coma to a conversion or psychogenic cause can be fatal to the patient as most organic causes of coma are critical and even life-threatening. All patients with coma should have an initial evaluation and stabilization of critical functions, including airway, breathing, and circulation. It is prudent for emergency physicians to have a broad differential diagnosis upon presentation with extensive laboratory and imaging evaluations, especially including CT and, if necessary, MRI. Two causes that deserve special attention to avoid misdiagnosis are trauma, especially of the cervical spine, and toxicologic. In essence, attributing coma to a neurologic conversion presentation is a diagnosis of exclusion after serious organic causes have been ruled out.

With this background, how then can the physician identify psychogenic coma? Initial evaluation should focus upon history. Factors that may suggest a functional cause include onset during a stressful event, oftentimes in the presence of others. Witnesses may describe a pattern of onset that prevented injury, such as slumping or sliding to the floor rather than falling in an uncontrolled manner.

Careful physical examination may also reveal evidence of a functional or conversion disorder cause of coma. In psychogenic coma, brainstem reflexes should be intact. Among the reflexes that should be normal in a psychogenic coma are pupillary response, doll's head eye movements, and corneal reflexes. Additional involuntary responses that should be present in a neurologic conversion disorder-induced coma include sphincter tone and plantar reflexes. However, responses to painful stimuli such as Achilles tendon squeeze or pinprick may elicit no response. In functional cases of coma, patients may manifest a Bell's phenomenon-like response, in which eyes roll superiorly with passive eyelid opening. In contrast, organic coma will usually leave the eyes in a neutral position. Finally, patients with pseudocoma may manifest resistance to painful stimuli or avoid injury with falling limbs (e.g., dropped raised arms not striking the face).

Ice water calorics are the most effective means of differentiating hysterical or functional causes of coma from organic coma. To do this test, draw ice water from a basin into a 30 cc syringe and inject it in one ear with the eyes held open. If the eyes deviate to the side of the injected ear and then jerk back to the midline (nystagmus), then this is an indication that both brainstem and hemispheres are fully functional. This test should be done in both ears. Amazingly, patients may not respond by awakening to this test, despite its intense discomfort. However, the induction of nausea, vomiting, or recovery from coma may occur due to the pain induced by this maneuver.

In the category of diagnostic technologies, an electroencephalogram (EEG) can be very useful. If EEG indicates normal cerebral function, this is highly suggestive of functional or hysterical coma. However, it should be known that some patients with brainstem damage-induced coma can have normal EEGs.

Once the diagnosis of coma caused by a neurologic conversion disorder is established, the next step is to induce "awakening." The physician should allow the patient to emerge from their coma with suggestion and encouragement. This allows the patient a "way out" without ridicule or condemnation. Patients with psychogenic coma should have a mental health consult to uncover, if possible, the underlying psychiatric issues that produced this unusual clinical picture.

28.6 Seizures (Psychogenic Nonepileptic Seizures)

Psychogenic nonepileptic seizures, or seizures felt to be due to a functional cause, are commonly encountered in the ED. Unfortunately, the relatively high prevalence of this condition does not simplify its identification and management in the ED. Among the difficulties encountered is that a significant percentage (10–50% in various studies) of patients with true epileptic seizures may concomitantly also manifest psychogenic seizures. Functional seizures can present either with motor symptoms or nonmotor symptoms (e.g., absence seizure-like). The occurrence of psychogenic seizures recedes with aging, declining in incidence in patients over age 35 and exceedingly rare after age 50. The evaluation of psychogenic seizures is also quite expensive, with one study noting that a typical patient may receive up to $112,000 in testing prior to the establishment of a functional diagnosis.

The existing literature suggests that underlying psychological trauma and stressors are important causes of psychogenic seizure events. However, similar triggers can also lead to epileptic seizures. Smaller studies have found that other factors associated with psychogenic seizures are female sex, elevated BMI, and a background inability to describe emotions (alexithymia). In the ED, it is important to emphasize that the presence of these factors does not definitively confirm the likelihood of psychogenic seizures. Instead, they contribute to a global picture that might suggest that psychogenic seizure is the etiology of the patient's presentation.

Nonepileptic seizures are generally characterized by hyperventilation, eyelid flutter, writhing truncal movements, pelvic thrusts, or spasms. Spells may last anywhere from a few seconds to minutes; there is usually no postictal confusion or stupor. Some patients

Table 28.2 Characteristics of psychogenic nonepilleptic seizures hat may differentiate from epileptic seizures

1. Variable pattern of presentation
2. Rapid recovery of consciousness (short or absent postictal period)
3. Prolonged convulsive period (epileptic seizures rarely are longer than 2 minutes)
4. Lack of amnesia of event
5. Lack of tongue biting and/or incontinence
6. Thrashing or thrusting movements of the head and pelvis
7. Lack of response to antiseizure medications
8. Movements of upper and lower extremities are not in phase
9. Pupillary reflexes remain intact during episode
10. Normal EEG during episodes

may actually communicate during the spell. Tongue biting is rare but incontinence of urine may occur. EEG is normal and spells rarely occur during prolonged EEG monitoring. However, EEG interpretation can be complex, with patients with psychogenic seizures being misdiagnosed as having epileptic seizures and vice versa. Patients may be suggestible, and the spell may be arrested by pressure applied to the neck or head. Table 28.2 provides a summary of characteristics that suggest a differentiation of psychogenic seizures from epileptic seizures.

Treatment of psychogenic seizures requires taking into account the psychological factors that underlie this condition. IV lorazepam may be helpful to alleviate anxiety and the use of other antiseizure medications may be instituted if there is any doubt regarding the nature of the spells. It is also important to give the patient the opportunity to emerge from the episode without embarrassment or shame. Encouragement that the episode is coming to an end or even the announced use of an agent that is in fact placebo (e.g., IV saline) can aid the resolution of the episode by giving the patient an out.

Once the diagnosis of a psychogenic nonepileptic seizure is made, the diagnosis can be discussed frankly with the patient and psychiatric consultation and care are necessary. There is evidence to suggest that with clarity of the diagnosis, utilization of acute care resources can be reduced as patients have more understanding of their condition and present less frequently to the ED.

28.7 Stroke/Pseudoparalysis, Hemiparesis, Sensory Loss

Given the potentially devastating consequences of failing to diagnose a stroke or other forms of paralysis, it is understandable that treating emergency physicians default to an aggressive evaluation of such patients in a rapid fashion. Yet it is of utmost importance to be able to distinguish psychogenic features from a true stroke, as treatments for these conditions are markedly different. Though stroke is the most concerning acute neurologic disorder falsely attributed in the presence of functional paralysis, hemiparesis, and/or sensory loss, each symptom deserves consideration in how emergency physicians assess whether patient presentations are due to hysteria or not.

Sensory symptoms are notoriously unreliable, but there are some clues that the examiner may use to sort out hysterical symptoms. Hemiparesthesia or numbness usually does not involve the tongue and, if real, would overlap the midline of the body. If there is anesthesia on one side of the body (no feeling at all), it is usually suggestive of hysterical numbness or loss of feeling. In addition, patients with hysterical sensory loss will often draw a discreet line of demarcation in the midline when organic sensory loss should start less discreetly one to two centimeters away from midline. Finally, loss of vibratory sense is rare and minimal with a stroke and, if the tuning fork is felt on one side of the face (frontal bone) and not the other, this may be a strong indicator of hysteria.

Suspected functional hemiparesis or limb weakness can be assessed in the ED with careful physical examination. The patient's concept of motor dysfunction may not conform to anatomical principles (i.e., the hand might be weak but not the arm). Weakness may be "give-way" – that is, strong at first and then with sudden collapse of the arm, or the leg may slip down on the bed suddenly (not smooth). The drop test, in which the patient's arm is raised above the face or midline of the body, may result in avoidance of striking the patient, suggesting a hysterical cause. Similarly, unexpected painful stimuli may result in movement of the paretic limb or limbs.

A classic physical examination maneuver to evaluate lower extremity weakness is the Hoover test. In this examination, the physician places his or her hand under the heel of the affected limb. With the other hand providing resistance, the physician asks the patient to flex or lift the unaffected limb. If counter-pressure is sensed from the affected limb's heel on the physician's hand, it is suggestion of a functional cause.

A careful examination of the face may also provide clues of a functional, rather than organic, cause to stroke-like symptoms. Torsion of the mouth in a twisted position is an odd finding and may conform to the patient's idea of what a stroke should look like. In contrast, a true stroke will generally not have such torsion, a sign of strength, and instead show evidence of facial weakness or droop.

Aphasia syndromes classically manifest with stroke. Yet hysteria also can cause aphasic symptoms that must be carefully distinguished from cerebrovascular etiologies. A history of a tragic event or stressor as a triggering event may be suggestive of a functional cause, but is not definitive. Conversion disorder-related aphasia may be seen in isolation, while organic aphasia is commonly coupled with other neurologic deficits. Fundamentally, however, it requires a careful assessment of the characteristics of the aphasia to determine if the cause is functional or organic. Functional aphasia may manifest through a stuttering initiation of speech followed by fluent expression. In contrast, aphasia due to stroke may have characteristics of fluency but show subtle changes suggestive of organic disease. For example, paraphasic (unintentional substitution of sounds or words in fluent speech) errors do not commonly occur in functional aphasia. Similarly, perseveration and anomia (inability to name familiar objects) are most often attributable to organic causes of aphasia rather than conversion disorder.

Given the time constraints with which emergency physicians work in assessing patients with acute weakness, aphasia, and possible stroke, it is understandable that the above physical examination findings may not be ascertained upon initial presentation. If there is any doubt whether stroke-like symptoms are functional, the emergency physician should image the patient as soon as possible with CT and possibly MRI. For patients with risk factors for stroke (atrial fibrillation, hypertension, diabetes, etc.), but evidence of hysterical signs or symptoms, a neurology consult would be appropriate to help reconcile diagnostic uncertainty. In the end, all of these physical examination techniques are merely clues and not diagnostically definitive in differentiating between organic or functional symptom causes.

28.8 Memory

Sudden loss of memory is a common symptom in the context of anxiety or a traumatic event. However, it can also be a symptom of organic disease, specifically transient global amnesia. For the emergency physician, the key is to distinguish between functional memory loss and transient global amnesia. Often, anxiety or psychologically induced memory loss is seen in elderly patients or a patient with a history of migraine who suddenly seems bewildered or anxious and queries repeatedly about what is happening or their location. Functional memory loss frequently follows an emotional upset and reflects an impact upon the memory center in the temporal lobes. A key distinguishing feature is that self-identity is always retained in transient global amnesia during the event. Sudden loss of identity is usually psychogenic or related to "fugue" states, where patients wander from their home, sometimes to great distances. These episodes are generally related to emotional issues or purposeful avoidance of authority. Patients with memory failure should be evaluated with brain imaging, and an EEG if a seizure is suspected. Given the difficulties in making a definitive etiologic diagnosis of memory loss in the ED, it may behoove emergency physicians to admit patients to a neurology service for further evaluation.

28.9 Movement Disorders and Gait Disturbances

Movement disorders and gait disturbances due to a conversion disorder can manifest quite dramatically in the ED. They can range from the most common (tremor) to more extreme (Parkinson-like disturbances and gait abnormalities). As thematically noted above, historical factors provide some clues as to the underlying disease process that may be causing the movement or gait disorder. An underlying stressful event as a trigger at the time of symptom onset may suggest a functional cause. Further historical factors pointing to a conversion disorder include spontaneous regression of symptoms, varying symptom presentations, and manifestation of the disorder at an unusual age. However, all of these factors are simply suggestive and do not definitively prove that a movement disorder is functional.

Hysterical truncal torsion or athetoid movements may be extremely difficult to distinguish from true torsion dystonia or choreoathetosis. Clandestine observation of the patient by medical staff when the patient is unaware is, of course, most valuable to discern inconsistencies in presentation. A careful interrogation to exclude family history or ingestion of medication with strong anticholinergic activity that may produce dystonia is paramount. Hysterical dystonia or choreoathetosis has no regular pattern and is often associated with bizarre gait disturbances. The literature suggests that the use of placebo may have an exaggerated effect on patients with hysterical choreoathetosis, perhaps by providing the patient an "out" from a functional condition, as with psychogenic seizures.

Hysterical gait disorders are characterized by imbalance and falling to either side, usually without injury. A number of different patterns of gait are described in the literature, suggestive of a functional gait disturbance. The most commonly encountered pattern is a dragging gait, with the patient exhibiting one leg internally or externally rotated and the foot not leaving the ground. Other types of patterns seen include a tightrope pattern with arms outstretched to allow balance or a crouching gait, which can also be seen in patients with conditions such as cerebral palsy. Astasia-abasia is a pattern in which strength and function seem preserved on lying examination but then manifest abnormality in gait with attempts at walking. The patient may pitch and start or pull or push one leg or the other without signs or history of injury. Patients who have no known psychiatric history and have the sudden inability to walk should have a careful neurological examination and imaging studies of the brain and spinal cord, as well as testing of urine and blood for intoxicants.

A final commonly encountered functional movement disorder is tremor. Distinguishing conversion disorder-related tremor from organic disease-induced tremor requires careful observation and physical examination. Functional tremor is often intentional and will disappear with restraint of the affected limb or transfer to the opposite arm. Similarly, hysteria-related tremor may change characteristics and have an abrupt onset or remission. The entrainment test is another important physical examination maneuver that can aid in distinguishing functional vs organic tremor. In this examination, the patient is asked with the unaffected limb to tap their finger at a rhythm of 3 Hz. The functional tremor in this test may stop or entrain to the same rhythm as that in the tested limb. The test has a low false positive rate, but not an equivalent false negative rate. As such, emergency physicians should not wholly rely on the results of this test to make a diagnosis of functional tremors. Another commonly encountered functional tremor may involve the heel of a patient tapping rhythmically with the foot in a plantar-flexed position. As tremor is rarely a sign of emergent diagnosis, emergency physicians, even with a high suspicion of a functional diagnosis, should refer patients to neurology for further outpatient evaluation.

28.10 Convergence Spasms (Spasms of Accommodation), Tics, and Habit Spasms

This strange hysterical phenomenon is seen in patients with conversion-related movement disorders. It mimics sixth cranial nerve palsies and is a forced conversion of the eyes to the midline with pupillary constriction. Attempted abduction of the eye shows the pupil remains miotic. What provokes this unusual phenomenon remains a mystery, but it is apparent that careful examination can elicit this finding and it is only infrequently seen in organic disease. To test for this condition, the examiner asks the patient to focus on his/her finger at an extreme lateral gaze for five seconds. The examiner then slowly moves their finger toward the midline and observes for convergence spasm with miosis. One study found that 69% of individuals with psychogenic movement disorders can manifest this condition in contrast to approximately one-third of individuals with organic movement disorders and healthy controls. Eliciting this finding can spare emergency physicians from unnecessary testing of patients for neurovascular and other anatomical causes of apparent sixth cranial nerve conditions.

Although no underlying pathologic lesions have ever been demonstrated, tics or facial spasms are generally considered to have an organic basis because they can be induced by medications or caused by encephalitis. Nevertheless, blepharospasm can be a nervous tic. As these conditions are rarely due to an emergent condition, most patients with tics can be discharged from the ED with outpatient follow-up.

28.11 Hysterical Blindness and Disorders of Vision

Sudden visual changes (blindness, diplopia) are emergent conditions that require rapid and careful evaluation in the ED. Yet there are important physical examination findings that suggest the presence of a functional cause to these quite distressing symptoms. The first step is to evaluate whether the patient is presenting with monocular or binocular blindness or diplopia. Hysterical monocular blindness can be uncovered by noting a normal pupillary response to light and fundoscopic examination while monocular diplopia is exceedingly rare and is largely ruled out by the same findings. With monocular hysterical blindness, the nystagmus response to an optokinetic tape or drum suggests a functional cause. Another maneuver is to hold a mirror in front of the patient and move it slowly at a relatively close distance. The eyes will involuntarily follow in functional blindness. Similarly, patients with functional blindness may assume that they should be unable to bring their fingers together in front of their face, but this is not mediated by vision.

Tubular vision is another ophthalmologic condition that has a broad differential diagnosis but may also be seen with hysteria. Organic tubular vision has an expanding conical visual field while psychogenic tubular vision does not expand with distance. This cannot be uncovered in the ED, and formal visual field testing is needed.

Ptosis and anisocoria are eye-related signs that can present in the ED. The former condition can be a sign of more serious neurologic conditions such as myasthenia gravis. A key distinguishing feature between true and functional ptosis is that true ptosis should spare the eyebrow. Some patients, especially medical personnel, may have access to mydriatic eye drops that when applied to one eye will produce anisocoria.

28.12 Hysterical Dysphonia

Hysterical dysphonia is a rare phenomenon characterized by whispering or mutism. As with other hysterical features, it often appears to be due to an emotional event. While mutism may be hysterical, dominant hemisphere strokes may result in mutism as well. Hysterical mutism may be uncovered by whispering to the patient and suggesting that they may whisper too. Indeed, a normal whisper or cough make less likely an organic cause of the dysphonia. Hysterical dysphonia is suggested by reflexively causing a guttural noise by stimulating the pharynx. Normal vocal cord function on direct visualization also suggests a functional cause to dysphonia or mutism.

28.13 Hysterical Deafness

Hysterical deafness is rare and is often associated with mutism. In the ED, one can test for this by eliciting the cochleo-orbital reflex by simply producing a loud sound in one ear and looking for an ipsilateral blink.

28.14 Conveying the Diagnosis of Hysteria

Once the diagnosis of hysteria is suggested based on a comprehensive history and physical examination, the next step for emergency physicians is to convey the diagnosis. This can be quite challenging for a number of reasons. First, in the chaotic ED environment it may seem simpler to state to the patient that they do not have an acute neurologic condition. However, that does a disservice to the patient, who is entitled to an honest assessment of his or her condition, and to the health system as a whole, where inappropriate resource utilization is

Table 28.3 Conveying the diagnosis of hysteria to a patient

1. Express directly empathy and that the condition is real.

2. Explain the organic conditions the patient does not have.

3. Give an actual diagnosis to the patient, not merely the absence of other diagnoses. It is appropriate to call the condition functional or conversion disorder-related.

4. State the high prevalence and treatability of functional conditions and that self-awareness is a key factor.

5. Specifically address how depression/anxiety can be triggers for these symptoms and introduce appropriate medication treatments.

6. Use direct written communication and materials to emphasize the real nature of the disease and that it is not malingering (feigned symptoms for personal gain) or imagined.

7. Facilitate appropriate referral to psychiatry or other psychological resources.

a serious concern. Second, there are specific treatments available to patients with functional disorders (e.g., counseling, antidepressant medications) that should be offered to individuals where appropriate. With this background, how can emergency physicians and consultant neurologists continue to engage patients in an empathetic manner while conveying that treatment will focus more prominently on a psychological, rather than neurological, cause?

Table 28.3 provides a framework for conveying the diagnosis of a conversion disorder with neurologic symptoms to a patient. In its essence, it emphasizes the importance of both directly conveying the diagnosis to the patient and appropriately referring that individual to psychiatric care. Stone et al. have done the most significant work on communicating the diagnosis of hysteria to patients, and the framework given here is based on their work

While this process will help convey the diagnosis of hysteria to ED patients, it is important to emphasize that most diagnostic techniques for functional disorders are inferential and not conclusive. It behooves emergency physicians to carefully consider whether their diagnosis of a conversion disorder with neurological symptoms is definitive enough to discharge the patient with appropriate follow-up. In addition, patients with clear functional disorders may still require inpatient evaluation and treatment. For example, a patient experiencing a psychogenic seizure with a prolonged "postictal" period may require hospitalization for recovery to baseline function and psychological counseling. In essence, making the diagnosis of hysteria does not absolve treating physicians of the necessity of evaluating the appropriate setting for continued treatment, including acute inpatient care.

28.15 Conclusion

Hysterical symptoms can seem mysterious and frustrating to emergency physicians. Instinctively, emergency physicians are trained to evaluate for acute conditions and institute rapid, appropriate treatment. Functional or conversion disorders often militate against that therapeutic pathway due to the difficulties with diagnosis and the lengthy time to treat appropriately. In addition, hysteria can present very closely in nature to organic neurologic disease, leading to considerable resource utilization by a process of diagnostic elimination rather than definitive conclusion. What is clear is that careful history and physical examination with appropriate assessment by consultant neurologists can provide highly suggestive evidence of the presence of a functional disorder and that, with appropriate counseling, patients can be treated expeditiously and well.

Pearls and Pitfalls

- Careful history-taking and physical examination are the most important diagnostic tools in assessing a potential functional disorder.
- Assuming a functional disorder because of the inability to ascertain a specific neurologic diagnosis can have serious consequences for the patient.
- Functional coma can often be ascertained by findings on neurologic examination and abetted by a normal EEG.
- Psychogenic nonepileptic seizures and epileptic seizures may occur in the same patient.
- The Hoover sign is helpful for distinguishing organic from functional lateralized lower extremity weakness.
- Sudden blindness can have diverse organic causes and must be evaluated thoroughly before consideration of a functional cause.

Bibliography

Carson A, Brown R, David A, et al. Functional (conversion) neurological symptoms: research since the millennium. *J Neurol Neurosurg Psychiatry* 2012;83:842–850.

Duncan R. Psychogenic nonepileptic seizures: diagnosis and initial management. *Expert Rev Neurother* 2010;10(12):1803–1809.

Fekete R, Baizabal-Carvallo J, Ha A, Davidson A, Jankovic J. Convergence spasm in conversion disorders: prevalence in psychogenic and other movement disorders compared with controls. *J Neurol Neurosurg Psychiatry* 2012;83:202–204.

Ganos C, Aguirremozcorta M, Batla A, et al. Psychogenic paroxysmal movement disorders: clinical features and diagnostic clues. *Parkinsonism Relat Disord* 2014;20:41–46.

Glick T, Workman T, Gaufberg S. Suspected conversion disorder: foreseeable risks and avoidable errors. *Acad Emerg Med* 2000;7:1272–1277.

Hingray C, Maillard L, Hubsch C, et al. Psychogenic nonepileptic seizures: characterization of two distinct patient profiles on the basis of trauma history. *Epilepsy Behav* 2011;22:532–536.

Kaplan M, Dwivedi A, Privitera M, et al. Comparisons of childhood trauma, alexithymia, and defensive styles in patients with psychogenic non-epileptic seizures vs. epilepsy: implications for the etiology of conversion disorder. *J Psychosomat Res* 2013;75:142–146.

Marquez A, Farias S, Apperson M, et al. Psychogenic nonepileptic seizures are associated with an increased risk of obesity. *Epilepsy Behav* 2004;5:88–93.

Merskey H. Conversion symptoms revised. *Semin Neurol* 1990;10(3):221–228.

Panagos P, Merchant R, Alunday R. Psychogenic seizures: a focused clinical review for the emergency medicine practitioner. *Postgrad Med* 2010;122 (1):34–38.

Parra J, Iriarte J, Kanner A. Are we overusing the diagnosis of psychogenic non-epileptic events? *Seizure* 1999;8:223–227.

Razvi S, Mulhern S, Duncan R. Newly diagnosed psychogenic nonepileptic seizures: health care demand prior to and following diagnosis at a first seizure clinic. *Epilepsy Behav* 2012;23:7–9.

Riggio S. Psychogenic seizures. *Emerg Med Clin N Am* 1994;12(4):1001–1012.

Scheidt C, Baumann K, Katzev M, et al. Differentiating cerebral ischemia from functional neurological symptom disorder: a psychosomatic perspective. *BMC Psychiatry* 2014;14:158–163.

Schwingenschu P, Katschnig P, Seiler S, et al. Moving toward "laboratory-supported" criteria for psychogenic tremor. *Move Disord* 2011;26(14):2509–2515.

Sevush S, Brooks J. Aphasia vs. functional disorder: factors in differential diagnosis. *Psychosomatics* 1983;24(9):847–848.

Shaibani A, Sabbagh M. Pseudoneurologic syndromes: recognition and diagnosis. *Am Fam Phys* 1998;57(10):2485–2494.

Siket M, Merchant R. Psychogenic seizures: a review and description of pitfalls in their acute diagnosis and management in the emergency department. *Emerg Med Clin N Am* 2011;29:73–81.

Stone J, Carson A. Functional neurologic symptoms: assessment and management. *Neurol Clin* 2011;29:1–18.

Stone J, Carson A, Duncan R, et al. Symptoms "unexplained by organic disease" in 1144 new neurology out-patients: how often does the diagnosis change at follow-up? *Brain* 2009;132:2878–2888.

Stone J, Carson A, Sharpe M. Functional symptoms in neurology: diagnosis and management. *ACNR* 2005;4(6): 8–11.

Stone J, Carson A, Sharpe M. Functional symptoms and signs in neurology: assessment and diagnosis. *J Neurol Neurosurg Psychiatry* 2005;76(Suppl I):i1–i12.

Stone J, Smyth R, Carson A, et al. Systemic review of misdiagnosis of conversion symptoms and "hysteria." *BMJ* 2005;331 (7523):989–993.

Stone J, Smyth R, Carson A, Warlow C, Sharpe M. La belle indifference in conversion symptoms and hysteria. *Br J Psychiatry* 2006;188:204–209.

Teasell R, Shapiro A. Misdiagnosis of conversion disorders. *Am J Phys Med Rehabil* 2002;81:236–240.

Young J, Rund D. Psychiatric considerations in patients with decreased levels of consciousness. *Emerg Med Clin N Am* 2010;28:595–609.

Ziv I, Djaldetti R, Zoldan Y, Avraham M, Melamed E. Diagnosis of "non-organic" limb paresis by a novel objective motor assessment: the quantitative Hoover's test. *J Neurol* 1998;245:797–802.

Index

Printed in the United States
by Baker & Taylor Publisher Services